DSM-5®
Handbook
of
Differential
Diagnosis

DSM-5®
Handbook of Differential Diagnosis

Michael B. First, M.D.
Professor of Clinical Psychiatry, Columbia University; and
Research Psychiatrist, Division of Clinical Phenomenology,
New York State Psychiatric Institute, New York, New York

AMERICAN
PSYCHIATRIC
ASSOCIATION
PUBLISHING

Note: The author has worked to ensure that all information in this book is accurate at the time of publication and consistent with general psychiatric and medical standards, and that information concerning drug dosages, schedules, and routes of administration is accurate at the time of publication and consistent with standards set by the U.S. Food and Drug Administration and the general medical community. As medical research and practice continue to advance, however, therapeutic standards may change. Moreover, specific situations may require a specific therapeutic response not included in this book. For these reasons and because human and mechanical errors sometimes occur, we recommend that readers follow the advice of physicians directly involved in their care or the care of a member of their family.

Books published by American Psychiatric Association Publishing represent the findings, conclusions, and views of the individual authors and do not necessarily represent the policies and opinions of American Psychiatric Association Publishing or the American Psychiatric Association.

If you wish to buy 50 or more copies of the same title, please go to www.appi.org/specialdiscounts for more information.

The author, Michael B. First, M.D., has no competing interests to disclose.

Manufactured in the United States of America on acid-free paper
17 16 5 4 3 2
First Edition

Typeset in Palatino LT Std and HelveticaNeue LT Std.

American Psychiatric Association Publishing
1000 Wilson Boulevard
Arlington, VA 22209-3901
www.appi.org

Library of Congress Cataloging-in-Publication Data
First, Michael B., 1956– author.
DSM-5 handbook of differential diagnosis / Michael B. First. — First edition.
p. ; cm.
Handbook of differential diagnosis
Includes index.
ISBN 978-1-58562-462-1 (pbk. : alk. paper)
I. American Psychiatric Association, issuing body. II. Title. III. Title: Handbook of differential diagnosis.
[DNLM: 1. Diagnostic and statistical manual of mental disorders. 5th ed. 2. Mental Disorders—diagnosis—Handbooks. 3. Diagnosis, Differential—Handbooks. WM 34]
RC473.D54
616.89'075—dc23

2013036943

British Library Cataloguing in Publication Data
A CIP record is available from the British Library.

To Leslee,
my bashert, for all the love and support
that made this book possible.

Contents

Preface xiii

1 **Differential Diagnosis Step by Step** 1

2 **Differential Diagnosis by the Trees** 17

2.1 Decision Tree for Poor School Performance 22

2.2 Decision Tree for Behavioral Problems in a Child or Adolescent 25

2.3 Decision Tree for Speech Disturbance 30

2.4 Decision Tree for Distractibility 35

2.5 Decision Tree for Delusions 38

2.6 Decision Tree for Hallucinations 44

2.7 Decision Tree for Catatonic Symptoms 49

2.8 Decision Tree for Elevated or Expansive Mood 52

2.9 Decision Tree for Irritable Mood 56

2.10 Decision Tree for Depressed Mood 61

2.11 Decision Tree for Suicidal Ideation or Behavior 67

2.12 Decision Tree for Psychomotor Retardation 72

2.13 Decision Tree for Anxiety 75

2.14 Decision Tree for Panic Attacks 80

2.15 Decision Tree for Avoidance Behavior 83

2.16 Decision Tree for Trauma or Psychosocial Stressors Involved in the Etiology 87

2.17 Decision Tree for Somatic Complaints or Illness/Appearance Anxiety 91

2.18 Decision Tree for Appetite Changes or Unusual Eating Behavior 94

2.19 Decision Tree for Insomnia 99

2.20 Decision Tree for Hypersomnolence 104

2.21 Decision Tree for Sexual Dysfunction in a Female 109

2.22 Decision Tree for Sexual Dysfunction in a Male 113

2.23 Decision Tree for Aggressive Behavior 116

2.24 Decision Tree for Impulsivity or Impulse-Control Problems 122

2.25 Decision Tree for Self-Injury or Self-Mutilation 126

2.26 Decision Tree for Excessive Substance Use 129

2.27 Decision Tree for Memory Loss 135

2.28 Decision Tree for Cognitive Impairment 139

2.29 Decision Tree for Etiological Medical Conditions 149

3 Differential Diagnosis by the Tables 157

Neurodevelopmental Disorders

3.1.1 Differential Diagnosis for Intellectual Disability (Intellectual Developmental Disorder) 162

3.1.2 Differential Diagnosis for Communication Disorders 164

3.1.3 Differential Diagnosis for Autism Spectrum Disorder 166

3.1.4 Differential Diagnosis for Attention-Deficit/Hyperactivity Disorder 168

3.1.5 Differential Diagnosis for Specific Learning Disorder 172

3.1.6 Differential Diagnosis for Tic Disorders 174

Schizophrenia Spectrum and Other Psychotic Disorders

3.2.1 Differential Diagnosis for Schizophrenia or Schizophreniform Disorder 175

3.2.2 Differential Diagnosis for Schizoaffective Disorder 177

3.2.3 Differential Diagnosis for Delusional Disorder 178

3.2.4 Differential Diagnosis for Brief Psychotic Disorder 180

3.2.5 Differential Diagnosis for Unspecified Catatonia 181

Bipolar and Related Disorders

3.3.1 Differential Diagnosis for Bipolar I Disorder 182

3.3.2 Differential Diagnosis for Bipolar II Disorder 185

3.3.3 Differential Diagnosis for Cyclothymic Disorder 188

Depressive Disorders

3.4.1 Differential Diagnosis for Major Depressive Disorder 189

3.4.2 Differential Diagnosis for Persistent Depressive Disorder (Dysthymia) 192

3.4.3 Differential Diagnosis for Premenstrual Dysphoric Disorder 194

3.4.4 Differential Diagnosis for Disruptive Mood Dysregulation Disorder 196

Anxiety Disorders

3.5.1 Differential Diagnosis for Separation Anxiety Disorder 198

3.5.2 Differential Diagnosis for Selective Mutism 201

3.5.3 Differential Diagnosis for Specific Phobia 202

3.5.4 Differential Diagnosis for Social Anxiety Disorder (Social Phobia) 204

3.5.5 Differential Diagnosis for Panic Disorder 208

3.5.6 Differential Diagnosis for Agoraphobia 210

3.5.7 Differential Diagnosis for Generalized Anxiety Disorder 212

Obsessive-Compulsive and Related Disorders

3.6.1 Differential Diagnosis for Obsessive-Compulsive Disorder 215

3.6.2 Differential Diagnosis for Body Dysmorphic Disorder 218

3.6.3 Differential Diagnosis for Hoarding Disorder 220

3.6.4 Differential Diagnosis for Trichotillomania (Hair-Pulling Disorder) 222

3.6.5 Differential Diagnosis for Excoriation (Skin-Picking) Disorder. 224

Trauma- and Stressor-Related Disorders

3.7.1 Differential Diagnosis for Posttraumatic Stress Disorder or Acute Stress Disorder 225

3.7.2 Differential Diagnosis for Adjustment Disorder. 227

Dissociative Disorders

3.8.1 Differential Diagnosis for Dissociative Amnesia. 229

3.8.2 Differential Diagnosis for Depersonalization/Derealization Disorder 231

Somatic Symptom and Related Disorders

3.9.1 Differential Diagnosis for Somatic Symptom Disorder 234

3.9.2 Differential Diagnosis for Illness Anxiety Disorder 236

3.9.3 Differential Diagnosis for Conversion Disorder (Functional Neurological Symptom Disorder) 239

3.9.4 Differential Diagnosis for Psychological Factors Affecting Other Medical Conditions 241

3.9.5 Differential Diagnosis for Factitious Disorder 243

Feeding and Eating Disorders

3.10.1 Differential Diagnosis for Avoidant/Restrictive Food Intake Disorder 244

3.10.2 Differential Diagnosis for Anorexia Nervosa 246

3.10.3 Differential Diagnosis for Bulimia Nervosa 249

3.10.4 Differential Diagnosis for Binge-Eating Disorder 251

Sleep-Wake Disorders

3.11.1 Differential Diagnosis for Insomnia Disorder 252

3.11.2 Differential Diagnosis for Hypersomnolence Disorder 255

Sexual Dysfunctions

3.12.1 Differential Diagnosis for Sexual Dysfunctions 258

Gender Dysphoria

3.13.1 Differential Diagnosis for Gender Dysphoria 260

Disruptive, Impulse-Control, and Conduct Disorders

3.14.1 Differential Diagnosis for Oppositional Defiant Disorder. 262

3.14.2 Differential Diagnosis for Intermittent Explosive Disorder. . . . 264

3.14.3 Differential Diagnosis for Conduct Disorder 266

Substance-Related and Addictive Disorders

3.15.1 Differential Diagnosis for Substance Use Disorders 268

3.15.2 Differential Diagnosis for Gambling Disorder 270

Neurocognitive Disorders

3.16.1 Differential Diagnosis for Delirium 271

3.16.2 Differential Diagnosis for Major or Mild Neurocognitive Disorder 273

Personality Disorders

3.17.1 Differential Diagnosis for Paranoid Personality Disorder 276

3.17.2 Differential Diagnosis for Schizoid Personality Disorder. 277

3.17.3 Differential Diagnosis for Schizotypal Personality Disorder 278

3.17.4 Differential Diagnosis for Antisocial Personality Disorder. . . . 279

3.17.5 Differential Diagnosis for Borderline Personality Disorder . . . 281
3.17.6 Differential Diagnosis for Histrionic Personality Disorder 282
3.17.7 Differential Diagnosis for Narcissistic Personality Disorder 283
3.17.8 Differential Diagnosis for Avoidant Personality Disorder 284
3.17.9 Differential Diagnosis for Dependent Personality Disorder 285
3.17.10 Differential Diagnosis for Obsessive-Compulsive Personality Disorder 286
3.17.11 Differential Diagnosis for Personality Change Due to Another Medical Condition 287

Paraphilic Disorders

3.18.1 Differential Diagnosis for Paraphilic Disorders 288

Appendix: DSM-5 Classification 291

Alphabetical Index of Decision Trees 319

Alphabetical Index of Differential Diagnosis Tables 321

Preface

Differential diagnosis is the bread and butter of our task as clinicians. Most patients do not come to the office saying, "I have major depressive disorder...give me an antidepressant" (although some do!). More typically, the patient consults us seeking some relief from particular symptoms such as depressed mood and fatigue (the "chief complaints" in the parlance of medicine) that are the source of clinically significant distress or impairment. When we are confronted with these presenting symptoms, our job is to cull from all of the myriad conditions included in DSM-5 those that could possibly account for them (e.g., for depressed mood and fatigue, the possibilities include Major Depressive Disorder, Persistent Depressive Disorder [Dysthymia], Bipolar I Disorder, Bipolar II Disorder, Schizoaffective Disorder, Depressive Disorder Due to Another Medical Condition, Substance/Medication-Induced Depressive Disorder, Adjustment Disorder, etc.). Once we have determined a list of candidates, our next job is to collect additional information—from personal history, other informants, treatment records, mental status examination, and laboratory investigations—that will allow a winnowing down of this differential diagnosis list to a single most likely contender, which becomes the initial diagnosis leading to an initial treatment plan. We must still keep an open mind, however, for the possibility that additional information that becomes available after the initial assessment is completed might justify a change in the diagnosis and possibly the treatment plan. For example, an initial diagnosis of recurrent Major Depressive Disorder might be changed to Bipolar I Disorder after a requested copy of the medical record for a past hospitalization reveals that what was reported by a patient as a past Major Depressive Episode was in fact a Manic Episode With Mixed Features.

This handbook should improve your skill in formulating a comprehensive differential diagnosis by presenting the problem from a number of different perspectives. Chapter 1, "Differential Diagnosis Step by Step," explores the differential diagnostic issues that must be considered in each and every patient being evaluated by providing a six-step diagnostic framework. In Chapter 2, "Differential Diagnosis by the Trees," the differential diagnosis is approached from the bottom up—that is, from a point of origin that begins with the patient's presenting symptom(s) such as depressed mood, delusions, and insomnia. Each of the 29 decision trees indicates which DSM-5 diagnoses must be considered in the differential diagnosis of that particular symptom, and offers decision points reflecting the thinking process involved in choosing from among the possible contenders. In Chapter 3, "Differential Diagnosis by the Tables," the differential diagnosis is approached from a later point in the diagnostic assessment process—that is, after you have reached a tentative diagnosis and want to ensure that all reasonable alternatives have received adequate consideration. This section contains 66 differential diagnosis tables, one for each of the most important DSM-5 disorders. To facilitate the linkage between the decision trees in Chapter 2 and the differential diagnosis tables in Chapter 3, each of the disorders included in the terminal branches of the decision trees indicates the corresponding differential diagnosis table. Additionally, appendixes to this handbook include the DSM-5 classification, which has been included to facilitate coding and to provide an overview of all the DSM-5 diagnoses that must be considered in formulating a differential diagnosis, as well as alphabetical indexes of the decision trees and differential diagnosis tables, which provide an alternate way to locate a particular decision tree or differential diagnostic table that may be of interest.

The information provided in the decision trees and the differential diagnosis tables is somewhat overlapping, but each format has its own strengths and may be more or less useful depending on the situation. The decision trees highlight the overall algorithmic rules that govern the classification of a particular symptom. Differential diagnosis tables are provided for most of the disorders in DSM-5 and indicate those disorders that share important features and thus should be considered and ruled out. They have the advantage of providing a head-to-head comparison of each disorder, highlighting both the points of similarity as well as the points of differentiation. Various readers will have different purposes for and different methods of using this handbook. Some individuals will be interested in a comprehensive overview of the process of making DSM-5 diagnoses and will find it rewarding to review the handbook cover to cover. Others will use the handbook more as a reference guide to assist in the differential diagnosis of a particular patient.

The art and science of psychiatric diagnosis is cursed and blessed by the fact that individuals are so much more complex than the diagnostic rules laid out in any set of decision trees or tables. Clinicians must always temper the temptation to apply the DSM-5 criteria or the decision trees and differential diagnosis tables in this handbook in a rote or cookbook fashion. The approaches outlined here are meant to enhance and not to replace the central role of clinical judgment and the wisdom of accumulated experience. On the other hand, clinicians who are not aware of the guidelines for differential diagnosis included in DSM-5 may become idiosyncratic in their diagnostic habits, undermining one of the central functions of the DSM-5, which is to facilitate communication of diagnostic information among clinicians and between clinicians and their patients and family members. It is useful to know and take advantage of the precision afforded by following the DSM-5 rules but not to be enslaved by them.

Acknowledgments

I would like to thank Allen Frances, M.D., and Harold Alan Pincus, M.D., my coauthors on the DSM-IV and DSM-IV-TR editions of the *Handbook of Differential Diagnosis,* for helping to provide a solid foundation for this book. I would also like to thank my wife, Leslee Snyder, for her careful proofreading of the manuscript. Finally, I would like to thank those at American Psychiatric Publishing who assisted in the production of this book: Rick Prather, Production Manager, who was responsible for redrawing the decision trees; Debra J. Berman, who did the initial copyediting; and especially Ann M. Eng, Senior Developmental Editor, whose meticulous editing of the decision trees and differential diagnosis tables has helped to ensure that I got all of the details right.

1

Differential Diagnosis Step by Step

The process of DSM-5 differential diagnosis can be broken down into six basic steps: 1) ruling out Malingering and Factitious Disorder, 2) ruling out a substance etiology, 3) ruling out an etiological medical condition, 4) determining the specific primary disorder(s), 5) differentiating Adjustment Disorder from the residual Other Specified and Unspecified conditions, and 6) establishing the boundary with no mental disorder. A thorough review of this chapter provides a useful framework for understanding and applying the decision trees presented in the next chapter.

Step 1: Rule Out Malingering and Factitious Disorder

The first step is to rule out Malingering and Factitious Disorder because if the patient is not being honest regarding the nature or severity of his or her symptoms, all bets are off regarding the clinician's ability to arrive at an accurate psychiatric diagnosis. Most psychiatric work depends on a good-faith collaborative effort between the clinician and the patient to uncover the nature and cause of the presenting symptoms. There are times, however, when everything may not be as it seems. Some patients may elect to deceive the clinician by producing or feigning the presenting symptoms. Two conditions in DSM-5 are characterized by feigning: Malingering and Factitious Disorder. These two conditions are differentiated based on the motivation for the deception. When the motivation is the achievement of a clearly recognizable goal (e.g., insurance compensation, avoiding legal or military responsibilities, obtaining drugs), the patient is considered to be Malingering. When the deceptive behavior is present even in the absence of obvious external rewards, the diagnosis is Factitious Disorder. Although the motivation for many individuals with Factitious Disorder is to assume the sick role, this criterion was dropped in DSM-5 because of the inherent difficulty in determining an individual's underlying motivation for his or her observed behavior.

The intent is certainly not to advocate that every patient should be treated as a hostile witness and that every clinician should become a cynical district attorney. However, the clinician's index of suspicion should be raised 1) when there are clear external incentives to the patient's being diagnosed with a psychiatric condition (e.g., disability determinations, forensic evaluations in criminal or civil cases, prison settings), 2) when the patient presents with a cluster of psychiatric symptoms that conforms more to a lay perception of mental illness rather than to a recognized clinical entity, 3) when the nature of the symptoms shifts radically from one clinical encounter to another, 4) when the patient has a presentation that mimics that of a role model (e.g., another patient on the unit, a mentally ill close family member), and 5) when the patient is characteristically manipulative or suggestible. Finally, it is useful for clinicians to become mindful of tendencies they might have toward being either excessively skeptical or excessively gullible.

Step 2: Rule Out Substance Etiology (Including Drugs of Abuse, Medications)

The first question that should always be considered in the differential diagnosis is whether the presenting symptoms arise from a substance that is exerting a direct effect on the central nervous system (CNS). Virtually any presentation encountered in a mental health setting can be caused by substance use. Missing a substance etiology is probably the single most common diagnostic error made in clinical practice. This error is particularly unfortunate because making a correct diagnosis has immediate treatment implications. For example, if the clinician determines that psychotic symptoms are due to Cocaine Intoxication, it usually does not make sense for the patient to immediately start taking an antipsychotic medication unless the psychotic symptoms are putting the patient (or others) in immediate danger. The determination of whether psychopathology is due to substance use often can be difficult because although substance use is fairly ubiquitous and a wide variety of different symptoms can be caused by substances, the fact that substance use and psychopathology occur together does not necessarily imply a cause-and-effect relationship between them.

Obviously, the first task is to determine whether the person has been using a substance. This entails careful history taking and physical examination for signs of Substance Intoxication or Substance Withdrawal. Because substance-abusing individuals are notorious for underestimating their intake, it is usually wise to consult with family members and obtain laboratory analysis of body fluids to ascertain recent usage of particular substances. It should be remembered that patients who use or are exposed to any of a variety of substances (not only drugs of abuse) can and often do present with psychiatric symptoms. Medication-induced psychopathology is more and more common, and very often missed, especially as the population ages and many individuals are taking multiple medications. Although it is less common, toxin exposure should be considered, especially for people whose occupations bring them into contact with potential toxins.

Once substance use has been established, the next task is to determine whether there is an etiological relationship between it and the psychiatric symptomatology. This requires distinguishing among three possible relationships between the substance use and the psychopathology: 1) the psychiatric symptoms result from the direct effects of the substance on the CNS (resulting in diagnosis of Substance-Induced Disorders in DSM-5; e.g., Cocaine-Induced Psychotic Disorder, Reserpine-Induced Depressive Disorder); 2) the substance use is a consequence (or associated feature) of having a primary psychiatric disorder (e.g., self-medication); and 3) the psychiatric symptoms and the substance use are independent. Each of these relationships is discussed in turn.

1. **In diagnosing a Substance-Induced Disorder, there are three considerations in determining whether there is a causal relationship between the substance use and the psychiatric symptomatology.** First, you must determine whether there is a close temporal relationship between the substance or medication use and the psychiatric symptoms. Then, you must consider the likelihood that the particular pattern of substance/medication use can result in the observed psychiatric symptoms. Finally, you should consider whether there are better alternative explanations (i.e., a non-substance/medication-induced cause) for the clinical picture.
   - *You should consider whether a temporal relationship exists between the substance/medication use and the onset or maintenance of the psychopathology.* The determination of whether there was a period of time when the psychiatric symptoms were present outside the context of substance/medication use is probably the best (although still fallible) method for evaluating the etiological relationship between substance/medication use and psychiatric symptoms. At the extremes, this is relatively straightforward. If the onset of the psychopathology clearly precedes the onset of the substance/medication use, then it is likely that a non-substance/medication-induced psychiatric condition is primary and the substance/medication use is secondary (e.g., as a form of self-medication) or is unrelated. Conversely, if the onset of the substance/medication use clearly and closely precedes the psychopathology, it lends greater credence to the likelihood of a Substance-Induced Disorder. Unfortunately, in practice this seemingly simple determination can be quite difficult because the onsets of the substance/medication use and the psychopathology may be more or less simultaneous or impossible to reconstruct retrospectively. In such situations, you will have to rely more on what happens to the psychiatric symptoms when the person is no longer taking the substance or medication. Psychiatric symptoms that occur in the context of Substance Intoxication, Substance Withdrawal, and medication use result from the effects of the substance or medication on neurotransmitter systems. Once these effects have been removed (by a period of abstinence after the withdrawal phase), the symptoms should spontaneously resolve. Persistence of the psychiatric symptomatology for a significant period of time beyond periods of intoxication or withdrawal or medication use suggests that the psychopathology is primary and not due to substance/medication use. The exceptions to this are Substance/Medication-Induced Major or

Mild Neurocognitive Disorder, in which by definition the cognitive symptoms must persist after the cessation of acute intoxication or withdrawal or medication use, and Hallucinogen Persisting Perception Disorder, in which following cessation of use of a hallucinogen, one or more of the perceptual symptoms that the individual experienced while intoxicated with the hallucinogen (e.g., geometric hallucinations, flashes of color, trails of images of moving objects, halos around objects) are reexperienced. The DSM-5 criteria for substance/medication-induced presentations suggest that psychiatric symptoms be attributed to substance use if they remit within 1 month of the cessation of acute intoxication, withdrawal, or medication use. It should be noted, however, that the need to wait 1 full month before making a diagnosis of a primary psychiatric disorder is only a guideline that must be applied with clinical judgment; depending on the setting, it might make sense to use a more extended duration or a shorter duration depending on your concern for avoiding false positives versus false negatives with respect to detecting a substance/medication-induced presentation. Some clinicians, particularly those who work in substance use treatment settings, are most concerned about the possibility of misdiagnosing a substance/medication-induced presentation as a primary mental disorder that is not caused by substance use and might prefer allowing 6–8 weeks of abstinence before considering the diagnosis to be a primary mental disorder. On the other hand, clinicians who work primarily in psychiatric settings may be more concerned that given the wide use of substances among patients seen in clinical settings, such a long waiting period is impractical and might result in an overdiagnosis of Substance-Induced Disorders and an underdiagnosis of primary mental disorders. Moreover, it must be recognized that the one-size-fits-all 1-month time frame applies to a wide variety of substances and medications with very different pharmacokinetic properties and a wide variety of possible consequent psychopathologies. Therefore, the time frame must be applied flexibly, considering the extent, duration, and nature of the substance/medication use.

Sometimes, it is simply not possible to determine whether there was a period of time when the psychiatric symptoms occurred outside of periods of substance/medication use. This may occur in the often-encountered situation in which the patient is too poor a historian to allow a careful determination of past temporal relationships. In addition, substance use and psychiatric symptoms can have their onset around the same time (often in adolescence), and both can be more or less chronic and continuous. In these situations, it may be necessary to assess the patient during a current period of abstinence from substance use or to stop the medication suspected of causing the psychiatric symptoms. If the psychiatric symptoms persist in the absence of substance/medication use, then the psychiatric disorder can be considered to be primary. If the symptoms remit during periods of abstinence, then the substance use is probably primary. It is important to realize that this judgment can only be made after waiting for enough time to elapse so as to be confident that the psychiatric symptoms are not a consequence of withdrawal. Ideally, the best setting for making this determination is in a facility where the patient's access to substances can be controlled and the patient's psychiatric symptomatology can be serially assessed. Of course, it is often impossible to observe a patient for as long as 4 weeks in a tightly controlled setting. Consequently, these judgments must be based on less controlled observation, and the clinician's confidence in the accuracy of the diagnosis should be more guarded.

- *In determining the likelihood that the pattern of substance/medication use can account for the symptoms, you must also consider whether the nature, amount, and duration of substance/medication use are consistent with the development of the observed psychiatric symptoms.* Only certain substances and medications are known to be causally related to particular psychiatric symptoms. Moreover, the amount of substance or medication taken and the duration of its use must be above a certain threshold for it to reasonably be considered the cause of the psychiatric symptomatology. For example, a severe and persisting depressed mood following the isolated use of a small amount of cocaine should probably not be considered to be attributed to the cocaine use, even though depressed mood is sometimes associated with Cocaine Withdrawal. Similarly, cannabis smoked in typical moderate doses rarely causes prominent psychotic symptoms. For individuals who are regular substance users, a significant change in the amount used (either a large increase or a decrease in amount sufficient to trigger withdrawal symptoms) may in some cases cause the development of psychiatric symptoms.
- *You should also consider other factors in the presentation that suggest that the presentation is not caused by a substance or medication.* These include a history of many similar episodes not related to substance/medication use, a strong family history of the particular primary disorder, or the presence of physical examination or laboratory findings suggesting that a medical condition might be involved. Considering factors other than substance/medication use as a cause for the presentation of psychiatric symptoms requires fine clinical judgment (and often waiting and seeing) to weigh the relative probabilities in these situations. For example, an individual may have heavy family loading for Anxiety Disorders and still have a cocaine-induced panic attack that does not necessarily presage the development of primary Panic Disorder.

2. **In some cases, the substance use can be the consequence or an associated feature (rather than the cause) of psychiatric symptomatology.** Not uncommonly, the substance-taking behavior can be considered a form of self-medication for the psychiatric condition. For example, an individual with a primary Anxiety Disorder might use alcohol excessively for its sedative and antianxiety effects. One interesting implication of using a substance to self-medicate is that individuals with particular psychiatric disorders often preferentially choose certain classes of substances. For example, patients with negative symptoms of Schizophrenia often prefer stimulants, whereas patients with Anxiety Disorders often prefer CNS depressants. The hallmark of a primary psychiatric disorder with secondary substance use is that the primary psychiatric disorder occurs first and/or exists at times during the person's lifetime when he or she is not using any substance. In the most classic situation, the period of comorbid psychiatric symptomatology and substance use is immediately preceded by a period of time when the person had the psychiatric symptomatology but was abstinent from the substance. For example, an individual currently with 5 months of heavy alcohol use and depressive symptomatology might report that the alcohol use started

in the midst of a Major Depressive Episode, perhaps as a way of counteracting insomnia. Clearly the validity of this judgment depends on the accuracy of the patient's retrospective reporting. Because such information is sometimes suspect, it may be useful to confer with other informants (e.g., family members) or review past records to document the presence of psychiatric symptoms occurring in the absence of substance use.

3. **In other cases, both the psychiatric disorder and the substance use can be initially unrelated and relatively independent of each other.** The high prevalence rates of both psychiatric disorders and Substance Use Disorders mean that by chance alone, some patients would be expected to have two apparently independent illnesses (although there may be some common underlying factor predisposing to the development of both the Substance Use Disorder and the psychiatric disorder). Of course, even if initially independent, the two disorders may interact to exacerbate each other and complicate the overall treatment. This independent relationship is essentially a diagnosis made by exclusion. When confronted with a patient having both psychiatric symptomatology and substance use, you should first rule out that one is causing the other. A lack of a causal relationship in either direction is more likely if there are periods when the psychiatric symptoms occur in the absence of substance use and if the substance use occurs at times unrelated to the psychiatric symptomatology.

After deciding that a presentation is due to the direct effects of a substance or medication, you must then determine which DSM-5 Substance-Induced Disorder best describes the presentation. DSM-5 includes a number of specific Substance/Medication-Induced Mental Disorders, along with Substance Intoxication and Substance Withdrawal. Please refer to 2.26 Decision Tree for Excessive Substance Use in Chapter 2, "Differential Diagnosis by the Trees," for a presentation of the steps involved in making this determination.

Step 3: Rule Out a Disorder Due to a General Medical Condition

After ruling out a substance/medication-induced etiology, the next step is to determine whether the psychiatric symptoms are due to the direct effects of a general medical condition. This and the previous step of the differential diagnosis make up what was traditionally considered the "organic rule-outs" in psychiatry, in which the clinician is asked to first consider and rule out "physical" causes of the psychiatric symptomatology. Although DSM no longer uses words such as *organic, physical,* and *functional,* to avoid the anachronistic mind-body dualism implicit in such terms, the need to first rule out substances and general medical conditions as specific causes of the psychiatric symptomatology remains crucial. For similar reasons, the phrase "due to a medical condition" is avoided in DSM because of the potential implication that psychiatric symptomatology and mental disorders are separate and distinct from the concept of "medical conditions." In fact, from a disease classification perspective, psychiatric disorders are but one chapter of the International Classification of Diseases (ICD), as are infectious diseases, neurological conditions, and so forth. When the phrase "due to a medical condition" is used, what is really meant is that the symptoms are due to a medical condition that is classified outside the ICD mental disorders chapter—that is, a nonpsychiatric medical condition. In DSM-5 and this handbook, therefore, the phrase "medical condition" is modified with adjectives such as *another, other,* or *general* to clarify that the etiological condition, like a mental disorder, is a medical condition but that it is differentiated from psychiatric medical conditions by virtue of being nonpsychiatric.

From a differential diagnostic perspective, ruling out a general medical etiology is one of the most important and difficult distinctions in psychiatric diagnosis. It is important because many individuals with general medical conditions have resulting psychiatric symptoms as a complication of the general medical condition and because many individuals with psychiatric symptoms have an underlying general medical condition. The treatment implications of this differential diagnostic step are also profound. Appropriate identification and treatment of the underlying general medical condition can be crucial in both avoiding medical complications and reducing the psychiatric symptomatology.

This differential diagnosis can be difficult for four reasons: 1) symptoms of some psychiatric disorders and of many general medical conditions can be identical (e.g., symptoms of weight loss and fatigue can be attributable to a Depressive or Anxiety Disorder or to a general medical condition); 2) sometimes the first presenting symptoms of a general medical condition are psychiatric (e.g., depression preceding other symptoms in pancreatic cancer or a brain tumor); 3) the relationship between the general medical condition and the psychiatric symptoms may be complicated (e.g., depression or anxiety as a psychological reaction to having the general medical condition vs. the medical condition being a cause of the depression or anxiety via its direct physiological effect on the CNS); and 4) patients are often seen in settings primarily geared for the identification and treatment of mental disorders in which there may be a lower expectation for, and familiarity with, the diagnosis of medical conditions.

Virtually any psychiatric presentation can be caused by the direct physiological effects of a general medical condition, and these are diagnosed in DSM-5 as one of the Mental Disorders Due to Another Medical Condition (e.g., Depressive Disorder Due to Hypothyroidism). It is no great trick to suspect the possible etiological role of a general medical condition if the patient is encountered in a general hospital or primary care outpatient setting. The real diagnostic challenge occurs in mental health settings in which the base rate of general medical conditions is much lower but nonetheless consequential. It is not feasible (nor cost-effective) to order every conceivable screening test on every patient. You should direct the history, physical examination, and laboratory tests toward the diagnosis of those general medical conditions that are most commonly encountered and most likely to account for the presenting psychiatric symptoms (e.g., thyroid function tests for depression, brain imaging for late-onset psychotic symptoms).

Once a general medical condition is established, the next task is to determine its etiological relationship, if any, to the psychiatric symptoms. There are five possible relationships: 1) the general medical condition causes the psychiatric symptoms through a direct physiological effect on the brain; 2) the general medical condition causes the psychiatric symptoms through a psychological mechanism (e.g., depressive symptoms in response to being diagnosed with cancer—diagnosed as Major Depressive Disorder or Adjustment Disorder); 3) medication taken for the general medical condition causes the psychiatric symptoms, in which case the diagnosis is a Medication-Induced Mental Disorder (see "Step 2: Rule Out Substance Etiology" in this chapter); 4) the psychiatric symptoms cause or adversely affect the general medical condition (e.g., in which case Psychological Factors Affecting Other Medical Condition may be indicated); and 5) the psychiatric symptoms and the general medical condition are coincidental (e.g., hypertension and Schizophrenia). In the real clinical world, however, several of these relationships may occur simultaneously with a multifactorial etiology (e.g., a patient treated with an antihypertensive medication who has a stroke may develop depression due to a combination of the direct effects of the stroke on the brain, the psychological reaction to the resultant paralysis, and a side effect of the antihypertensive medication).

There are two clues suggesting that psychopathology is caused by the direct physiological effect of a general medical condition. Unfortunately, neither of these is infallible, and clinical judgment is always necessary.

- *The first clue involves the nature of the temporal relationship and requires consideration of whether the psychiatric symptoms begin following the onset of the general medical condition, vary in severity with the severity of the general medical condition, and disappear when the general medical condition resolves.* When all of these relationships can be demonstrated, a fairly compelling case can be made that the general medical condition has caused the psychiatric symptoms; however, such a clue does not establish that the relationship is physiological (the temporal covariation could also be due to a psychological reaction to the general medical condition). Also, sometimes the temporal relationship is not a good indicator of underlying etiology. For instance, psychiatric symptoms may be the first harbinger of the general medical condition and may precede by months or years any other manifestations. Conversely, psychiatric symptoms may be a relatively late manifestation occurring months or years after the general medical condition has been well established (e.g., depression in Parkinson's disease).
- *The second clue that a general medical condition should be considered in the differential diagnosis is if the psychiatric presentation is atypical in symptom pattern, age at onset, or course.* For example, the presentation cries out for a medical workup when severe memory or weight loss accompanies a relatively mild depression or when severe disorientation accompanies psychotic symptoms. Similarly, the first onset of a manic episode in an elderly patient may suggest that a general medical condition is involved in the etiology. However, atypicality does not in and of itself indicate a general medical etiology because the heterogeneity of primary psychiatric disorders leads to many "atypical" presentations.

Nonetheless, the most important bottom line with regard to this task in the differential diagnosis is not to miss possibly important underlying general medical conditions. Establishing the nature of the causal relationship often requires careful evaluation, longitudinal follow-up, and trials of treatment.

Finally, if you have determined that a general medical condition is responsible for the psychiatric symptoms, you must determine which of the DSM-5 Mental Disorders Due to Another Medical Condition best describes the presentation. DSM-5 includes a number of such disorders, each differentiated by the predominant symptom presentation. Please refer to 2.29 Decision Tree for Etiological Medical Conditions in Chapter 2, "Differential Diagnosis by the Trees," for a presentation of the steps involved in making this determination.

Step 4: Determine the Specific Primary Disorder(s)

Once substance use and general medical conditions have been ruled out as etiologies, the next step is to determine which among the primary DSM-5 mental disorders best accounts for the presenting symptomatology. Many of the diagnostic groupings in DSM-5 (e.g., Schizophrenia Spectrum and Other Psychotic Disorders, Anxiety Disorders, Dissociative Disorders) are organized around common presenting symptoms precisely to facilitate this differential diagnosis. The decision trees in Chapter 2 provide the decision points needed for choosing among the primary mental disorders that might account for each presenting symptom. Once you have selected what appears to be the most likely disorder, you may wish to review the pertinent differential diagnosis table in Chapter 3, "Differential Diagnosis by the Tables," to ensure that all other likely contenders in the differential diagnosis have been considered and ruled out.

Step 5: Differentiate Adjustment Disorders From the Residual Other Specified or Unspecified Disorders

Many clinical presentations (particularly in outpatient and primary care settings) do not conform to the particular symptom patterns, or they fall below the established severity or duration thresholds to qualify for one of the specific DSM-5 diagnoses. In such situations, if the symptomatic presentation is severe enough to cause clinically significant impairment or distress and represents a biological or psychological dysfunction in the individual, a diagnosis of a mental disorder is still warranted and the differential comes down to either an Adjustment Disorder or one of the residual Other Specified or Unspecified categories. If the clinical judgment is made that the symptoms have developed as a maladaptive response to a psychosocial stressor, the diagnosis would be an Adjustment Disorder. If it is judged that a stressor is not responsible for the development of the clinically significant symptoms, then the relevant Other Specified or Unspecified category may be diagnosed, with the choice of the appropriate residual category depending on which DSM-5 diagnostic grouping best covers the symptomatic presentation. For example, if the patient's presentation is characterized by depressive symptoms that do not meet the criteria for any of the disorders included in the DSM-5 chapter "Depressive Disorders," then Other Specified Depressive Disorder or Unspecified Depressive Disorder is diagnosed (rules regarding which of these two categories to use are provided in the next paragraph). Because stressful situations are a daily feature of most people's lives, the judgment in this step is centered more on whether a stressor is etiological rather than on whether a stressor is present.

DSM-5 offers two versions of residual categories: Other Specified Disorder and Unspecified Disorder. As the names suggest, the differentiation between the two depends on whether the clinician chooses to specify the reason that the symptomatic presentation does not meet the criteria for any specific category in that diagnostic grouping. If the clinician wants to indicate the specific reason, the name of the disorder ("Other Specified Disorder") is followed by the reason why the presentation does not conform to any of the specific disorder definitions. For example, if a patient has a clinically significant symptomatic presentation characterized by 4 weeks of depressed mood, most of the day nearly every day, which is accompanied by only two additional depressive symptoms (e.g., insomnia and fatigue), the clinician would record Other Specified Depressive Disorder, Depressive Episode With Insufficient Symptoms. If the clinician chooses not to indicate the specific reason why the presentation does not conform to any of the specific disorder definitions, the Unspecified Disorder designation is used. For example, if the clinician declines to indicate the reason why the depressive presentation does not fit any of the specified categories, the diagnosis Unspecified Depressive Disorder is made instead. The clinician might choose the unspecified option if there is insufficient information to make a more specific diagnosis and the clinician expects that additional information may be forthcoming, or if the clinician decides it is in the patient's best interest not to be specific about the reason (e.g., to avoid offering potentially stigmatizing information about the patient).

Step 6: Establish the Boundary With No Mental Disorder

Generally, the last step in each of the decision trees is to establish the boundary between a disorder and no mental disorder. This decision is by no means the least important or easiest to make. Taken individually, many of the symptoms included in DSM-5 are fairly ubiquitous and are not by themselves indicative of the presence of a mental disorder. During the course of their lives, most people may experience periods of anxiety, depression, sleeplessness, or sexual dysfunction that may be considered as no more than an expected part of the human condition. To be explicit that not every such individual qualifies for a diagnosis of a mental disorder, DSM-5 includes with most criteria sets a criterion that is usually worded more or less as follows: "The disturbance causes clinically significant distress or impairment in social, occupational, or other important areas of functioning." This criterion requires that any psychopathology must lead to clinically significant problems in order to warrant a mental disorder diagnosis. For example, a diagnosis of Male Hypoactive Sexual Desire Disorder, which includes the requirement that the low sexual desire causes clinically significant distress in the individual, would not be made in a man with low sexual desire who is not currently in a relationship and who is not particularly bothered by the low desire.

Unfortunately, but necessarily, DSM-5 makes no attempt to define the term *clinically significant.* The boundary between disorder and normality can be set only by clinical judgment and not by any hard-and-fast rules. What may seem clinically significant is undoubtedly influenced by the cultural context, the setting in which the individual is seen, clinician bias, patient bias, and the availability of resources. "Minor" depression may seem much more clinically significant in a primary care setting than in a psychiatric emergency room or state hospital where the emphasis is on the identification and treatment of far more impairing conditions.

In clinical mental health settings, the judgment regarding whether a presentation is clinically significant is often a nonissue; the fact that the individual has sought help automatically makes it "clinically significant." More challenging are situations in which the symptomatic picture is discovered in the course of treating another mental disorder or a medical condition, which, given the high comorbidity among mental disorders and between mental disorders and medical conditions, is not an uncommon occurrence. Generally, as a rule of thumb, if the comorbid psychiatric presentation warrants clinical attention and treatment, it is considered to be clinically significant.

Finally, some conditions that can impair functioning, such as Uncomplicated Bereavement, may still not qualify for the use of an Other Specified or Unspecified Disorder category because they do not represent an internal psychological or biological dysfunction in the individual, as is required in the DSM-5 definition of a mental disorder. Such "normal" but impairing symptomatic presentations may be worthy of clinical attention, but they do not qualify as a mental disorder and should be diagnosed with a category (usually a V or Z code, corresponding to ICD-9-CM or ICD-10-CM, respectively) from the DSM-5 Section II chapter "Other Conditions That May Be a Focus of Clinical Attention," which is included after the mental disorders chapters.

Differential Diagnosis and Comorbidity

Differential diagnosis is generally based on the notion that the clinician is choosing a single diagnosis from among a group of competing, mutually exclusive diagnoses to best explain a given symptom presentation. For example, in a patient who presents with delusions, hallucinations, and manic symptoms, the question is whether the best diagnosis is Schizophrenia, Schizoaffective Disorder, or Bipolar Disorder With Psychotic Features; only one of these can be given to describe the current presentation. Very often, however, DSM-5 diagnoses are not mutually exclusive, and the assignment of more than one DSM-5 diagnosis to a given patient is both allowed and necessary to adequately describe the presenting symptoms. Thus, multiple decision trees may need to be consulted to adequately cover all of the important clinically significant aspects of the patient's presentation. For example, a patient who presents with multiple unexpected panic attacks, significant depression, binge eating, and excessive substance use would require a consideration of the following decision trees: panic attacks (2.14), depressed mood (2.10), appetite changes or unusual eating behavior (2.18), and excessive substance use (2.26). Moreover, because of comorbidity within diagnostic groupings, multiple passes through a particular decision tree may be required to cover all possible diagnoses. For example, it is well recognized that if a patient has one Anxiety Disorder (e.g., Social Anxiety Disorder [Social Phobia]), he or she is more likely to have other comorbid Anxiety Disorders (e.g., Separation Anxiety Disorder, Panic Disorder). The anxiety decision tree (2.13), however, helps to differentiate among the various Anxiety Disorders, and therefore a pass through the tree will result in the diagnosis of only one of the Anxiety Disorders. Multiple passes through the anxiety tree, answering the key questions differently each time depending on which anxiety symptom is the current focus, are needed to capture the comorbidity.

The use of multiple diagnoses is in itself neither good nor bad as long as the implications are understood. A naïve and mistaken view of comorbidity might assume that a patient assigned more than one descriptive diagnosis actually has multiple independent conditions. This is certainly not the only possible relationship. In fact, there are six different ways in which two so-called comorbid conditions may be related to one another: 1) condition A may cause or predispose to condition B; 2) condition B may cause or predispose to condition A; 3) an underlying condition C may cause or predispose to both conditions A and B; 4) conditions A and B may, in fact, be part of a more complex unified syndrome that has been artificially split in the diagnostic system; 5) the relationship between conditions A and B may be artifactually enhanced by definitional overlap; and 6) the comorbidity is the result of a chance co-occurrence that may be particularly likely for those conditions that have high base rates. The particular nature of the relationships is often very difficult to determine. The major point to keep in mind is that "having" more than one DSM-5 diagnosis does not mean that there is more than one underlying pathophysiological process. Instead, DSM-5 diagnoses should be considered descriptive building blocks that are useful for communicating diagnostic information.

How to Use the Handbook: Case Example

To demonstrate how to use the diagnostic tools provided in this handbook to determine a differential diagnosis, consider the following case, adapted from *DSM-5 Clinical Cases*, edited by John W. Barnhill, M.D. (pp. 32–34).[1]

> John is a 25-year-old single, unemployed white man who has been seeing a psychiatrist for several years for management of psychosis, depression, anxiety, and abuse of marijuana and alcohol.
>
> After an apparently normal childhood, John began to show dysphoric mood, anhedonia, low energy, and social isolation by age 15. At about the same time, John began to drink alcohol and smoke marijuana every day. In addition, he developed recurrent panic attacks, marked by a sudden onset of palpitations, diaphoresis, and thoughts that he was going to die. When he was at his most depressed and panicky, he twice received a combination of sertraline 100 mg/day and psychotherapy. In both cases, his most intense depressive symptoms lifted within a few weeks, and he discontinued the sertraline after a few months. Between episodes of severe depression, he was generally seen as sad, irritable, and amotivated. His school performance declined around tenth grade and remained marginal through the rest of high school. He did not attend college, which had been his parents' expectation, but instead lived at home and did odd jobs in the neighborhood.
>
> Around age 20, John developed a psychotic episode in which he had the conviction that he had murdered people when he was 6 years old. Although he could not remember who these people were or the circumstances, he was absolutely convinced that it had happened, something that was confirmed by continuous voices accusing him of being a murderer. He also became convinced that other people would punish him for what happened when he was 6 years old and thus he also feared for his life. Over the next 2 or 3 weeks, he became guilt ridden and preoccupied with the idea that he should kill himself by slashing

---

[1]Adapted with permission from Heckers S: "Sad and Psychotic," in *DSM-5 Clinical Cases*. Edited by Barnhill JW. Washington, DC, American Psychiatric Publishing, 2014, pp. 32–34. Copyright © 2014 American Psychiatric Association.

his wrists, culminating in his being psychiatrically hospitalized because of his parents' concerns that he would act on these delusions. Although his affect on admission was anxious, within a couple of days he also became very depressed with accompanying symptoms of dysphoria, prominent anhedonia, poor sleep, and decreased appetite and concentration. With the combined use of antipsychotic and antidepressant medications, both the depression and psychotic symptoms remitted after an additional 4 weeks. Thus, the total duration of the psychotic episode was approximately 7 weeks, 4 of which were also characterized by the depressive episode. He was hospitalized with the same pattern of symptoms two additional times before age 22, starting out with a couple of weeks of delusions and hallucinations related to his conviction that he had murdered someone when he was a child, followed by severe depression lasting an additional month. Both of those relapses occurred while he was apparently adhering to reasonable dosages of antipsychotic medication. For the past 3 years, John has been adherent to clozapine and has been without any further episodes of hallucinations, delusions, or depression.

John began to abuse marijuana and alcohol at age 15. Before the onset of psychosis at age 20, he smoked several joints of marijuana almost daily and binge drank on weekends with occasional blackouts. After the onset of psychosis, his marijuana use decreased significantly, yet he continued to have two more psychotic episodes through age 22 (as described above). He started attending Alcoholics Anonymous and Narcotics Anonymous groups, achieved sobriety from marijuana and alcohol at age 23, and has since remained sober.

This case presents with both prominent psychotic symptoms (delusions and hallucinations) and mood symptoms (depression). Thus, the clinician can start the differential diagnosis process with any of the following decision trees: delusions (2.5), hallucinations (2.6), or depressed mood (2.10). Given the especially prominent nature of the delusions, we first start with the delusions decision tree (2.5). The first question, whether the beliefs are a manifestation of a culturally or religiously sanctioned belief system, can be answered "no" because John's fixed belief that he murdered people when he was age 6 is not a manifestation of any sanctioned belief system and is thus appropriately considered to be a delusion. The next question, regarding whether his delusions are due to the physiological effects of a substance, must be seriously considered given the fact that his delusions first emerged at age 20 during a time when he was smoking several joints of marijuana almost daily. To answer this question, we need to consider Step 2 of the six differential diagnosis steps presented earlier in this chapter, which provides guidance on how to rule out a substance etiology. In determining whether there is a causal relationship between the marijuana use and the delusions, we need to determine whether all three of the following conditions are true: 1) that there is a close temporal relationship between marijuana use and the onset and maintenance of the delusions, 2) that the pattern of marijuana use is consistent (in terms of dosage and duration) with the development of delusions, and 3) that there is no alternative (i.e., non-substance/medication-induced) explanation for the delusions. Although it is not common for marijuana to cause florid delusions, heavy marijuana use in some vulnerable individuals can result in delusions during Marijuana Intoxication, so the second condition (i.e., substance use is heavy and/or prolonged enough to induce the symptom) is met. In evaluating the first condition, however, although the delusions emerged during heavy marijuana use, the fact that the delusions persisted in the hospital when John was abstinent from marijuana and then subsequently reoccurred when his marijuana use was minimal indicates that the delusions cannot be explained as a manifestation of his marijuana use. Thus, the answer to the second question in the delusions decision tree, regarding whether there is a cannabis etiology for the delusions, is "no." The absence of any reported general medical conditions in John also rules out a medical etiology, and therefore the answer to the following question is also "no."

After ruling out cultural and religious, substance/medication-induced, and general medical etiologies for John's delusions, we then must differentiate among the primary psychotic and mood disorders as possible explanations for the delusions. The next question, which asks whether the delusions have occurred only in the context of an episode of elevated, expansive, or irritable mood, is answered "no" because of the absence of a history of manic or hypomanic symptoms. The subsequent question, about whether the delusions have occurred only in the context of an episode of depressed mood, is also answered "no" because the delusions also occurred at times when John was not experiencing a depressive episode (i.e., each psychotic episode is characterized by a several-week period of delusions before the development of the severe depressive symptoms).

The next block of questions in the delusions tree provides the differential diagnosis of non-mood-restricted delusions. The question inquiring whether the delusions last for 1 month or more is answered "yes" (i.e., each time the delusions have occurred, they lasted for several weeks), moving us for the first time to the right in the decision tree to consider the differential between Schizophrenia, Schizophreniform Disorder, Schizoaffective Disorder, Delusional Disorder, and Bipolar or Major Depressive Disorder With Psychotic Features. The subsequent question about whether the delusions are accompanied by other psychotic symptoms characteristic of Schizophrenia (i.e., hallucinations, disorganized speech, grossly disorganized or catatonic behavior, or negative symptoms) is also answered "yes" given that in John's case the delusions of having murdered a person when he was a child are accompanied by accusatory auditory hallucinations. The next question (i.e., whether there is a history of Major Depressive or Manic Episodes) is answered "yes" given the history of recurrent Major Depressive Episodes, as is the following question (i.e., whether during an uninterrupted period of illness the psychotic symptoms occur concurrently with the mood episodes) because the delusions and hallucinations continued to persist after the Major Depressive Episodes emerged, thus indicating a period of overlap.

The next question, which provides the crucial differential diagnostic distinction between Schizoaffective Disorder and Schizophrenia, asks whether, during an uninterrupted period of illness, the mood episodes have been present for a *minority* of the total duration of the active and residual phases of the illness. In John's case, each of the psychotic episodes was present for approximately 7–8 weeks, with about 4 of those weeks characterized by the simultaneous occurrence of a severe Major Depressive Episode. Therefore, it is *not* the case that the mood episodes were present for only a minority of the time during an uninterrupted episode of illness (they were in fact present for a majority of the time), so the question is answered "no," ruling out the diagnoses of both Schizophrenia and Schizophreniform Disorder. The next question, regarding whether delusions and hallucinations have occurred for at least 2 weeks in the absence of a Major Depressive Episode or Manic Episode, is answered "yes" (i.e., for the first 3 or 4 weeks of the psychotic episode, John was anxious but not suffering from significant depressed mood), bringing us to the terminal branch of the delusions decision tree (2.5) and the diagnosis of Schizoaffective Disorder. It should be noted that given the complete co-occurrence of the delusions and hallucinations during the psychotic episodes, had we started with the hallucinations tree (2.6) instead of the delusions tree, we would have gone through almost the exact same sequence of steps to arrive at the diagnosis of Schizoaffective Disorder, given the similarity of the branching structure of the delusions and hallucinations trees.

Alternatively, we could have approached this case from the perspective of John's severe depressive symptoms and instead started with the depressed mood decision tree (2.10). The first question in this tree inquires about a substance etiology for the depressive symptoms. Applying the same principles discussed above with regard to the relationship between John's marijuana use and his delusions, this question can also be answered in the negative because although the marijuana use is sufficient to cause depressed mood, the fact that John continued to experience episodes of severe depression after he stopped his heavy use of marijuana indicates that, like the delusions, his depression cannot be considered to have been induced by the marijuana use. The next question asks whether the depression is due to the physiological effects of a general medical condition, and that question can also be answered "no" because of the absence of any history of medical problems. The next question asks whether the depressed mood was part of a Major Depressive Episode. The answer to that question is "yes" given that the depressive periods that developed after the onset of delusions and hallucinations were characterized by approximately 4 weeks of dysphoric mood, prominent anhedonia, poor sleep, decreased appetite, and reduced concentration, thus meeting syndromal criteria for a Major Depressive Episode. Note that the decision tree does not end at this point but that the diagnostic flow continues onward because Major Depressive Episode is not a codable diagnostic entity in DSM-5 but instead comprises one of the building blocks for the diagnoses of Bipolar I or Bipolar II Disorder, Major Depressive Disorder, and Schizoaffective Disorder. The next question, about the presence of clinically significant manic or hypomanic symptoms, is answered "no," bringing us to a consideration of the relationship between the Major Depressive Episodes and the psychotic symptoms. The question about whether there is a history of delusions or hallucinations is answered "yes," bringing us to the critical question as to whether the psychotic symptoms occur exclusively during Manic or Major Depressive Episodes. In John's case, the psychotic symptoms have *not* occurred exclusively during the Major Depressive Episodes (i.e., the delusions and hallucinations occurred on their own for 3–4 weeks prior to the onset of the depressive episode), so the answer to this question is "no." At this point in the depressed mood decision tree (2.10), rather than being offered additional questions, we are told that a Schizophrenia Spectrum or Other Psychotic Disorder is present and are instructed to go to the delusions tree (2.5) or hallucinations tree (2.6) for the differential diagnosis, resulting in the diagnosis of Schizoaffective Disorder.

After arriving at the diagnosis of Schizoaffective Disorder through the use of the decision trees, we can refer to the DSM-5 classification in the Appendix to get the diagnostic code for Schizoaffective Disorder and/or we can review the differential diagnosis table for Schizoaffective Disorder in Chapter 3 (Table 3.2.2) to confirm that the key contenders to a diagnosis of Schizoaffective Disorder have been appropriately ruled out. The two main diagnostic contenders in this case are Schizophrenia and Major Depressive Disorder With Psychotic Features. Accordingly, the differential diagnosis table for Schizoaffective Disorder notes that Schizophrenia is differentiated from Schizoaffective Disorder by virtue of the fact that Schizophrenia is characterized by mood episodes that "have been present for a minority of the total duration of the active and residual periods of the illness." In John's case, each episode of the illness was characterized by a Major Depressive Episode being present for more than half of the time (i.e., about 4 weeks) of the total duration (i.e., 7–8 weeks), thus ruling out the diagnosis of Schizophrenia. Moreover, the table also notes that Schizoaffective Disorder is differentiated from Major Depressive Disorder With Psychotic Features by virtue of the fact that Major Depressive Disorder With Psychotic Features is characterized by psychotic symptoms that occur exclusively during Major Depressive Episodes. In John's case, the psychotic symptoms were not confined exclusively to the depressive episodes, ruling out the diagnosis of Major Depressive Disorder With Psychotic Features.

2

Differential Diagnosis by the Trees

Differential diagnosis is at the heart of every initial clinical encounter and is the beginning of every treatment plan. The clinician must determine which disorders are possible candidates for consideration and then choose from among them the disorder (or disorders) that best accounts for the presenting symptoms. The biggest problem encountered in differential diagnosis is the tendency for premature closure in coming to a final diagnosis. Studies in cognitive science have indicated that clinicians typically decide on the diagnosis within the first 5 minutes of meeting the patient and then spend the rest of the time during their evaluation interpreting (and often misinterpreting) elicited information through this diagnostic bias. Forming initial impressions can be valuable in helping to suggest which questions need to be asked and which hypotheses need to be tested. Unfortunately, however, first impressions are sometimes wrong—particularly because the patient's current state may not be a true reflection of the longitudinal course. Accurate diagnosis requires a methodical consideration of all possible contenders in the differential diagnosis.

Perhaps the best way to avoid prematurely jumping to a diagnostic conclusion is to approach the problem from the bottom up: by generating the differential diagnosis based on the presenting symptoms. This section of the handbook, which includes 29 symptom-oriented decision trees, facilitates this process. Each decision tree starts with a particular presenting symptom and then provides decision points for determining which diagnosis may best account for it. For any given patient, several trees may (and often do) apply. In many instances, following the branches within the different pertinent decision trees will lead to the same diagnosis, suggesting that the presenting symptoms constitute a single syndrome. In other instances, more than one diagnosis may be indicated.

The first step in using these decision trees is to determine which ones apply to the clinical presentation. The listings of the decision trees included in this handbook are organized in three different ways to facilitate finding the relevant decision trees. Two lists are provided at the end of this introduction to Chapter 2. The first itemizes the decision trees in order of the DSM-5 diagnostic groupings (trees related to neurodevelopmental presentations are listed first, trees related to psychotic presentations second, and so forth). The second list is organized by mental status examination domain (trees related to mood/affect, trees related to behavior, and so forth). Finally, at the end of this handbook, an alphabetical index of the decision trees is included, as well as an alphabetical index of the differential diagnosis tables covered in Chapter 3.

Each decision tree is laid out in a standardized fashion. The presenting symptom for each tree is shown in bold text in a box at the upper left. The boxes on the far right, the diagnostic end points, are indicated by shading and a thick border; these show all of the disorders that need to be considered in the differential diagnosis of the presenting symptom. The numerical codes in parentheses refer to the corresponding differential diagnostic table in Chapter 3. Intermediate boxes are decision points that indicate how different disorders are ruled in or ruled out. You should consider the statement in the decision box and then follow the "Y" branch if the answer is "yes" and the "N" branch if the answer is "no." Occasional intermediate boxes are not decision points per se but represent intermediate diagnostic conclusions, and thus lack the "Y" and "N" choices. For example, the Decision Tree for Elevated or Expansive Mood (2.8) includes intermediate boxes in which the presence of a Manic Episode or Hypomanic Episode is asserted, reflecting the fact that Manic Episode and Hypomanic Episode are building blocks for the diagnoses of Bipolar I and Bipolar II Disorders.

You should always keep in mind that the decision trees are no more than an overview of the DSM-5 diagnostic system and a guide to differential diagnosis. Clinical judgment is always required in the evaluation of each decision point. Moreover, when you have arrived at a diagnostic end point in a tree (i.e., a "final diagnosis"), it is important to review the actual DSM-5 criteria set for the disorder in question to ensure that the full criteria for that disorder have in fact been met. This confirmation is necessary for two reasons. First, the decision trees contain only summarized versions of the DSM-5 diagnostic criteria rather than the complete text of the criteria. Second, the decision trees only include selected criteria from the criteria sets—that is, those diagnostic criteria that differentiate between the various DSM-5 disorders. A review of the complete DSM-5 diagnostic criteria sets is needed to ensure that the case meets the full set of required diagnostic features and course requirements (e.g., persistence, minimum duration); for the most part, these are not included in the decision trees.

Many of the decision trees follow a standard format that mirrors the stepwise thought process used in making a differential diagnosis presented in Chapter 1 of this handbook. The first consideration is whether the particular symptom is the result of the direct effects of substance use (including medication) or a general medical condition (Steps 2 and 3 in Chapter 1). The next steps in the decision tree typically cover the primary mental disorders that may account for the symptom (Step 4). The final decision points in most of the decision trees provide the differential diagnosis for those presentations that do not conform to or that fall below the threshold for a specific DSM-5 diagnosis. These decision points thus differentiate among Adjustment Disorder, a residual Other Specified or Unspecified Disorder category, and no mental disorder at all (Steps 5 and 6). The important step of determining whether the presenting symptom has been feigned (as in Malingering or Factitious Disorder) has not been included in most of the decision trees because, as discussed in Step 1 in Chapter 1, that task potentially applies to the evaluation of all presenting symptoms but only in certain contexts and settings (e.g., forensic).

As noted above, the order of the 29 decision trees in this handbook corresponds roughly to the organization of the DSM-5 disorders. The following lists show the decision trees organized by 1) DSM-5 diagnostic grouping and 2) mental status examination domain.

Decision trees organized by DSM-5 diagnostic grouping

Neurodevelopmental presentations
2.1 Poor school performance
2.2 Behavioral problems in a child or adolescent
2.3 Speech disturbance
2.4 Distractibility

Schizophrenia and other psychotic presentations
2.5 Delusions
2.6 Hallucinations
2.7 Catatonic symptoms

Bipolar presentations
2.8 Elevated or expansive mood
2.9 Irritable mood

Depressive presentations
2.10 Depressed mood
2.11 Suicidal ideation or behavior
2.12 Psychomotor retardation

Anxiety presentations
2.13 Anxiety
2.14 Panic attacks
2.15 Avoidance behavior

Trauma- and stressor-related presentations
2.16 Trauma or psychosocial stressors involved in the etiology

Somatic symptom presentations
2.17 Somatic complaints or illness/appearance anxiety

Feeding and eating presentations
2.18 Appetite changes or unusual eating behavior

Sleep-wake presentations
2.19 Insomnia
2.20 Hypersomnolence

Decision trees organized by DSM-5 diagnostic grouping *(continued)*

Sexual dysfunction presentations

2.21 Sexual dysfunction in a female

2.22 Sexual dysfunction in a male

Disruptive, impulse-control, and conduct presentations

2.23 Aggressive behavior

2.24 Impulsivity or impulse-control problems

2.25 Self-injury or self-mutilation

Substance-related presentations

2.26 Excessive substance use

Neurocognitive presentations

2.27 Memory loss

2.28 Cognitive impairment

Etiological medical presentations

2.29 Etiological medical conditions

Decision trees organized by mental status examination domain

Mood/affect

2.8 Elevated or expansive mood

2.9 Irritable mood

2.10 Depressed mood

2.13 Anxiety

2.14 Panic attacks

Behavior

2.2 Behavioral problems in a child or adolescent

2.7 Catatonic symptoms

2.11 Suicidal ideation or behavior

2.12 Psychomotor retardation

2.15 Avoidance behavior

2.23 Aggressive behavior

2.24 Impulsivity or impulse-control problems

2.25 Self-injury or self-mutilation

2.26 Excessive substance use

Cognition

2.4 Distractibility

2.27 Memory loss

2.28 Cognitive impairment

Thought form/speech

2.3 Speech disturbance

Decision trees organized by mental status examination domain *(continued)*

Thought content
2.5 Delusions
2.11 Suicidal ideation or behavior

Perceptual disturbance
2.6 Hallucinations

Somatic symptoms
2.14 Panic attacks
2.17 Somatic complaints or illness/appearance anxiety

Personality features
2.24 Impulsivity or impulse-control problems
2.25 Self-injury or self-mutilation

Sleep/eating/sex
2.18 Appetite changes or unusual eating behavior
2.19 Insomnia
2.20 Hypersomnolence
2.21 Sexual dysfunction in a female
2.22 Sexual dysfunction in a male

Functioning
2.1 Poor school performance

Etiological factors
2.16 Trauma or psychosocial stressors involved in the etiology
2.26 Excessive substance use
2.29 Etiological medical conditions

2.1 Decision Tree for Poor School Performance

Poor school performance is an all-too-common and very nonspecific aspect of childhood and adolescence. On the one hand, clinicians should certainly not assume that every poor student has a mental disorder underlying his or her poor academic performance. On the other hand, most (if not all) mental disorders occurring in children are likely to have a negative impact on school performance, and, not infrequently, difficulty in school is the chief complaint.

The evaluation for the causes of poor school performance will usually include testing for overall IQ and for deficits in specific academic skills (e.g., reading, mathematics, writing, expressive and receptive language). A definitive diagnosis of a DSM-5 neurodevelopmental disorder requires that the learning or communication difficulties be substantially and quantifiably below what would be expected given the individual's age and that they substantially interfere with school, work, or social functioning. The next step is a careful assessment for the presence of the various psychiatric disorders that have impaired school performance as a consequence. This entails a careful history (supplemented by reports from parents, teachers, and pediatricians), clinical observation, and an evaluation of the role of substance use. For example, are there significant deficits in the social use of verbal and nonverbal communication (as in Autism Spectrum Disorder and Social [Pragmatic] Communication Disorder)? Are there clinically significant symptoms of inattention and/or hyperactive-impulsive behavior occurring in two or more different settings (as in Attention-Deficit/Hyperactivity Disorder)? Are there frequent uncontrollable temper tantrums on top of a baseline of persistent anger and irritability (as in Disruptive Mood Dysregulation Disorder)? Is there a pattern of antisocial behaviors such as truancy (as in Conduct Disorder)? Is there school refusal based on an inability to separate from attachment figures (as in Separation Anxiety Disorder)? Is there clinically significant depressed mood (as in Major Depressive Disorder)? Because neurodevelopmental disorders and other mental disorders frequently co-occur, it is important to evaluate for all possibilities in the tree (which may require going through the tree several times) and to make whichever diagnoses are appropriate.

The presence of a psychiatric disorder does not guarantee that it is the cause of problematic school performance. Other factors (e.g., poor work habits, excessive TV watching or video game playing, lack of motivation, poor schooling, disruptive home or community environment) may also play a significant role. Occasionally, the psychiatric disorder (e.g., Adjustment Disorder, Oppositional Defiant Disorder, Major Depressive Disorder) may be more the result of poor school performance than its cause.

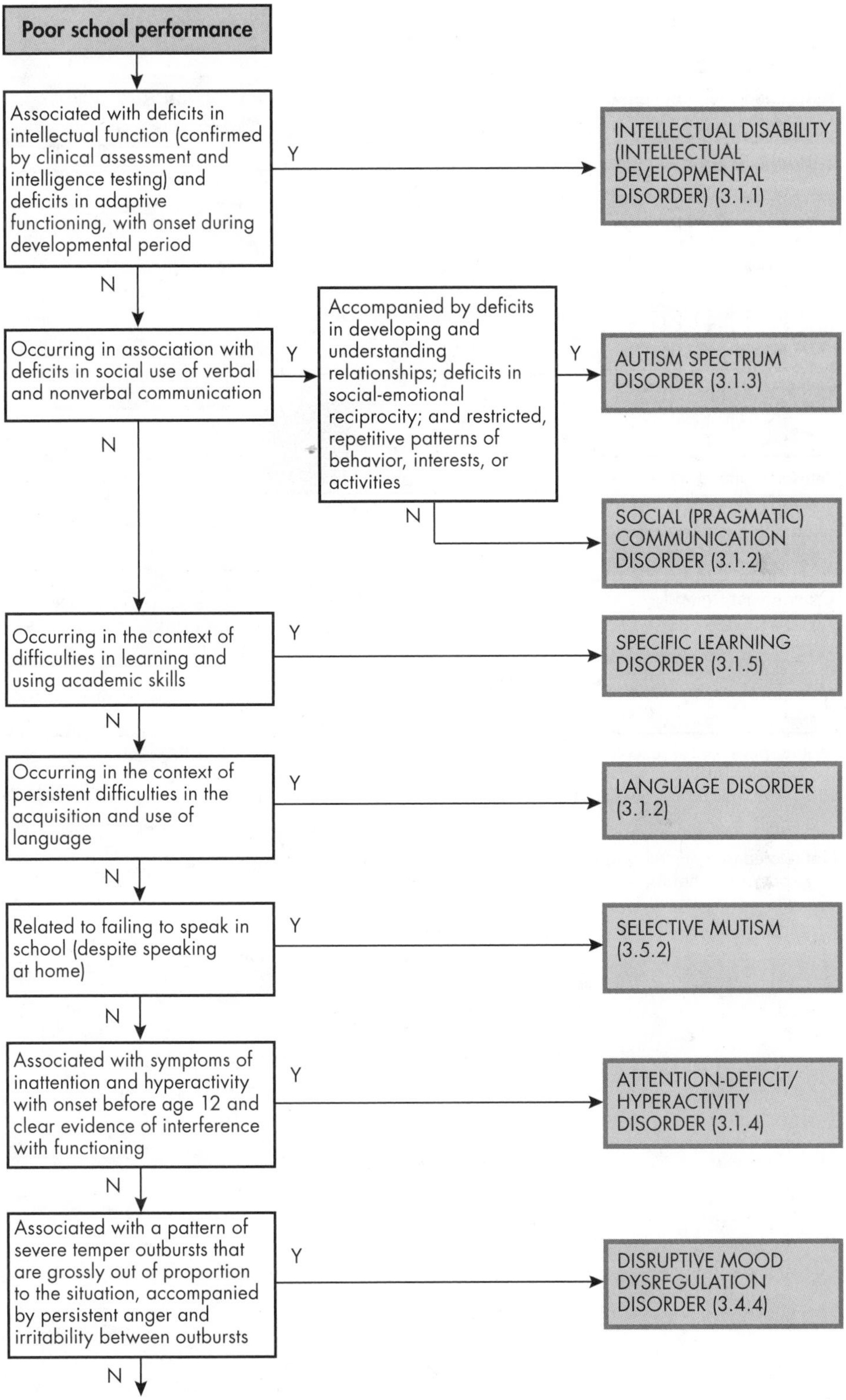
Poor school performance
Associated with deficits in intellectual function (confirmed by clinical assessment and intelligence testing) and deficits in adaptive functioning, with onset during developmental period
Y
INTELLECTUAL DISABILITY (INTELLECTUAL DEVELOPMENTAL DISORDER) (3.1.1)
N
Occurring in association with deficits in social use of verbal and nonverbal communication
Y
Accompanied by deficits in developing and understanding relationships; deficits in social-emotional reciprocity; and restricted, repetitive patterns of behavior, interests, or activities
Y
AUTISM SPECTRUM DISORDER (3.1.3)
N
SOCIAL (PRAGMATIC) COMMUNICATION DISORDER (3.1.2)
N
Occurring in the context of difficulties in learning and using academic skills
Y
SPECIFIC LEARNING DISORDER (3.1.5)
N
Occurring in the context of persistent difficulties in the acquisition and use of language
Y
LANGUAGE DISORDER (3.1.2)
N
Related to failing to speak in school (despite speaking at home)
Y
SELECTIVE MUTISM (3.5.2)
N
Associated with symptoms of inattention and hyperactivity with onset before age 12 and clear evidence of interference with functioning
Y
ATTENTION-DEFICIT/ HYPERACTIVITY DISORDER (3.1.4)
N
Associated with a pattern of severe temper outbursts that are grossly out of proportion to the situation, accompanied by persistent anger and irritability between outbursts
Y
DISRUPTIVE MOOD DYSREGULATION DISORDER (3.4.4)
N

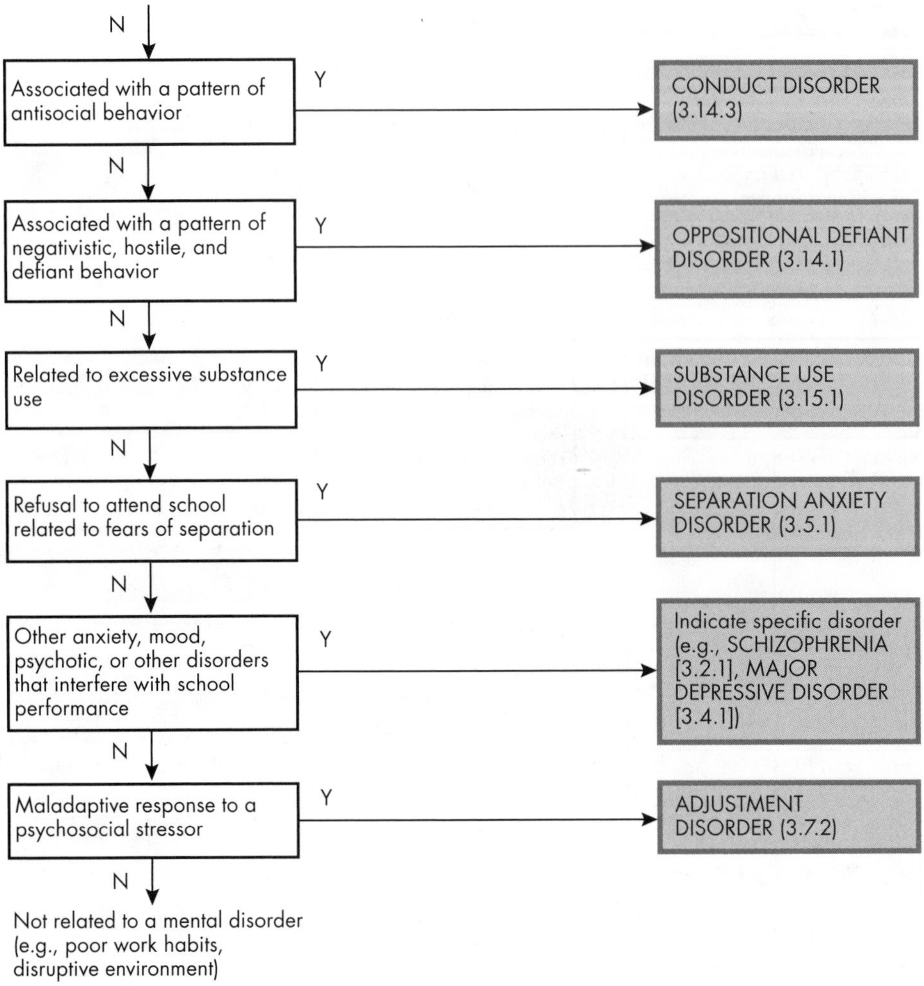
N
Associated with a pattern of antisocial behavior
Y
CONDUCT DISORDER (3.14.3)
N
Associated with a pattern of negativistic, hostile, and defiant behavior
Y
OPPOSITIONAL DEFIANT DISORDER (3.14.1)
N
Related to excessive substance use
Y
SUBSTANCE USE DISORDER (3.15.1)
N
Refusal to attend school related to fears of separation
Y
SEPARATION ANXIETY DISORDER (3.5.1)
N
Other anxiety, mood, psychotic, or other disorders that interfere with school performance
Y
Indicate specific disorder (e.g., SCHIZOPHRENIA [3.2.1], MAJOR DEPRESSIVE DISORDER [3.4.1])
N
Maladaptive response to a psychosocial stressor
Y
ADJUSTMENT DISORDER (3.7.2)
N
Not related to a mental disorder (e.g., poor work habits, disruptive environment)

2.2 Decision Tree for Behavioral Problems in a Child or Adolescent

A common reason for referring a child or adolescent to a mental health professional is to request an evaluation and possible treatment for a reported behavioral problem. It goes without saying, however, that many behavioral problems occurring in children or adolescents are not due to a mental disorder. In some instances, the behavioral problems are not of sufficient severity or duration to warrant such a diagnosis. In others, the problem is more of a disturbance in the family relationship than a problem emanating primarily from the child. Finally, there are some very serious behavioral problems (e.g., shooting, mugging, rape) that occur for reasons outside the domain of the mental disorders covered in DSM-5 (e.g., financial gain, status, revenge).

Behavioral problems with an onset in early childhood are most often associated with Attention-Deficit/Hyperactivity Disorder, Oppositional Defiant Disorder, Disruptive Mood Dysregulation Disorder, Autism Spectrum Disorder, Stereotypic Movement Disorder, and Intellectual Disability (Intellectual Developmental Disorder). The differential among these is usually straightforward and is determined by a consideration of the accompanying symptoms.

A first onset of behavioral problems during adolescence strongly suggests that substances may play an important role. The behavioral problems may result from the direct effect of the substance on the brain (as in Substance Intoxication), may be a by-product of a Substance Use Disorder (e.g., illegal activities associated with procurement), or may be motivated by gain (e.g., a plan to get rich quick as a drug dealer). Other disorders that often have an onset in later childhood or early adolescence include the Adolescent-Onset Type of Conduct Disorder (which has a better prognosis than Childhood-Onset Type occurring before age 10), Major Depressive Disorder, Bipolar Disorder, Schizophrenia, Kleptomania, and Pyromania. Conduct Disorder that has an onset in childhood (i.e., before age 10) is particularly worrisome and is associated with a higher incidence of violence, poorer peer relationships, and an increased likelihood for the child to develop into an adult with Antisocial Personality Disorder.

Behavioral problems occurring in response to a psychosocial stressor suggest either 1) a diagnosis of Posttraumatic Stress Disorder or Acute Stress Disorder, if the stressor is of a particularly traumatic nature and the behavioral problems are accompanied by intrusion symptoms associated with the traumatic events, avoidance of reminders of the event, and a change in cognition, mood, and arousal; or 2) a diagnosis of Adjustment Disorder.

If the behavioral problems are not covered by any of the decision points so far and the problems are clinically significant and represent a psychological or biological dysfunction in the individual, a residual category—Other Specified Disruptive, Impulse-Control, and Conduct Disorder or Unspecified Disruptive, Impulse-Control, and Conduct Disorder—would apply, the choice depending on whether the clinician wishes to record the symptomatic presentation on the chart (in which case Other Specified Disruptive, Impulse-Control, and Conduct Disorder would be used, followed by the specific reason) or not (in which case Unspecified Disruptive, Impulse-Control, and Conduct Disorder would be used). Otherwise, the behavioral problems would be considered problematic but not indicative of a mental disorder, possibly justifying the V code or Z code (dependent on whether ICD-9-CM or ICD-10-CM is applicable, respectively) for Child or Adolescent Antisocial Behavior, which is listed in "Other Conditions That May Be a Focus of Clinical Attention" in DSM-5.

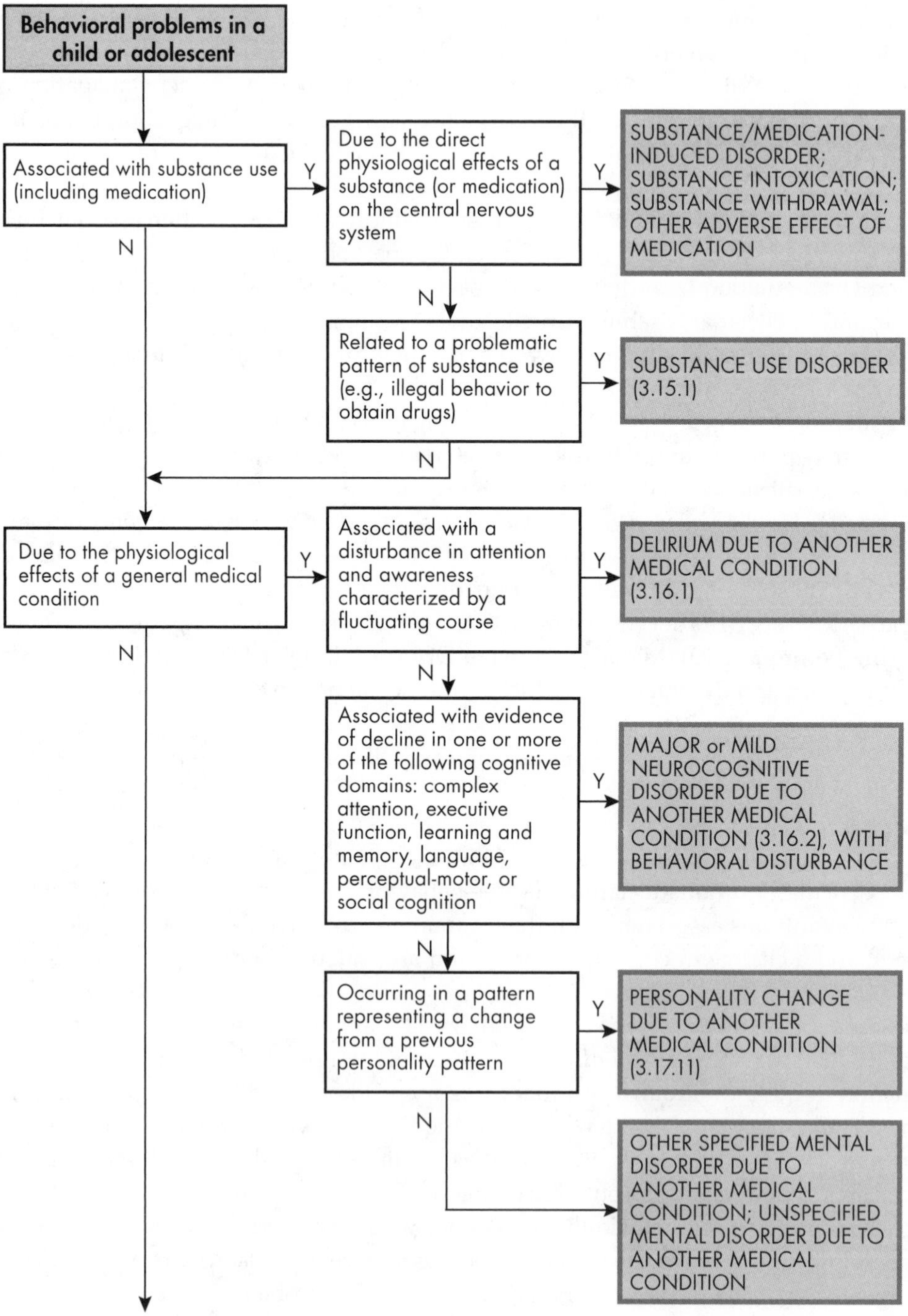

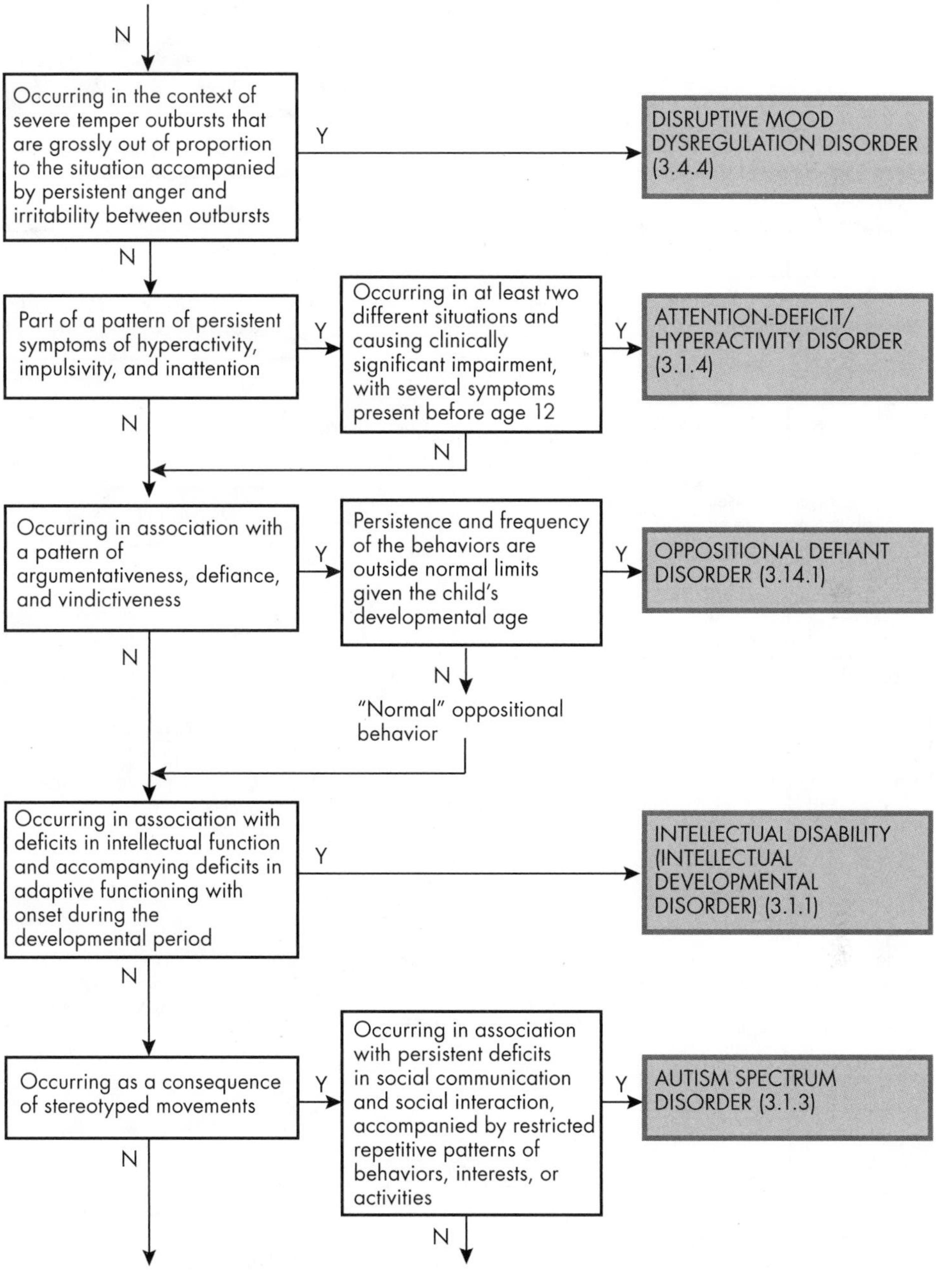
N
Occurring in the context of severe temper outbursts that are grossly out of proportion to the situation accompanied by persistent anger and irritability between outbursts
Y
DISRUPTIVE MOOD DYSREGULATION DISORDER (3.4.4)
N
Part of a pattern of persistent symptoms of hyperactivity, impulsivity, and inattention
Y
Occurring in at least two different situations and causing clinically significant impairment, with several symptoms present before age 12
Y
ATTENTION-DEFICIT/ HYPERACTIVITY DISORDER (3.1.4)
N
N
Occurring in association with a pattern of argumentativeness, defiance, and vindictiveness
Y
Persistence and frequency of the behaviors are outside normal limits given the child's developmental age
Y
OPPOSITIONAL DEFIANT DISORDER (3.14.1)
N
"Normal" oppositional behavior
N
Occurring in association with deficits in intellectual function and accompanying deficits in adaptive functioning with onset during the developmental period
Y
INTELLECTUAL DISABILITY (INTELLECTUAL DEVELOPMENTAL DISORDER) (3.1.1)
N
Occurring as a consequence of stereotyped movements
Y
Occurring in association with persistent deficits in social communication and social interaction, accompanied by restricted repetitive patterns of behaviors, interests, or activities
Y
AUTISM SPECTRUM DISORDER (3.1.3)
N
N

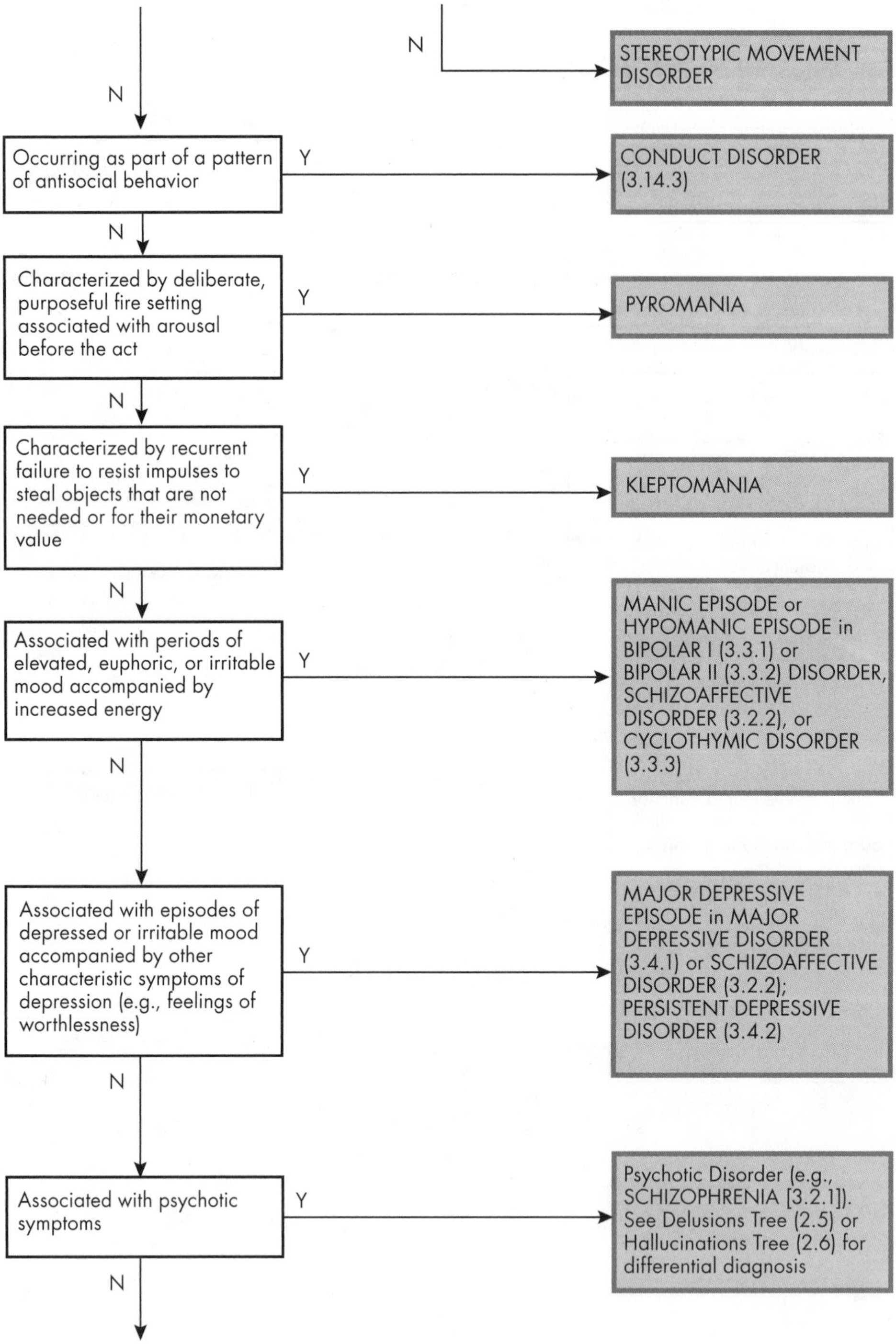
N
STEREOTYPIC MOVEMENT DISORDER
N
Occurring as part of a pattern of antisocial behavior
Y
CONDUCT DISORDER (3.14.3)
N
Characterized by deliberate, purposeful fire setting associated with arousal before the act
Y
PYROMANIA
N
Characterized by recurrent failure to resist impulses to steal objects that are not needed or for their monetary value
Y
KLEPTOMANIA
N
Associated with periods of elevated, euphoric, or irritable mood accompanied by increased energy
Y
MANIC EPISODE or HYPOMANIC EPISODE in BIPOLAR I (3.3.1) or BIPOLAR II (3.3.2) DISORDER, SCHIZOAFFECTIVE DISORDER (3.2.2), or CYCLOTHYMIC DISORDER (3.3.3)
N
Associated with episodes of depressed or irritable mood accompanied by other characteristic symptoms of depression (e.g., feelings of worthlessness)
Y
MAJOR DEPRESSIVE EPISODE in MAJOR DEPRESSIVE DISORDER (3.4.1) or SCHIZOAFFECTIVE DISORDER (3.2.2); PERSISTENT DEPRESSIVE DISORDER (3.4.2)
N
Associated with psychotic symptoms
Y
Psychotic Disorder (e.g., SCHIZOPHRENIA [3.2.1]). See Delusions Tree (2.5) or Hallucinations Tree (2.6) for differential diagnosis
N

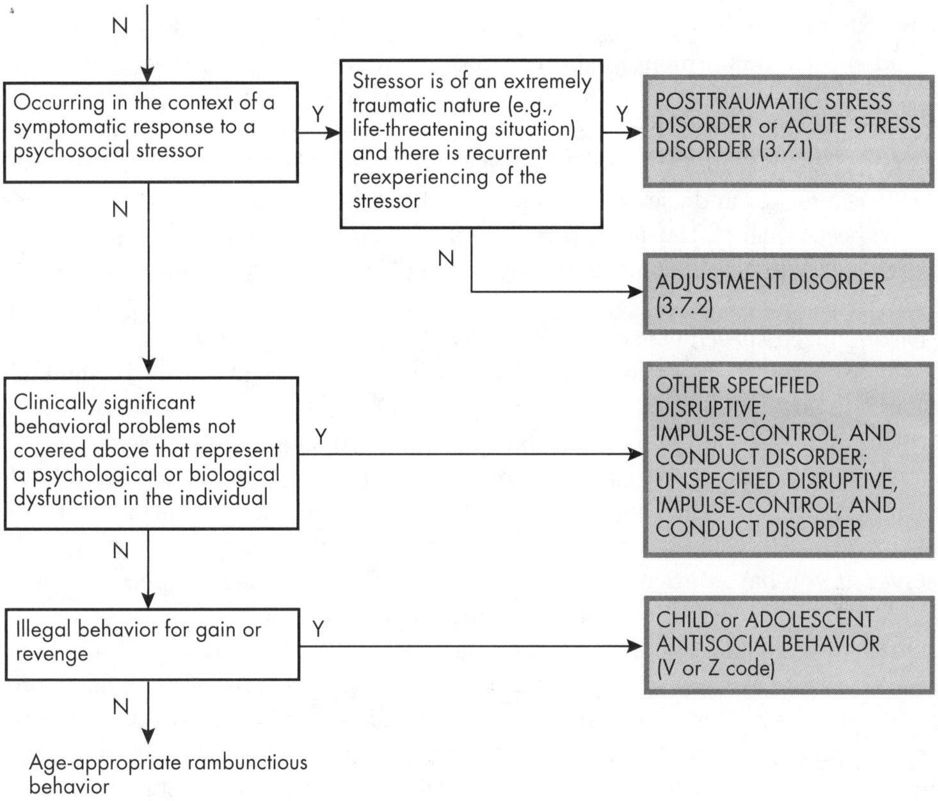
N
Occurring in the context of a symptomatic response to a psychosocial stressor
Y
Stressor is of an extremely traumatic nature (e.g., life-threatening situation) and there is recurrent reexperiencing of the stressor
Y
POSTTRAUMATIC STRESS DISORDER or ACUTE STRESS DISORDER (3.7.1)
N
ADJUSTMENT DISORDER (3.7.2)
N
Clinically significant behavioral problems not covered above that represent a psychological or biological dysfunction in the individual
Y
OTHER SPECIFIED DISRUPTIVE, IMPULSE-CONTROL, AND CONDUCT DISORDER; UNSPECIFIED DISRUPTIVE, IMPULSE-CONTROL, AND CONDUCT DISORDER
N
Illegal behavior for gain or revenge
Y
CHILD or ADOLESCENT ANTISOCIAL BEHAVIOR (V or Z code)
N
Age-appropriate rambunctious behavior

2.3 Decision Tree for Speech Disturbance

The decision tree for speech disturbance covers three types of disturbed speech: disorganized speech, impairment in speech production, and unusual speech. *Disorganized speech* is characterized by the individual's switching from one topic to another without a discernible connection or providing answers to questions that are only obliquely related or unrelated to the question. *Impaired speech production* may be related to problems with the acquisition and use of language, with the ability to articulate words intelligibly, or with speech fluency. *Unusual speech* includes deficits in understanding and following the social rules of verbal communication, slowed or pressured speech, or repetitive or stereotyped speech.

Disorganized speech is one of the most challenging symptoms to diagnose because there is no standard by which to judge when speech is "disorganized." This judgment depends in part on your ability to comprehend and on the patient's pattern of speech production. Furthermore, no one speaks in logically coherent and syntactically correct sentences all the time. Many clinicians and trainees have a tendency to overcall mildly illogical speech as clinically significant "loosening of associations." The kinds of "disorganized speech" covered in this decision tree should be obvious even to the most casual observer. If you have difficulty deciding whether or not a patient's speech is disorganized, then it should probably not be considered pathological.

Once it is established that the individual has disorganized, impaired, or unusual speech, the next challenge is to determine which of the many possible mental disorders best accounts for it. This usually requires an evaluation of the context and the accompanying symptoms. Speech disturbance that is due to a general medical condition may be diagnosed as aphasia, Delirium, or a Major or Mild Neurocognitive Disorder, depending on which other symptoms are present. The speech disturbance in Delirium is accompanied by a disturbance of attention and awareness, whereas the speech disturbance in Major or Mild Neurocognitive Disorder is accompanied by other cognitive deficits. Aphasia (impairment in the understanding or transmission of ideas by language due to injury or disease of the brain centers involved in language) that occurs in the absence of other cognitive symptoms can be diagnosed using the ICD-9-CM symptom code 784.3 (or ICD-10-CM symptom code R47.01).

Disorganized speech is a common manifestation of substance use. Usually a diagnosis of Substance Intoxication or Substance Withdrawal will suffice, but severely disorganized speech suggests a diagnosis of Substance Intoxication Delirium or Substance Withdrawal Delirium or an underlying Substance/Medication-Induced Major Neurocognitive Disorder. The differential diagnosis of disorganized speech in a Manic Episode versus Schizophrenia has been the subject of considerable discussion. The disorganized speech in an episode of Schizophrenia (e.g., so-called loosening of associations) presumably is distinguished from the "flight of ideas" in mania based on the observer's ability to follow the train of thought. Theoretically at least, one can discern how the patient got from one topic to the next in a flight of ideas, whereas the derailments in the speech of patients with Schizophrenia are much less understandable. Although this distinction may be helpful in the most classic cases, at the boundary there are many instances in which it is difficult or impossible to distinguish between loosening of associations and flight of ideas. Similarly, whereas rapid or pressured speech is often characteristic of mania, the speech of an excited or agitated patient with Schizophrenia may also be overwhelming. Therefore, it is best to base the differential diagnosis between Schizophrenia and Manic Episodes on the accompanying symptoms and overall course rather than on an isolated evaluation of the speech pattern.

The decision tree also includes the differential diagnosis for several disorders that are characterized by impaired speech first presenting during development. A diagnosis of a Language Disorder may be warranted if an individual has symptoms such as difficulty understanding words, sentences, or specific types of words; a markedly limited vocabulary; and/or difficulty producing sentences. Difficulties with speech sound production that interfere with intelligibility may warrant a diagnosis of Speech Sound Disorder. Problems in the fluency and time patterning of speech that are inappropriate for age and language skills suggest a diagnosis of Childhood-Onset Fluency Disorder (Stuttering). In Autism Spectrum Disorder and Social (Pragmatic) Communication Disorder, there are deficits in the social use of verbal and nonverbal communication. These problems may be manifested by the person having difficulties with understanding and following social rules of verbal and nonverbal communication in naturalistic contexts, struggles with changing language according to the needs of the listener or situation, and problems following rules for conversations and storytelling. Inappropriate vocal outbursts that occur in the context of otherwise normal speech suggest a Tic Disorder.

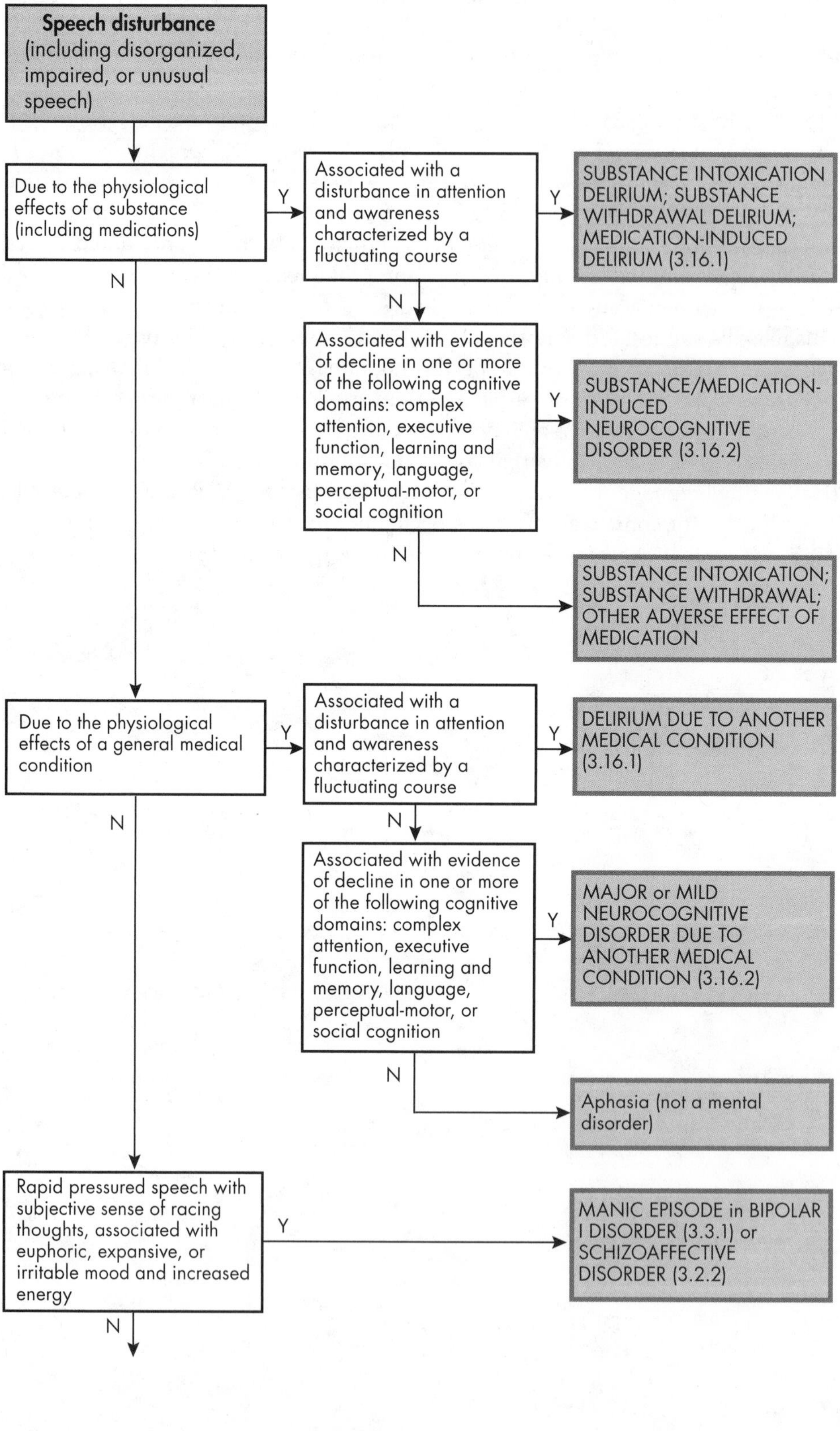
Speech disturbance (including disorganized, impaired, or unusual speech)
Due to the physiological effects of a substance (including medications)
Y
Associated with a disturbance in attention and awareness characterized by a fluctuating course
Y
SUBSTANCE INTOXICATION DELIRIUM; SUBSTANCE WITHDRAWAL DELIRIUM; MEDICATION-INDUCED DELIRIUM (3.16.1)
N
Associated with evidence of decline in one or more of the following cognitive domains: complex attention, executive function, learning and memory, language, perceptual-motor, or social cognition
Y
SUBSTANCE/MEDICATION-INDUCED NEUROCOGNITIVE DISORDER (3.16.2)
N
SUBSTANCE INTOXICATION; SUBSTANCE WITHDRAWAL; OTHER ADVERSE EFFECT OF MEDICATION
N
Due to the physiological effects of a general medical condition
Y
Associated with a disturbance in attention and awareness characterized by a fluctuating course
Y
DELIRIUM DUE TO ANOTHER MEDICAL CONDITION (3.16.1)
N
Associated with evidence of decline in one or more of the following cognitive domains: complex attention, executive function, learning and memory, language, perceptual-motor, or social cognition
Y
MAJOR or MILD NEUROCOGNITIVE DISORDER DUE TO ANOTHER MEDICAL CONDITION (3.16.2)
N
Aphasia (not a mental disorder)
N
Rapid pressured speech with subjective sense of racing thoughts, associated with euphoric, expansive, or irritable mood and increased energy
Y
MANIC EPISODE in BIPOLAR I DISORDER (3.3.1) or SCHIZOAFFECTIVE DISORDER (3.2.2)
N

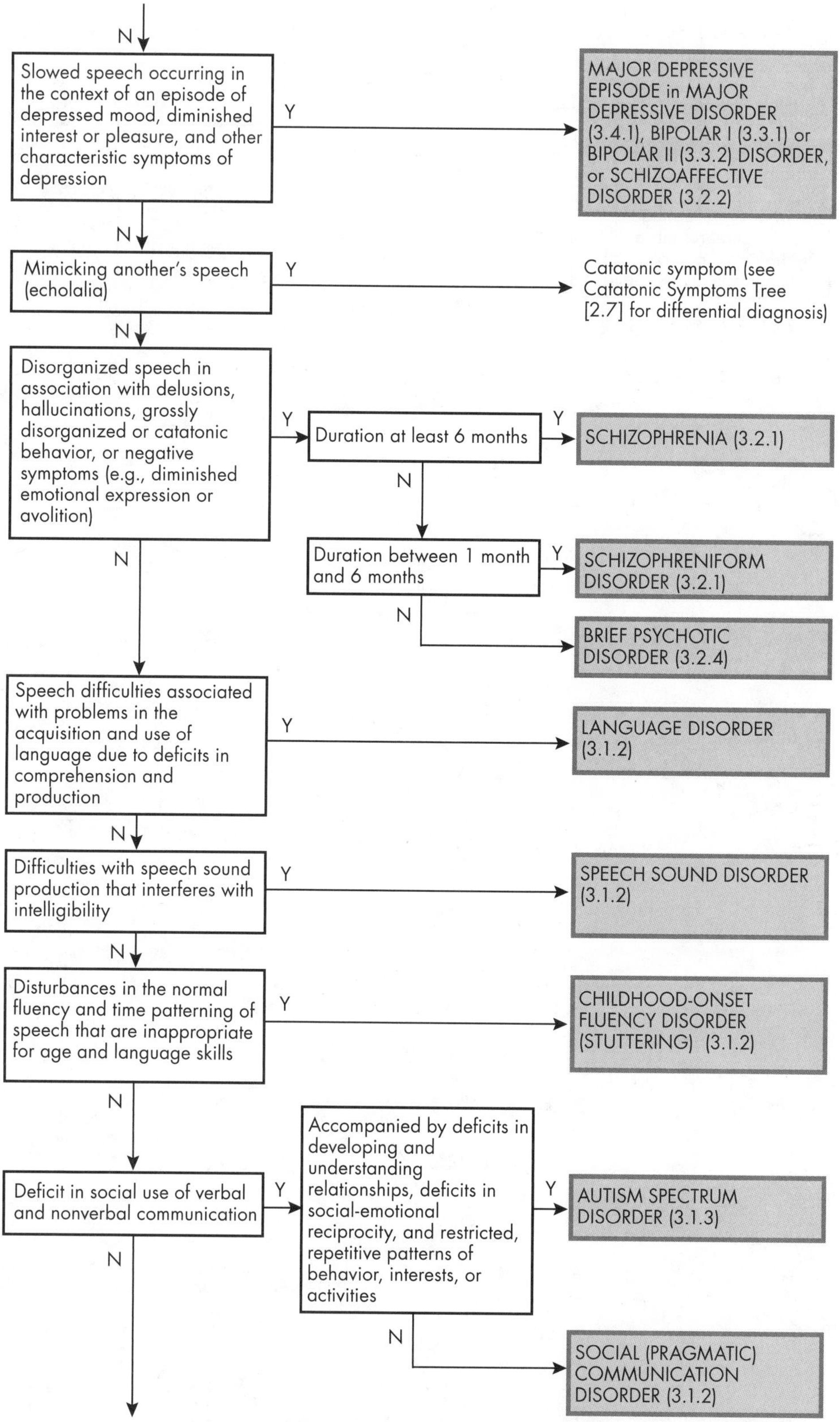
N
Slowed speech occurring in the context of an episode of depressed mood, diminished interest or pleasure, and other characteristic symptoms of depression
Y
MAJOR DEPRESSIVE EPISODE in MAJOR DEPRESSIVE DISORDER (3.4.1), BIPOLAR I (3.3.1) or BIPOLAR II (3.3.2) DISORDER, or SCHIZOAFFECTIVE DISORDER (3.2.2)
N
Mimicking another's speech (echolalia)
Y
Catatonic symptom (see Catatonic Symptoms Tree [2.7] for differential diagnosis)
N
Disorganized speech in association with delusions, hallucinations, grossly disorganized or catatonic behavior, or negative symptoms (e.g., diminished emotional expression or avolition)
Y
Duration at least 6 months
Y
SCHIZOPHRENIA (3.2.1)
N
Duration between 1 month and 6 months
Y
SCHIZOPHRENIFORM DISORDER (3.2.1)
N
BRIEF PSYCHOTIC DISORDER (3.2.4)
N
Speech difficulties associated with problems in the acquisition and use of language due to deficits in comprehension and production
Y
LANGUAGE DISORDER (3.1.2)
N
Difficulties with speech sound production that interferes with intelligibility
Y
SPEECH SOUND DISORDER (3.1.2)
N
Disturbances in the normal fluency and time patterning of speech that are inappropriate for age and language skills
Y
CHILDHOOD-ONSET FLUENCY DISORDER (STUTTERING) (3.1.2)
N
Deficit in social use of verbal and nonverbal communication
Y
Accompanied by deficits in developing and understanding relationships, deficits in social-emotional reciprocity, and restricted, repetitive patterns of behavior, interests, or activities
Y
AUTISM SPECTRUM DISORDER (3.1.3)
N
SOCIAL (PRAGMATIC) COMMUNICATION DISORDER (3.1.2)
N

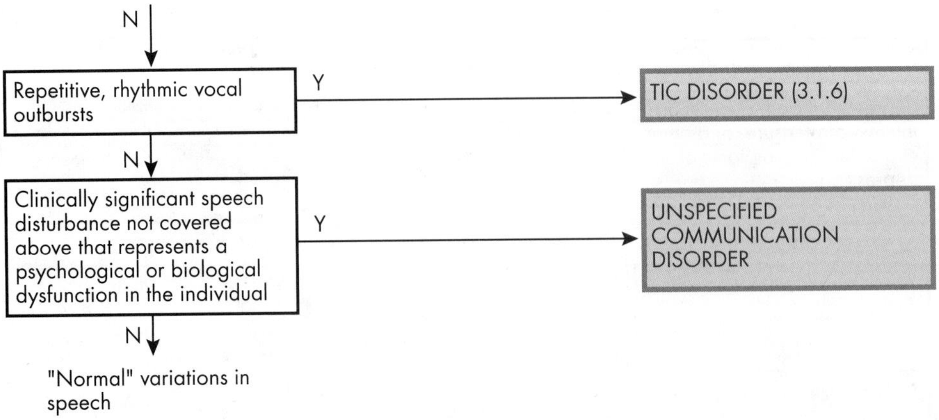
N
Repetitive, rhythmic vocal outbursts
Y
TIC DISORDER (3.1.6)
N
Clinically significant speech disturbance not covered above that represents a psychological or biological dysfunction in the individual
Y
UNSPECIFIED COMMUNICATION DISORDER
N
"Normal" variations in speech

2.4 Decision Tree for Distractibility

Distractibility refers to an inability to filter out extraneous stimuli when attempting to concentrate on a particular task or activity. This is a very nonspecific symptom that occurs in a wide variety of mental disorders, as well as in individuals without any mental disorder. The differential diagnosis rests on the age at onset, severity, the symptoms with which the distractibility is associated, and whether it results from a reaction to an external stressor. Clinically significant inattention with an onset in early childhood suggests a diagnosis of Attention-Deficit/Hyperactivity Disorder. Inattention with onset in adolescence suggests a variety of possible disorders, including recurrent Substance Intoxication or Substance Withdrawal, Major Depressive or Bipolar Disorder, and Schizophrenia. When inattention has a first onset later in life, it is especially important to consider the possible etiological role of a medication, drug of abuse, or general medical condition.

You should consider a diagnosis of Delirium when inattention is severe and is associated with other cognitive or perceptual symptoms (e.g., disorientation, hallucinations). The hallmark of Delirium is a disturbance of attention and awareness—the patient is unable to appreciate or respond appropriately to the external environment, to filter out irrelevant stimuli, and to follow instructions or reply to questions. Because Delirium is often a medical emergency, it is crucial to identify (and then correct) the underlying etiological factors that may be related to a general medical condition, substance use (including medication side effects), or some combination of these.

Distractibility is rarely the presenting symptom in disorders other than Attention-Deficit/Hyperactivity Disorder and Delirium. The evaluation of the differential diagnosis depends on what the accompanying features are (e.g., elevated mood in Manic Episode, excessive worry and anxiety in Generalized Anxiety Disorder, persistent psychotic symptoms in Schizophrenia). It is also always useful to determine whether the patient has experienced psychosocial stressors that may be causing or increasing distractibility.

Finally, everybody has differing abilities to filter out extraneous stimuli from the environment. Moreover, the nature and level of stimulation characteristic of the environment can increase or reduce any individual's ability to maintain attention. Whether a particular manifestation of distractibility constitutes an aspect of a mental disorder or should be considered within the normal range depends on its severity and persistence, and on whether it causes clinically significant distress or impairment.

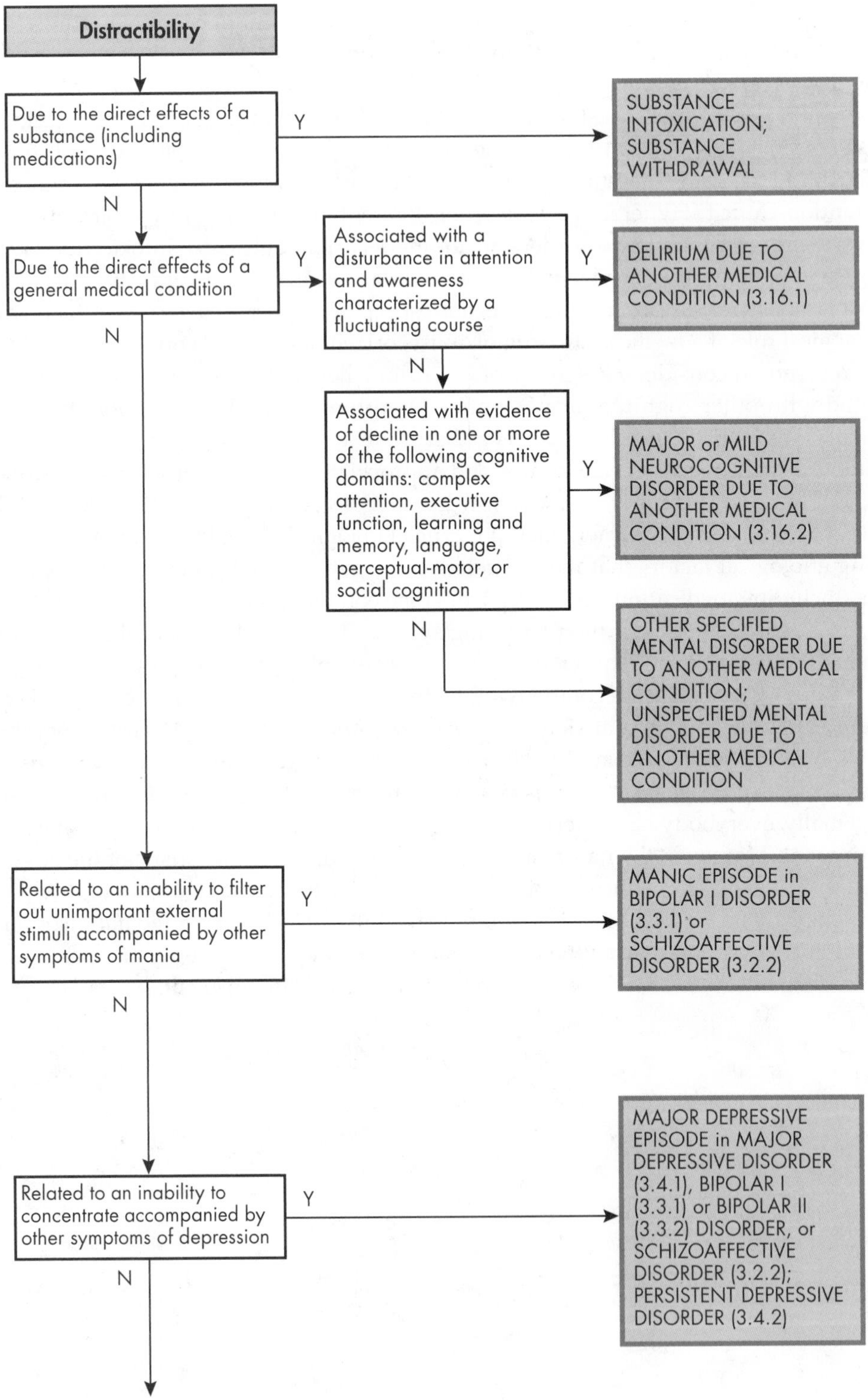
Distractibility
Due to the direct effects of a substance (including medications)
Y
SUBSTANCE INTOXICATION; SUBSTANCE WITHDRAWAL
N
Due to the direct effects of a general medical condition
Y
Associated with a disturbance in attention and awareness characterized by a fluctuating course
Y
DELIRIUM DUE TO ANOTHER MEDICAL CONDITION (3.16.1)
N
Associated with evidence of decline in one or more of the following cognitive domains: complex attention, executive function, learning and memory, language, perceptual-motor, or social cognition
Y
MAJOR or MILD NEUROCOGNITIVE DISORDER DUE TO ANOTHER MEDICAL CONDITION (3.16.2)
N
OTHER SPECIFIED MENTAL DISORDER DUE TO ANOTHER MEDICAL CONDITION; UNSPECIFIED MENTAL DISORDER DUE TO ANOTHER MEDICAL CONDITION
N
Related to an inability to filter out unimportant external stimuli accompanied by other symptoms of mania
Y
MANIC EPISODE in BIPOLAR I DISORDER (3.3.1) or SCHIZOAFFECTIVE DISORDER (3.2.2)
N
Related to an inability to concentrate accompanied by other symptoms of depression
Y
MAJOR DEPRESSIVE EPISODE in MAJOR DEPRESSIVE DISORDER (3.4.1), BIPOLAR I (3.3.1) or BIPOLAR II (3.3.2) DISORDER, or SCHIZOAFFECTIVE DISORDER (3.2.2); PERSISTENT DEPRESSIVE DISORDER (3.4.2)
N

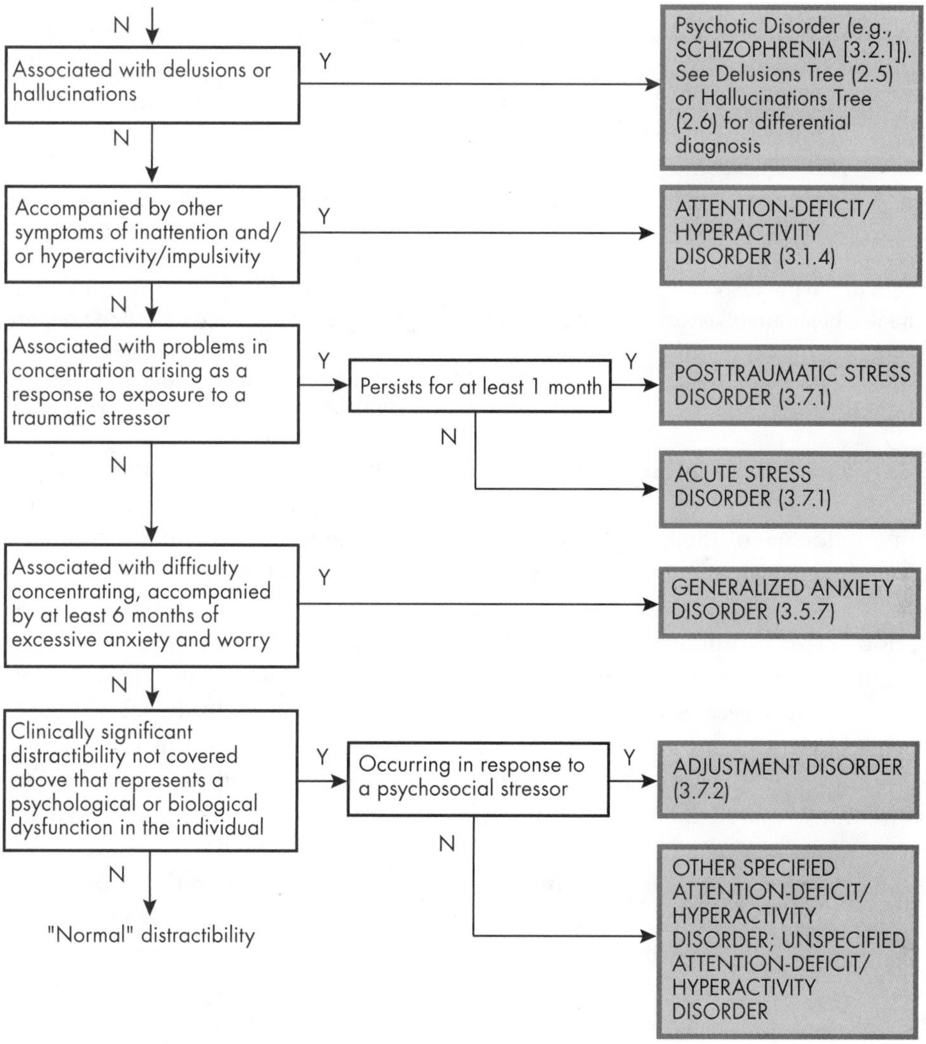
N
Associated with delusions or hallucinations
Y
Psychotic Disorder (e.g., SCHIZOPHRENIA [3.2.1]). See Delusions Tree (2.5) or Hallucinations Tree (2.6) for differential diagnosis
N
Accompanied by other symptoms of inattention and/or hyperactivity/impulsivity
Y
ATTENTION-DEFICIT/HYPERACTIVITY DISORDER (3.1.4)
N
Associated with problems in concentration arising as a response to exposure to a traumatic stressor
Y
Persists for at least 1 month
Y
POSTTRAUMATIC STRESS DISORDER (3.7.1)
N
ACUTE STRESS DISORDER (3.7.1)
N
Associated with difficulty concentrating, accompanied by at least 6 months of excessive anxiety and worry
Y
GENERALIZED ANXIETY DISORDER (3.5.7)
N
Clinically significant distractibility not covered above that represents a psychological or biological dysfunction in the individual
Y
Occurring in response to a psychosocial stressor
Y
ADJUSTMENT DISORDER (3.7.2)
N
OTHER SPECIFIED ATTENTION-DEFICIT/HYPERACTIVITY DISORDER; UNSPECIFIED ATTENTION-DEFICIT/HYPERACTIVITY DISORDER
N
"Normal" distractibility

2.5 Decision Tree for Delusions

A common error regarding the differential diagnosis for delusions is to assume that a belief that is unusual (at least from the clinician's perspective) is necessarily a delusion. Such misattributions can be avoided through a careful application of the DSM-5 glossary definition of *delusion:*

> A false belief based on incorrect inference about external reality that is firmly held despite what almost everyone else believes and despite what constitutes incontrovertible and obvious proof or evidence to the contrary. The belief is not ordinarily accepted by other members of the person's culture or subculture (e.g., it is not an article of religious faith). When a false belief involves a value judgment, it is regarded as a delusion only when the judgment is so extreme as to defy credibility. Delusional conviction can sometimes be inferred from an overvalued idea (in which case the individual has an unreasonable belief or idea but does not hold it as firmly as is the case with a delusion). (p. 819)

Several aspects of this definition are helpful to keep in mind when attempting to determine whether a patient is delusional. Delusional convictions are impervious to compelling evidence of their implausibility, and the person remains totally convinced of their veracity, rejecting alternative explanations out of hand. In deciding whether a belief is fixed and false enough to be considered a delusion, you must first determine that a serious error in inference and reality testing has occurred and then determine the strength of the conviction. It may be helpful to ask the patient to talk at length about his or her conviction because it is often only in the specific details of the belief that the errors of inference become apparent. In evaluating the strength of the delusional conviction, you should present alternative explanations (e.g., the possibility that the phone hang-ups are due to people dialing a wrong number). The patient who cannot even acknowledge the possibility of these explanations is most likely to be delusional. It should be noted that the evaluation of whether a religious belief is delusional is especially challenging because religious beliefs cannot be subject to the typical test of whether the belief is "true" or "false" and thus cannot be challenged with incontrovertible evidence or proof to the contrary. In such situations the clinician must consider the parameters of the belief system that is characteristic of the person's religion and determine if the person's beliefs deviate markedly from what would be considered "normal" within the context of his or her religion. If you are unfamiliar with the beliefs characteristic of the individual's cultural or religious background, consultation with other individuals who are familiar with the patient's culture or religion is often necessary to avoid misdiagnosing a religious belief as a delusion. As noted in the first step of this decision tree, fixed beliefs that are sanctioned by that person's culture or religion should not be considered to be delusions.

Once it is determined that a delusion is present, your next task is to determine which from among the many possible DSM-5 disorders best accounts for it. The particular content and form of a delusion are much less important in making the diagnosis than is the context in which it occurs. The most common diagnostic error here is to overlook the critically important role of substances (including medications) and general medical conditions in the etiology of delusions. In younger individuals presenting with delusions, it is important to do a careful history and drug screening to rule out the role of drugs of abuse. First onset of delusional thinking at a late age should always raise a red flag for a possible underlying general medical condition or a medication side effect.

Once substance and general medical etiologies have been ruled out, the next task is to determine whether clinically significant mood symptoms are also present. The presence of a Manic or Major Depressive Episode raises the possibility that the delusions are part of a Bipolar I Disorder With Psychotic Features, Bipolar II Disorder With Psychotic Features, Major Depressive Disorder With Psychotic Features, or Schizoaffective Disorder. The differential diagnosis in this case depends on the temporal relationship between the delusions and the mood episodes. If the delusions are confined exclusively to the mood episodes, then the diagnosis is Bipolar I Disorder With Psychotic Features, Bipolar II Disorder With Psychotic Features, or Major Depressive Disorder With Psychotic Features. On the other hand, if delusions and other psychotic symptoms also occur before or after the mood episodes, the diagnosis might be Schizophrenia, Schizophreniform Disorder, Delusional Disorder, or Schizoaffective Disorder, depending on the overlap between the mood episodes and delusions, and the relative duration of the mood episodes versus the delusions. The diagnosis is Schizophrenia, Schizophreniform Disorder, or Delusional Disorder if either there is no period of overlap between mood episodes and delusions or, if there is a period of overlap, the mood episodes have been present for only a minority of the total duration of the psychotic illness (e.g., several months of mood episodes during a chronic psychotic disturbance lasing years). In contrast, the diagnosis is Schizoaffective Disorder if the mood episodes overlap with the delusions and the mood episodes are present for the majority of the total duration of the psychotic disturbance (e.g., a 2-year psychotic disturbance with 1½ years of mood symptoms). Note that in those cases of Schizophrenia, Schizophreniform Disorder, or Delusional Disorder in which there are mood episodes that either 1) do not overlap with the psychotic symptoms or 2) are present for only a minority of the time relative to the total duration of a psychotic disturbance, a comorbid diagnosis of Bipolar I, Bipolar II, or Major Depressive Disorder may also be given. This is a change from DSM-IV-TR, in that the hierarchy between Schizophrenia–Schizophreniform Disorder–Delusional Disorder and Bipolar Disorder–Major Depressive Disorder has been eliminated in DSM-5, making it permissible for an individual to be diagnosed with comorbid 1) Schizophrenia, Schizophreniform Disorder, or Delusional Disorder and 2) Bipolar or Major Depressive Disorder.

Once you have ruled out significant mood episodes, the differential diagnosis depends on symptom pattern and duration. The distinction between Schizophrenia and Delusional Disorder is usually based on the presence in Schizophrenia of one or more additional characteristic symptoms (e.g., hallucinations, disorganized speech, grossly disorganized or catatonic behavior, negative symptoms). The duration of the episode is what distinguishes Schizophrenia (over 6 months' duration), Schizophreniform Disorder (1–6 months' duration), and Brief Psychotic Disorder (less than 1 month).

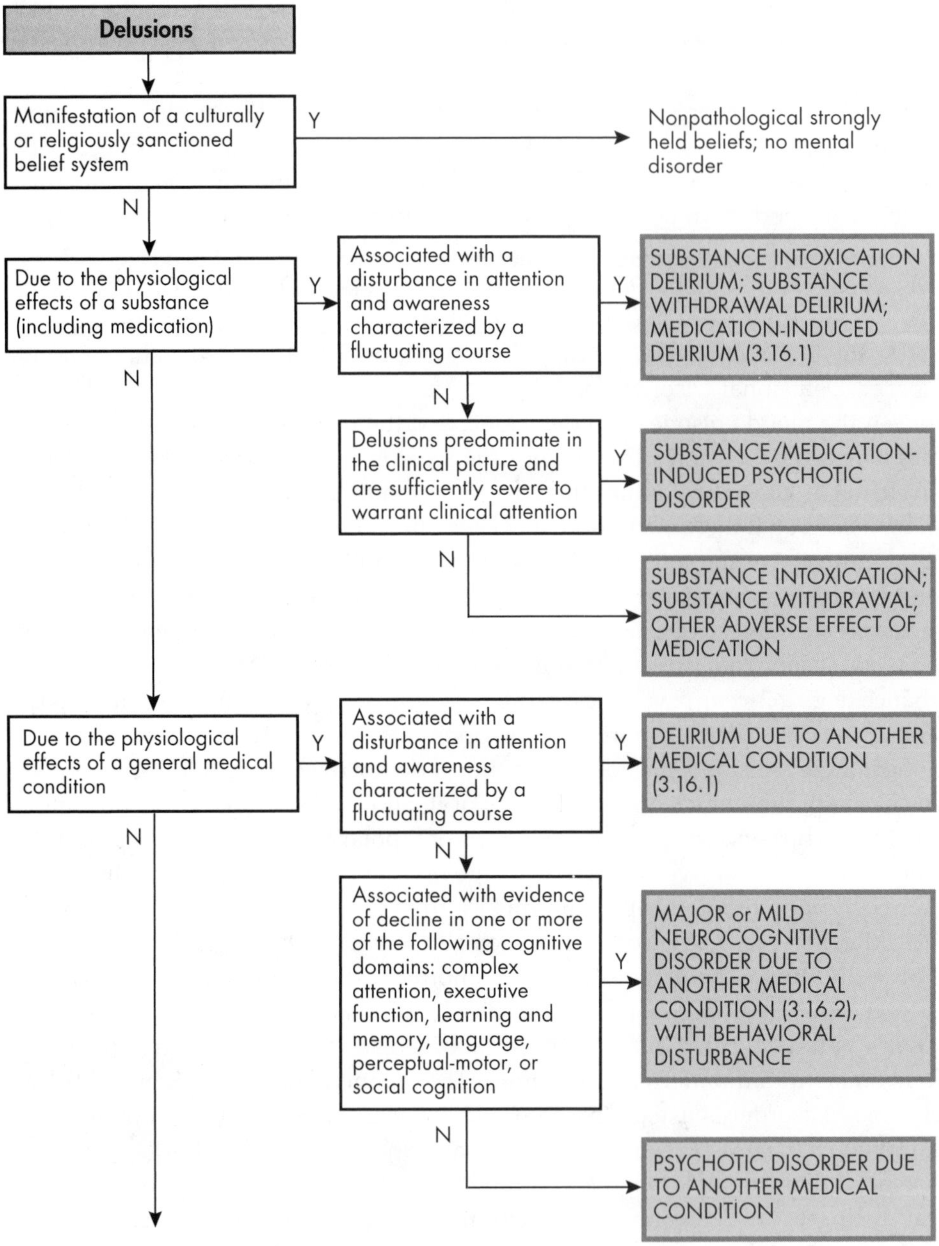
Delusions
Manifestation of a culturally or religiously sanctioned belief system
Y
Nonpathological strongly held beliefs; no mental disorder
N
Due to the physiological effects of a substance (including medication)
Y
Associated with a disturbance in attention and awareness characterized by a fluctuating course
Y
SUBSTANCE INTOXICATION DELIRIUM; SUBSTANCE WITHDRAWAL DELIRIUM; MEDICATION-INDUCED DELIRIUM (3.16.1)
N
Delusions predominate in the clinical picture and are sufficiently severe to warrant clinical attention
Y
SUBSTANCE/MEDICATION-INDUCED PSYCHOTIC DISORDER
N
SUBSTANCE INTOXICATION; SUBSTANCE WITHDRAWAL; OTHER ADVERSE EFFECT OF MEDICATION
N
Due to the physiological effects of a general medical condition
Y
Associated with a disturbance in attention and awareness characterized by a fluctuating course
Y
DELIRIUM DUE TO ANOTHER MEDICAL CONDITION (3.16.1)
N
Associated with evidence of decline in one or more of the following cognitive domains: complex attention, executive function, learning and memory, language, perceptual-motor, or social cognition
Y
MAJOR or MILD NEUROCOGNITIVE DISORDER DUE TO ANOTHER MEDICAL CONDITION (3.16.2), WITH BEHAVIORAL DISTURBANCE
N
PSYCHOTIC DISORDER DUE TO ANOTHER MEDICAL CONDITION
N

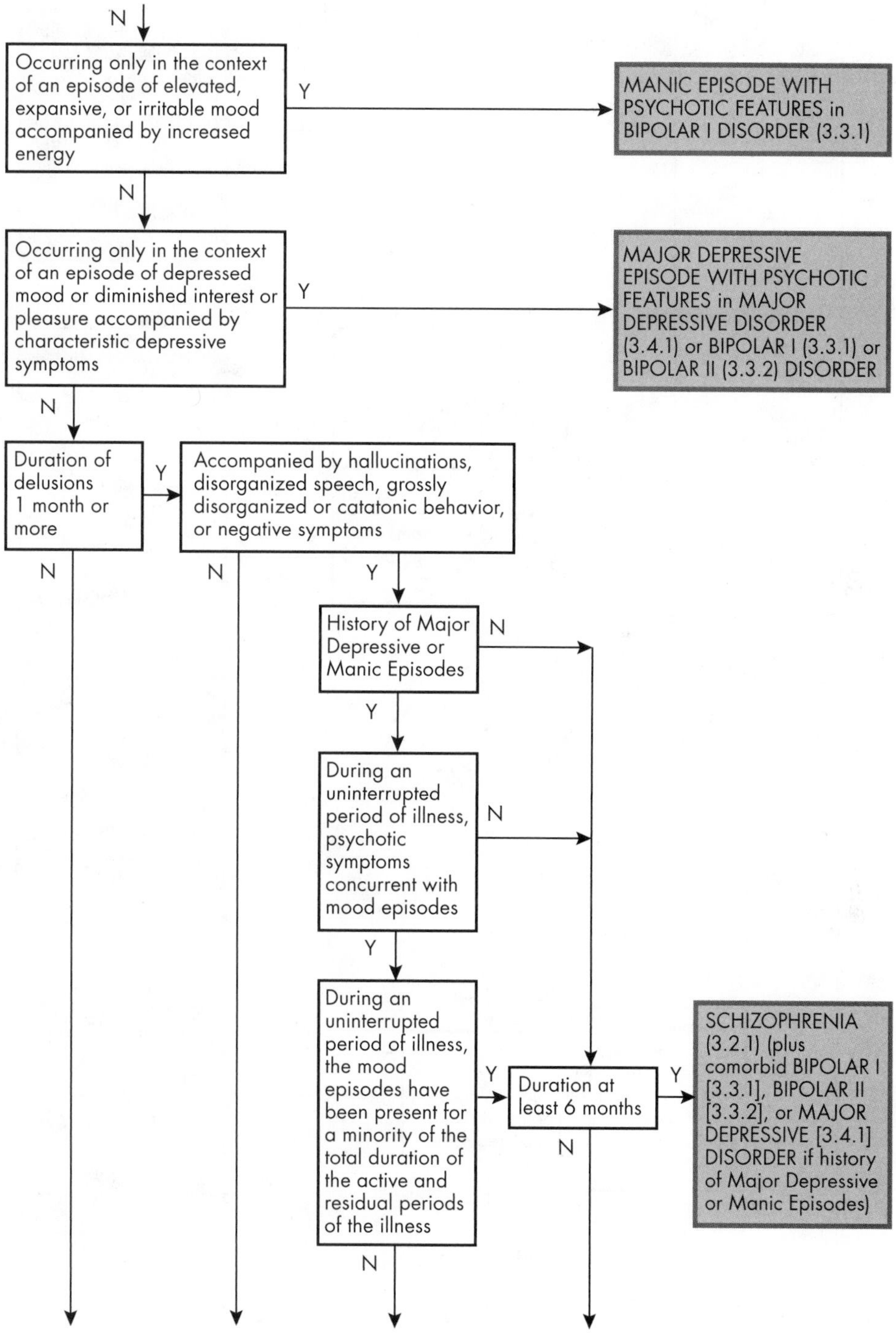
N
Occurring only in the context of an episode of elevated, expansive, or irritable mood accompanied by increased energy
Y
MANIC EPISODE WITH PSYCHOTIC FEATURES in BIPOLAR I DISORDER (3.3.1)
N
Occurring only in the context of an episode of depressed mood or diminished interest or pleasure accompanied by characteristic depressive symptoms
Y
MAJOR DEPRESSIVE EPISODE WITH PSYCHOTIC FEATURES in MAJOR DEPRESSIVE DISORDER (3.4.1) or BIPOLAR I (3.3.1) or BIPOLAR II (3.3.2) DISORDER
N
Duration of delusions 1 month or more
Y
Accompanied by hallucinations, disorganized speech, grossly disorganized or catatonic behavior, or negative symptoms
N
N
Y
History of Major Depressive or Manic Episodes
N
Y
During an uninterrupted period of illness, psychotic symptoms concurrent with mood episodes
N
Y
During an uninterrupted period of illness, the mood episodes have been present for a minority of the total duration of the active and residual periods of the illness
Y
Duration at least 6 months
Y
SCHIZOPHRENIA (3.2.1) (plus comorbid BIPOLAR I [3.3.1], BIPOLAR II [3.3.2], or MAJOR DEPRESSIVE [3.4.1] DISORDER if history of Major Depressive or Manic Episodes)
N
N

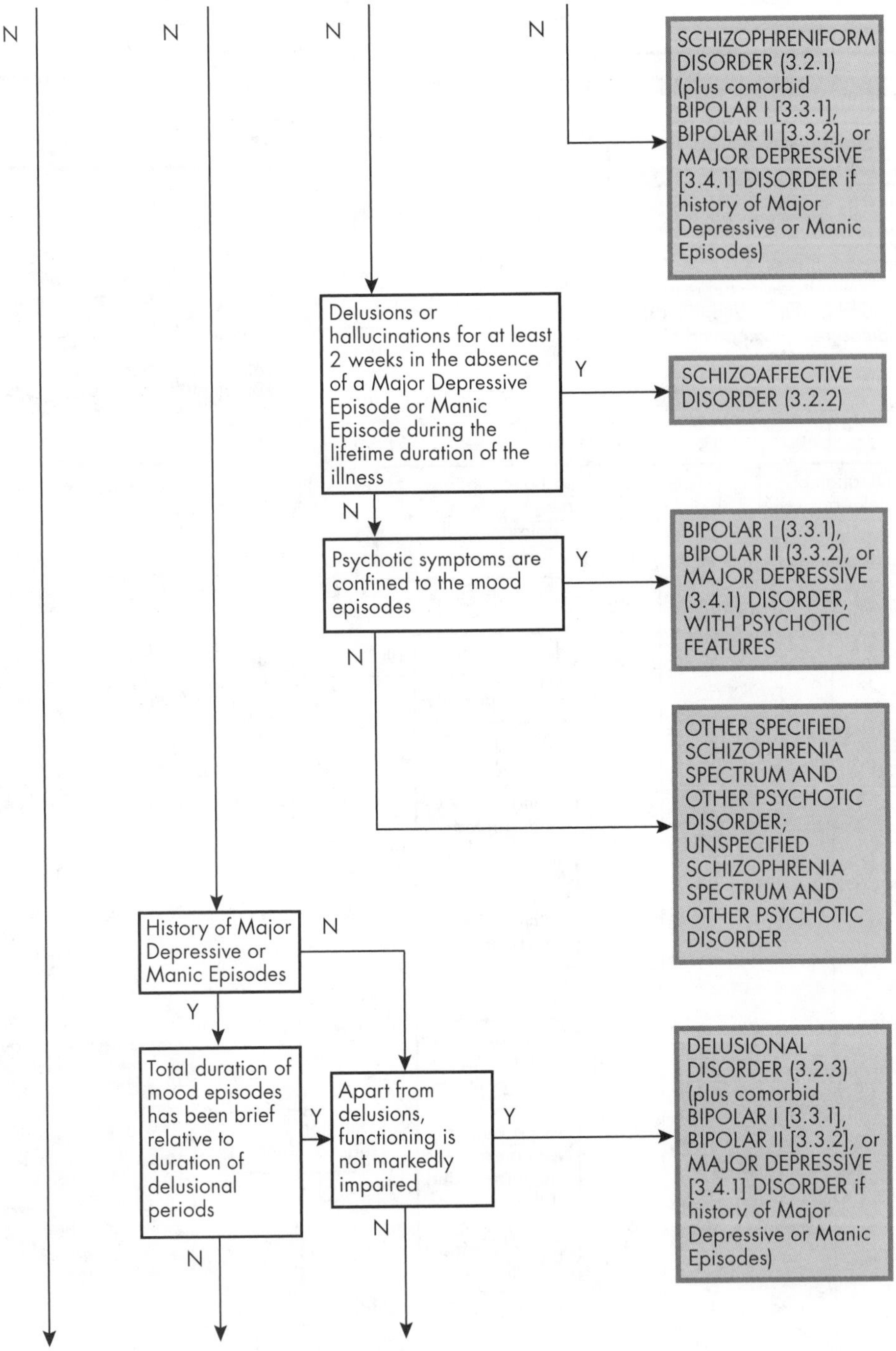
N
N
N
N
SCHIZOPHRENIFORM DISORDER (3.2.1) (plus comorbid BIPOLAR I [3.3.1], BIPOLAR II [3.3.2], or MAJOR DEPRESSIVE [3.4.1] DISORDER if history of Major Depressive or Manic Episodes)
Delusions or hallucinations for at least 2 weeks in the absence of a Major Depressive Episode or Manic Episode during the lifetime duration of the illness
Y
SCHIZOAFFECTIVE DISORDER (3.2.2)
N
Psychotic symptoms are confined to the mood episodes
Y
BIPOLAR I (3.3.1), BIPOLAR II (3.3.2), or MAJOR DEPRESSIVE (3.4.1) DISORDER, WITH PSYCHOTIC FEATURES
N
OTHER SPECIFIED SCHIZOPHRENIA SPECTRUM AND OTHER PSYCHOTIC DISORDER; UNSPECIFIED SCHIZOPHRENIA SPECTRUM AND OTHER PSYCHOTIC DISORDER
History of Major Depressive or Manic Episodes
N
Y
Total duration of mood episodes has been brief relative to duration of delusional periods
Y
Apart from delusions, functioning is not markedly impaired
Y
DELUSIONAL DISORDER (3.2.3) (plus comorbid BIPOLAR I [3.3.1], BIPOLAR II [3.3.2], or MAJOR DEPRESSIVE [3.4.1] DISORDER if history of Major Depressive or Manic Episodes)
N
N

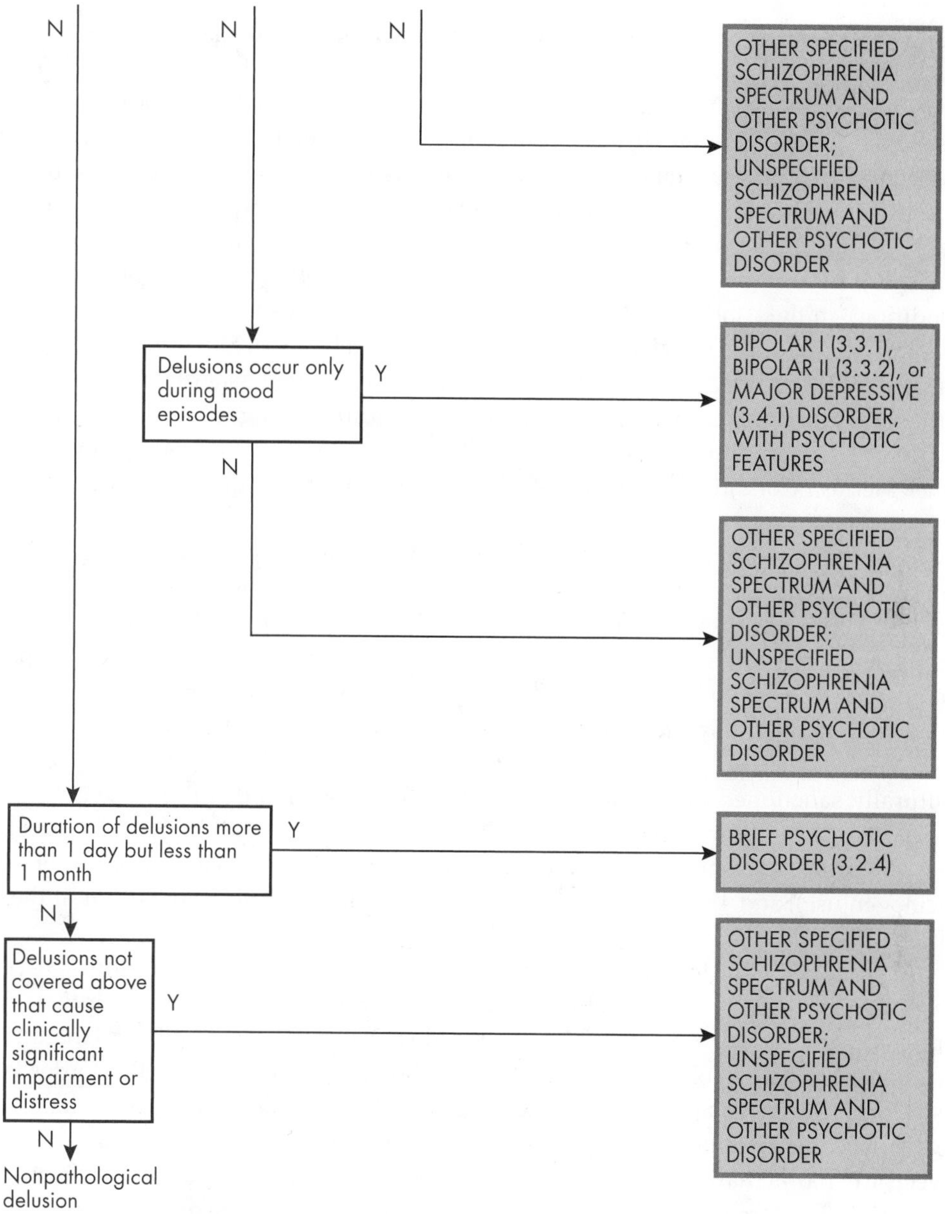
N
N
N
OTHER SPECIFIED SCHIZOPHRENIA SPECTRUM AND OTHER PSYCHOTIC DISORDER; UNSPECIFIED SCHIZOPHRENIA SPECTRUM AND OTHER PSYCHOTIC DISORDER
Delusions occur only during mood episodes
Y
BIPOLAR I (3.3.1), BIPOLAR II (3.3.2), or MAJOR DEPRESSIVE (3.4.1) DISORDER, WITH PSYCHOTIC FEATURES
N
OTHER SPECIFIED SCHIZOPHRENIA SPECTRUM AND OTHER PSYCHOTIC DISORDER; UNSPECIFIED SCHIZOPHRENIA SPECTRUM AND OTHER PSYCHOTIC DISORDER
Duration of delusions more than 1 day but less than 1 month
Y
BRIEF PSYCHOTIC DISORDER (3.2.4)
N
Delusions not covered above that cause clinically significant impairment or distress
Y
OTHER SPECIFIED SCHIZOPHRENIA SPECTRUM AND OTHER PSYCHOTIC DISORDER; UNSPECIFIED SCHIZOPHRENIA SPECTRUM AND OTHER PSYCHOTIC DISORDER
N
Nonpathological delusion

2.6 Decision Tree for Hallucinations

Hallucinations are sensory perceptions without external stimulation. When trying to determine the etiology of a hallucination, you need to consider the sensory modality involved (i.e., whether the hallucination is auditory, visual, gustatory, olfactory, or tactile). As a rule of thumb, visual, gustatory, and olfactory hallucinations are especially suggestive of an etiological substance or general medical condition and demand a careful medical workup. Similarly, a late age at first onset of hallucinations in any modality suggests the need for an especially careful medical workup. Hallucinations can occur in the context of a Delirium (either substance- or medication-induced or due to a general medical condition), in the context of a Major or Mild Neurocognitive Disorder Due to Another Medical Condition (in which case the specifier "With Behavioral Disturbance" should be used), in the absence of accompanying cognitive impairment as a direct physiological consequence of a substance or general medical condition (diagnosed respectively as a Substance/Medication-Induced Psychotic Disorder or a Psychotic Disorder Due to Another Medical Condition), or as a typical feature of an intoxication or withdrawal syndrome.

After ruling out a general medical condition or substance as an etiological factor, you must then consider whether the hallucination is indicative of a psychotic disorder. There are four circumstances in which "hallucinations" should not count toward the diagnosis of a psychotic disorder: 1) those that occur in the context of conversion (so-called pseudohallucinations), which tend to affect multiple sensory modalities at the same time and to have psychologically meaningful content presented to the clinician in the form of an interesting story; 2) hallucinatory experiences that are part of a religious ritual or are a culturally sanctioned experience (e.g., hearing the voice of a dead relative giving advice); 3) those substance-induced hallucinations that occur with intact reality testing (e.g., an individual who is aware that the perceptual disturbances are due to recent hallucinogen use); and 4) hypnopompic or hypnagogic hallucinations that occur at the beginning or end of sleep episodes.

The next task is to determine whether clinically significant mood symptoms are present and, if so, the relationship between the hallucinations and the mood symptoms. The presence of a Manic or Major Depressive Episode raises the possibility that the hallucinations are part of a Bipolar I Disorder With Psychotic Features, Bipolar II Disorder With Psychotic Features, Major Depressive Disorder With Psychotic Features, or Schizoaffective Disorder. The differential diagnosis here depends on the temporal relationship between the hallucinations and the mood episodes. If the hallucinations are confined exclusively to the mood episodes, then the diagnosis is Bipolar I Disorder With Psychotic Features, Bipolar II Disorder With Psychotic Features, or Major Depressive Disorder With Psychotic Features. Such hallucinations can be mood congruent (e.g., castigating accusatory voices in an individual with depression) or mood incongruent (i.e., hallucinations that have nothing to do with the prevailing mood).

On the other hand, if hallucinations and other psychotic symptoms also occur before or after the mood episodes, the diagnosis might be Schizophrenia, Schizophreniform Disorder, or Schizoaffective Disorder, depending on the overlap between the mood episodes and hallucinations, and the relative duration of the mood episodes versus the total duration of the psychotic disturbance. The diagnosis is Schizophrenia or Schizophreniform Disorder if there is no period of overlap between mood episodes and the hallucinations or, if there is a period of overlap, the mood episodes have been present for only a minority of the total duration of the psychotic illness (e.g., several months of mood episodes during a chronic psychotic disturbance lasting years). By contrast, the diagnosis is Schizoaffective Disorder if the mood episodes overlap with the hallucinations and the mood episodes are present for a majority of the total time of the disturbance (e.g., a 2-year psychotic disturbance with 1½ years of mood symptoms). Note that in those cases of Schizophrenia or Schizophreniform Disorder in which either 1) there are mood episodes that do not overlap with the psychotic symptoms or 2) all mood episodes are present for a minority of the time relative to the total duration of the psychotic disturbance, a comorbid diagnosis of Bipolar Disorder or Major Depressive Disorder may also be given. This is a change from DSM-IV-TR, in that the hierarchy between Schizophrenia and Bipolar Disorder/Major Depressive Disorder has been eliminated in DSM-5, making it permissible to have comorbidity between Schizophrenia and Bipolar or Major Depressive Disorder.

Illusions differ from hallucinations; an illusion involves a misperception of an actual stimulus. When illusions occur in the absence of hallucinations, they do not count toward a diagnosis of a psychotic disorder and instead suggest Delirium, Substance Intoxication or Substance Withdrawal, Schizotypal Personality Disorder, or no mental disorder.

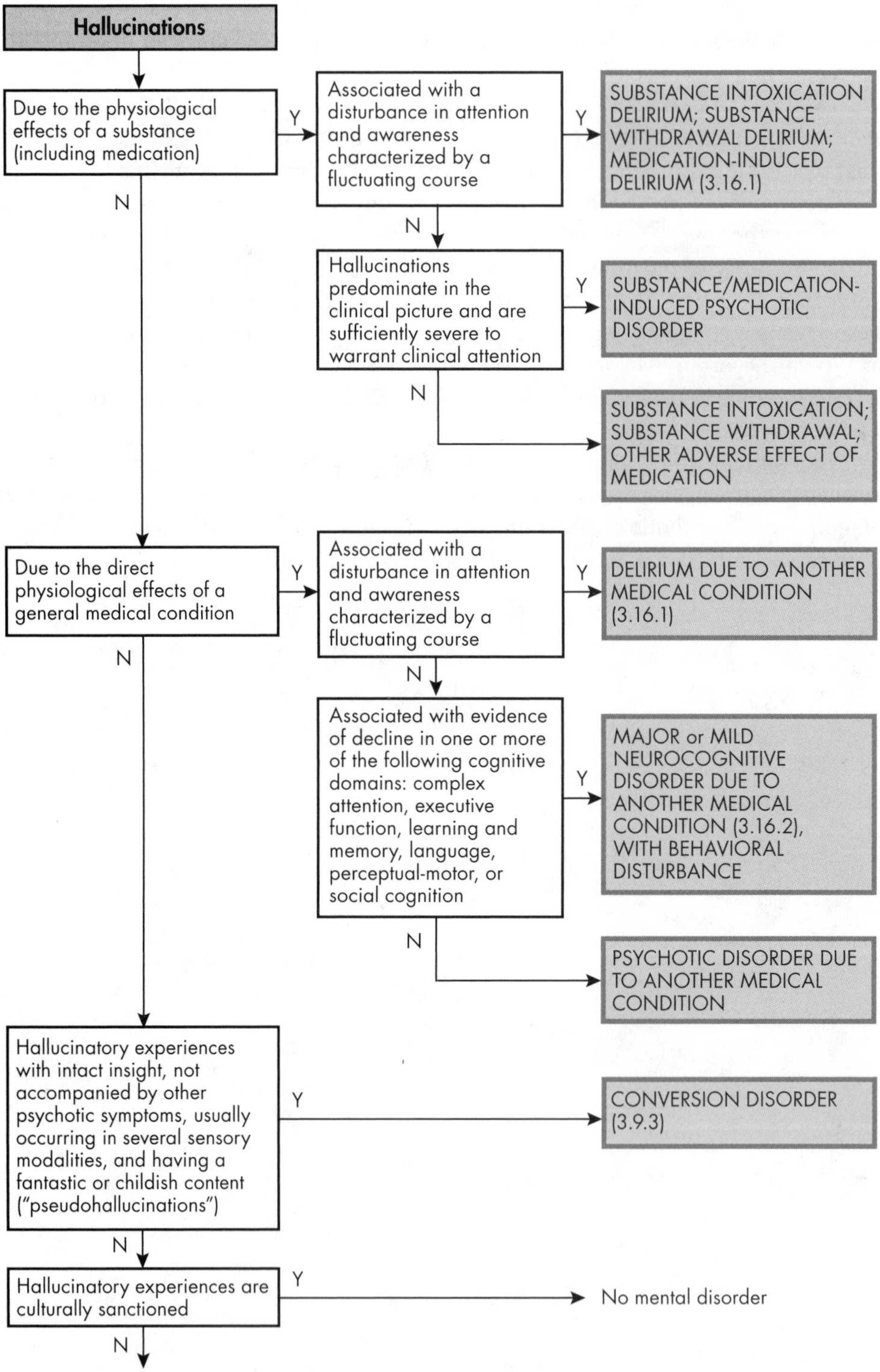
Hallucinations
Due to the physiological effects of a substance (including medication)
Y
Associated with a disturbance in attention and awareness characterized by a fluctuating course
Y
SUBSTANCE INTOXICATION DELIRIUM; SUBSTANCE WITHDRAWAL DELIRIUM; MEDICATION-INDUCED DELIRIUM (3.16.1)
N
Hallucinations predominate in the clinical picture and are sufficiently severe to warrant clinical attention
Y
SUBSTANCE/MEDICATION-INDUCED PSYCHOTIC DISORDER
N
SUBSTANCE INTOXICATION; SUBSTANCE WITHDRAWAL; OTHER ADVERSE EFFECT OF MEDICATION
N
Due to the direct physiological effects of a general medical condition
Y
Associated with a disturbance in attention and awareness characterized by a fluctuating course
Y
DELIRIUM DUE TO ANOTHER MEDICAL CONDITION (3.16.1)
N
Associated with evidence of decline in one or more of the following cognitive domains: complex attention, executive function, learning and memory, language, perceptual-motor, or social cognition
Y
MAJOR or MILD NEUROCOGNITIVE DISORDER DUE TO ANOTHER MEDICAL CONDITION (3.16.2), WITH BEHAVIORAL DISTURBANCE
N
PSYCHOTIC DISORDER DUE TO ANOTHER MEDICAL CONDITION
N
Hallucinatory experiences with intact insight, not accompanied by other psychotic symptoms, usually occurring in several sensory modalities, and having a fantastic or childish content ("pseudohallucinations")
Y
CONVERSION DISORDER (3.9.3)
N
Hallucinatory experiences are culturally sanctioned
Y
No mental disorder
N

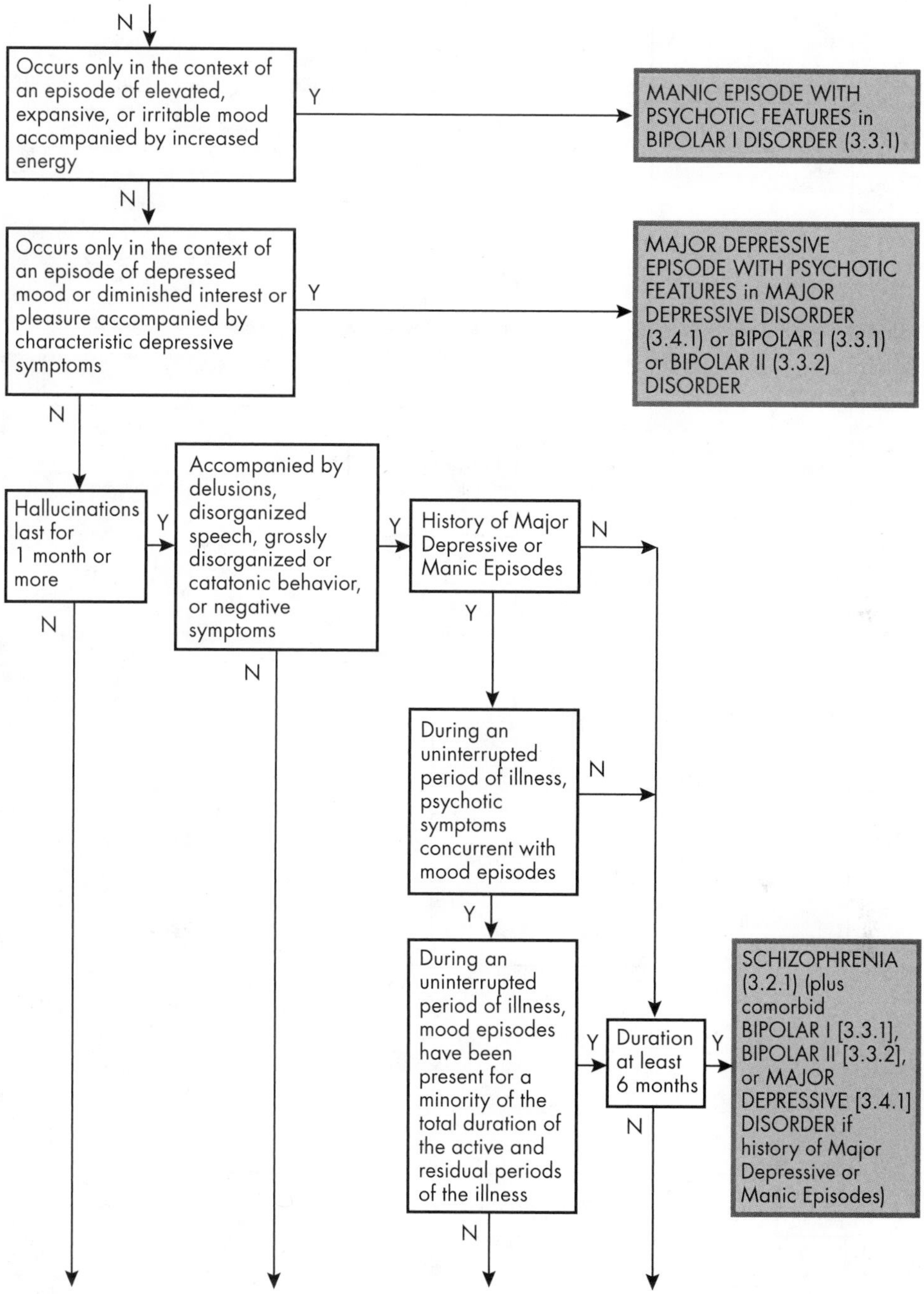
N
Occurs only in the context of an episode of elevated, expansive, or irritable mood accompanied by increased energy
Y
MANIC EPISODE WITH PSYCHOTIC FEATURES in BIPOLAR I DISORDER (3.3.1)
N
Occurs only in the context of an episode of depressed mood or diminished interest or pleasure accompanied by characteristic depressive symptoms
Y
MAJOR DEPRESSIVE EPISODE WITH PSYCHOTIC FEATURES in MAJOR DEPRESSIVE DISORDER (3.4.1) or BIPOLAR I (3.3.1) or BIPOLAR II (3.3.2) DISORDER
N
Hallucinations last for 1 month or more
Y
Accompanied by delusions, disorganized speech, grossly disorganized or catatonic behavior, or negative symptoms
Y
History of Major Depressive or Manic Episodes
N
Y
During an uninterrupted period of illness, psychotic symptoms concurrent with mood episodes
N
Y
During an uninterrupted period of illness, mood episodes have been present for a minority of the total duration of the active and residual periods of the illness
Y
Duration at least 6 months
Y
SCHIZOPHRENIA (3.2.1) (plus comorbid BIPOLAR I [3.3.1], BIPOLAR II [3.3.2], or MAJOR DEPRESSIVE [3.4.1] DISORDER if history of Major Depressive or Manic Episodes)
N
N
N
N

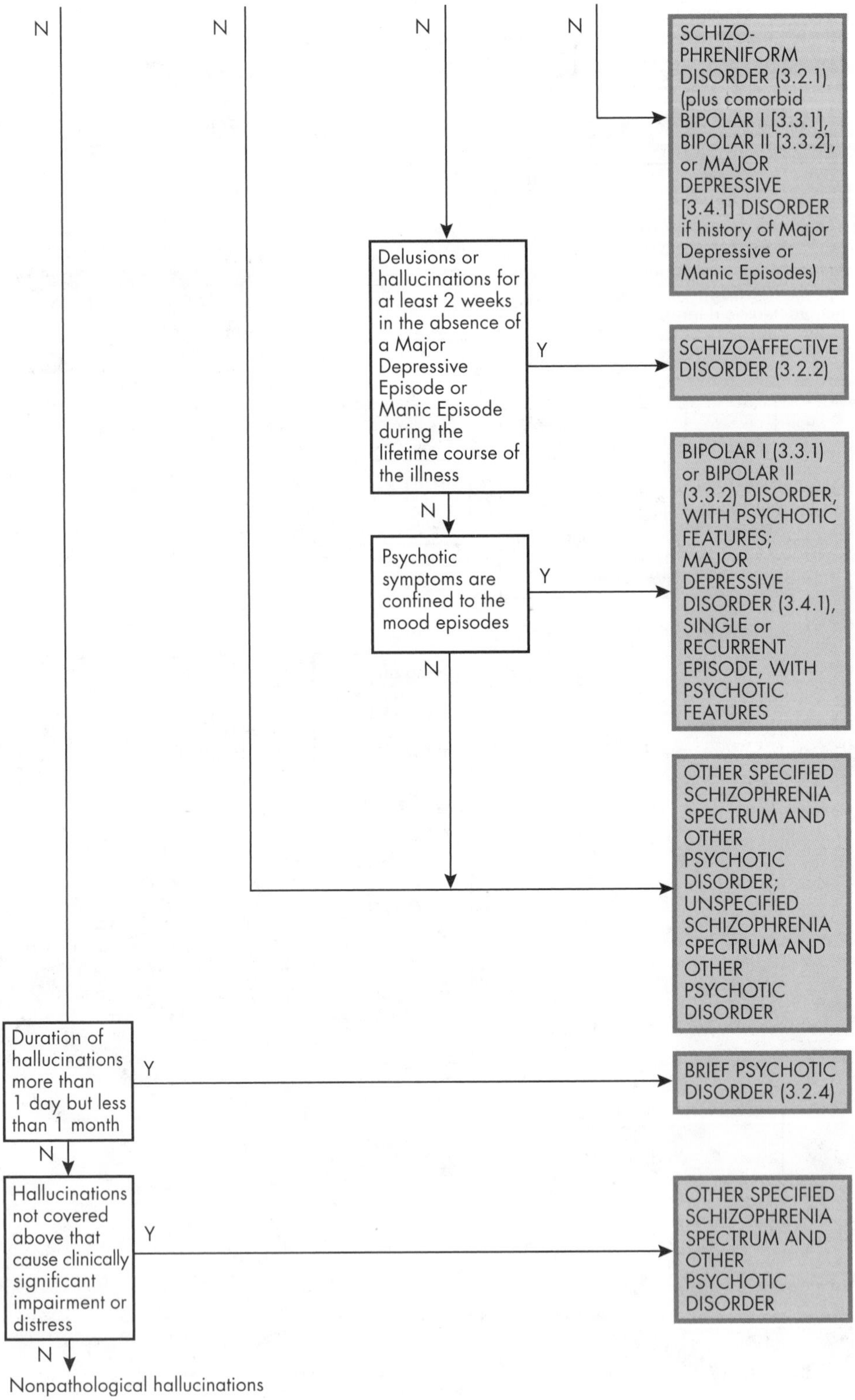
N
N
N
N
SCHIZO-PHRENIFORM DISORDER (3.2.1) (plus comorbid BIPOLAR I [3.3.1], BIPOLAR II [3.3.2], or MAJOR DEPRESSIVE [3.4.1] DISORDER if history of Major Depressive or Manic Episodes)
Delusions or hallucinations for at least 2 weeks in the absence of a Major Depressive Episode or Manic Episode during the lifetime course of the illness
Y
SCHIZOAFFECTIVE DISORDER (3.2.2)
N
Psychotic symptoms are confined to the mood episodes
Y
BIPOLAR I (3.3.1) or BIPOLAR II (3.3.2) DISORDER, WITH PSYCHOTIC FEATURES; MAJOR DEPRESSIVE DISORDER (3.4.1), SINGLE or RECURRENT EPISODE, WITH PSYCHOTIC FEATURES
N
OTHER SPECIFIED SCHIZOPHRENIA SPECTRUM AND OTHER PSYCHOTIC DISORDER; UNSPECIFIED SCHIZOPHRENIA SPECTRUM AND OTHER PSYCHOTIC DISORDER
Duration of hallucinations more than 1 day but less than 1 month
Y
BRIEF PSYCHOTIC DISORDER (3.2.4)
N
Hallucinations not covered above that cause clinically significant impairment or distress
Y
OTHER SPECIFIED SCHIZOPHRENIA SPECTRUM AND OTHER PSYCHOTIC DISORDER
N
Nonpathological hallucinations

2.7 Decision Tree for Catatonic Symptoms

The catatonic symptoms covered here include stupor (i.e., no psychomotor activity, no active relating to environment), catalepsy (i.e., passive induction of a posture held against gravity), waxy flexibility (i.e., slight, even resistance to positioning by examiner), mutism (i.e., no, or very little, verbal response), negativism (i.e., opposing or not responding to instructions or external stimuli), posturing (i.e., spontaneous and active maintenance of a posture against gravity), mannerisms (i.e., odd, circumstantial caricatures of normal actions), stereotypy (i.e., repetitive, abnormally frequent, non-goal-directed movements), agitation (not influenced by external stimuli), grimacing, echolalia (i.e., mimicking another's speech), and echopraxia (i.e., mimicking another's movements).

The initial task is to determine whether the "syndrome" of catatonia is present. This can be difficult because a number of the individual items resemble other types of symptoms characteristic of DSM-5 disorders (e.g., catatonic excitement may resemble psychomotor agitation in a Manic or Major Depressive Episode, catatonic stupor may resemble extreme psychomotor retardation in a Major Depressive Episode or Delirium, catatonic mutism may resemble alogia and avolition in Schizophrenia). The judgment about these distinctions is based in part on the context in which the symptom occurs (i.e., the presence of multiple catatonic symptoms vs. the presence of symptoms characteristic of the other disorder) and on its presentation (i.e., individuals with catatonic symptoms appear to be oblivious to external environmental stimuli, although they may later report accurately about what was happening around them).

If catatonic symptoms are present but do not constitute the syndrome of catatonia, a substance- or medication-induced etiology for such symptoms should first be considered. If the symptoms are due to the direct physiological effect of substance use, such as from Phencyclidine Intoxication, a diagnosis of Substance Intoxication or Substance Withdrawal would apply. If the catatonic-like symptoms are judged to be due to the use of a neuroleptic medication, then one of the neuroleptic-induced movement disorders (i.e., Neuroleptic Malignant Syndrome, Neuroleptic-Induced Dystonia, or Neuroleptic-Induced Parkinsonism) would apply.

Once the syndrome of catatonia has been established, the next step is to determine the etiology. A catatonic syndrome can be due to the direct physiological effects of a neurological or other medical condition (in which case Catatonic Disorder Due to Another Medical Condition is diagnosed), can be a manifestation of a Manic Episode or Major Depressive Episode (in which case catatonia associated with Bipolar I Disorder, Bipolar II Disorder, or Major Depressive Disorder would be diagnosed), or can occur in the context of other psychotic symptoms such as delusions, hallucinations, or disorganized speech (in which case Catatonia Associated With [the appropriate psychotic disorder] would be diagnosed).

If the clinically significant catatonic symptoms are present, are not covered by one of the decision points so far, and represent a psychological or biological dysfunction in the individual (thus meeting the definitional requirements of a mental disorder), the residual category Unspecified Catatonia would apply. Otherwise, the motoric symptoms would be considered part of the normal repertoire of changes in psychomotor activity or behavior and not indicative of a mental disorder.

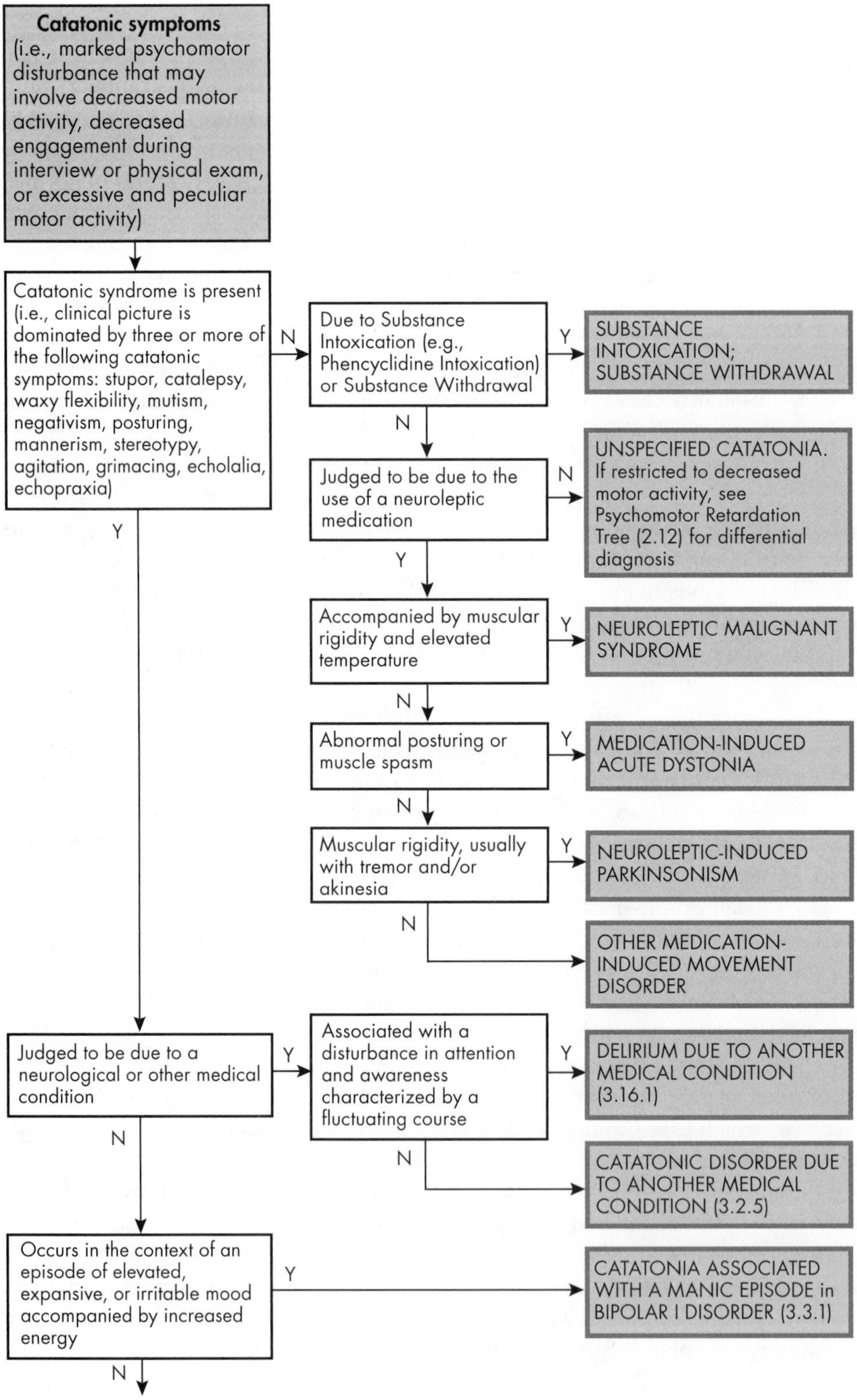
Catatonic symptoms
(i.e., marked psychomotor disturbance that may involve decreased motor activity, decreased engagement during interview or physical exam, or excessive and peculiar motor activity)
Catatonic syndrome is present (i.e., clinical picture is dominated by three or more of the following catatonic symptoms: stupor, catalepsy, waxy flexibility, mutism, negativism, posturing, mannerism, stereotypy, agitation, grimacing, echolalia, echopraxia)
N
Due to Substance Intoxication (e.g., Phencyclidine Intoxication) or Substance Withdrawal
Y
SUBSTANCE INTOXICATION; SUBSTANCE WITHDRAWAL
N
Judged to be due to the use of a neuroleptic medication
N
UNSPECIFIED CATATONIA. If restricted to decreased motor activity, see Psychomotor Retardation Tree (2.12) for differential diagnosis
Y
Accompanied by muscular rigidity and elevated temperature
Y
NEUROLEPTIC MALIGNANT SYNDROME
N
Abnormal posturing or muscle spasm
Y
MEDICATION-INDUCED ACUTE DYSTONIA
N
Muscular rigidity, usually with tremor and/or akinesia
Y
NEUROLEPTIC-INDUCED PARKINSONISM
N
OTHER MEDICATION-INDUCED MOVEMENT DISORDER
Y
Judged to be due to a neurological or other medical condition
Y
Associated with a disturbance in attention and awareness characterized by a fluctuating course
Y
DELIRIUM DUE TO ANOTHER MEDICAL CONDITION (3.16.1)
N
CATATONIC DISORDER DUE TO ANOTHER MEDICAL CONDITION (3.2.5)
N
Occurs in the context of an episode of elevated, expansive, or irritable mood accompanied by increased energy
Y
CATATONIA ASSOCIATED WITH A MANIC EPISODE in BIPOLAR I DISORDER (3.3.1)
N

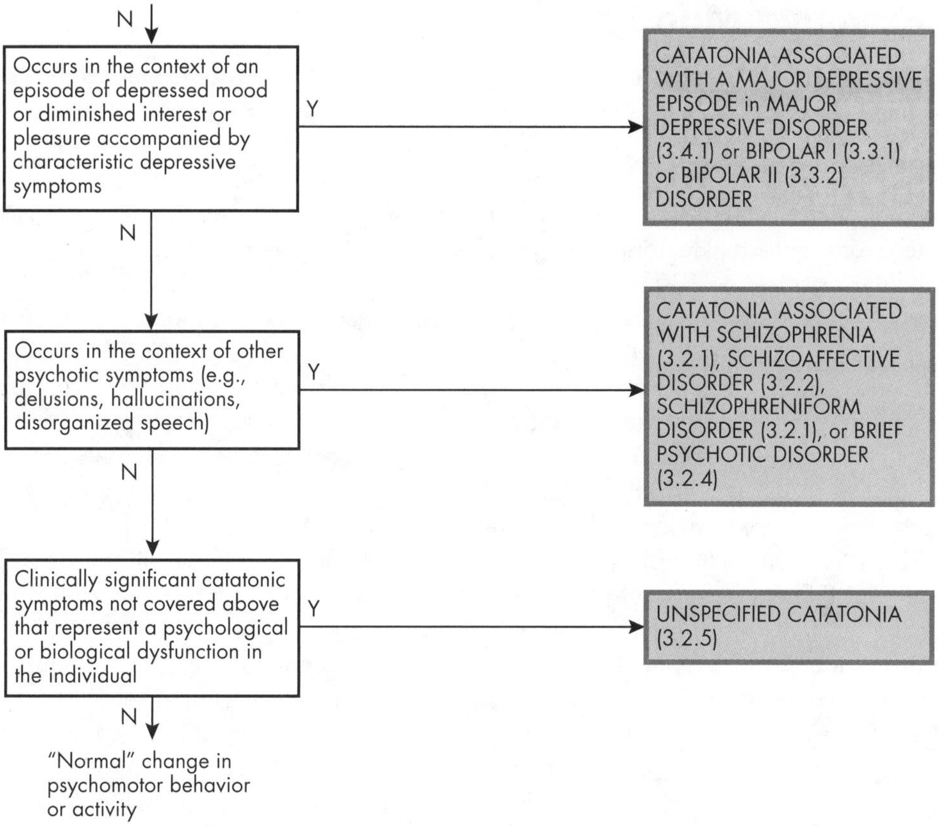
N
Occurs in the context of an episode of depressed mood or diminished interest or pleasure accompanied by characteristic depressive symptoms
Y
CATATONIA ASSOCIATED WITH A MAJOR DEPRESSIVE EPISODE in MAJOR DEPRESSIVE DISORDER (3.4.1) or BIPOLAR I (3.3.1) or BIPOLAR II (3.3.2) DISORDER
N
Occurs in the context of other psychotic symptoms (e.g., delusions, hallucinations, disorganized speech)
Y
CATATONIA ASSOCIATED WITH SCHIZOPHRENIA (3.2.1), SCHIZOAFFECTIVE DISORDER (3.2.2), SCHIZOPHRENIFORM DISORDER (3.2.1), or BRIEF PSYCHOTIC DISORDER (3.2.4)
N
Clinically significant catatonic symptoms not covered above that represent a psychological or biological dysfunction in the individual
Y
UNSPECIFIED CATATONIA (3.2.5)
N
"Normal" change in psychomotor behavior or activity

2.8 Decision Tree for Elevated or Expansive Mood

Most people have experienced at least some periods of elevated or expansive mood in their lives, usually in response to a particularly wonderful event or experience such as falling in love, having a child, graduating from school, landing a coveted job, being victorious at a sporting event, or winning money at a game of chance. These mood states become a concern only when they are *abnormally* elevated or expansive and are disconnected from contextual factors, in which the individual feels persistently euphoric for no particular reason.

The first step in the differential diagnosis is to ensure that the mood disturbance is not caused by substance/medication use or a general medical condition. The clinician's first reflex, particularly for any late onset of these symptoms, should be to conduct a thorough medical workup and to evaluate whether the individual is using any medication (or drugs of abuse) that may produce mood changes as a side effect. In younger individuals, there is always a strong possibility that the changes in mood are caused by the effects of Substance Intoxication or Substance Withdrawal.

The next step is to determine whether the elevated mood is part of a Manic or Hypomanic Episode. Such episodes are not coded separately in DSM-5 but instead form the building blocks for the bipolar disorders. It should be noted that the symptomatic definitions of Manic and Hypomanic Episodes are essentially the same. The boundary between them depends on a clinical judgment as to the severity and impairment caused by the mood disturbance. By definition, a Hypomanic Episode does not cause marked impairment or distress and may even be compatible with improved social and job performance. The bipolar disorders are made up of combinations of Manic, Hypomanic, and Major Depressive Episodes. Bipolar I Disorder consists of one or more Manic Episodes and (optionally) one or more Major Depressive Episodes. The term *bipolar* is used even for individuals who have had only unipolar Manic Episodes (with no depressive episodes) because the vast majority of such individuals will eventually go on to have Major Depressive Episodes, and their course, family loading, and treatment issues are equivalent to those who have had both Manic and Major Depressive Episodes. Bipolar II Disorder consists of one or more Major Depressive Episodes with intercurrent Hypomanic Episodes.

If the individual has a lifetime history of delusions or hallucinations, you must also be sure to differentiate Bipolar I or Bipolar II Disorder With Psychotic Features from other psychotic disorders such as Schizophrenia, Delusional Disorder, or Schizoaffective Disorder. If psychotic symptoms are confined to Manic or Major Depressive Episodes, then the diagnosis is Bipolar I or Bipolar II Disorder With Psychotic Features. If, however, there have been clinically significant delusions or hallucinations that extend beyond the mood episodes, then a non-mood-related psychotic disorder will have to be diagnosed to account for the psychotic symptoms. In these cases, you should refer to the delusions tree (2.5) or hallucinations tree (2.6) for the differential diagnosis.

Cyclothymic Disorder is a relatively uncommon bipolar spectrum disorder characterized by the alternation between periods of hypomania and depression that are less severe than a Manic, Hypomanic, or Major Depressive Episode. Finally, because for most people, periods of elevated and expansive mood are intermittently common during gambling (i.e., at least when a person is winning), it is important *not* to diagnose such symptoms as evidence of mania if they are confined to sessions of gambling. However, given that some individuals might engage in (often reckless) gambling behavior during Manic Episodes, the combination of gambling and euphoric mood does not necessarily rule out a diagnosis of Bipolar Disorder.

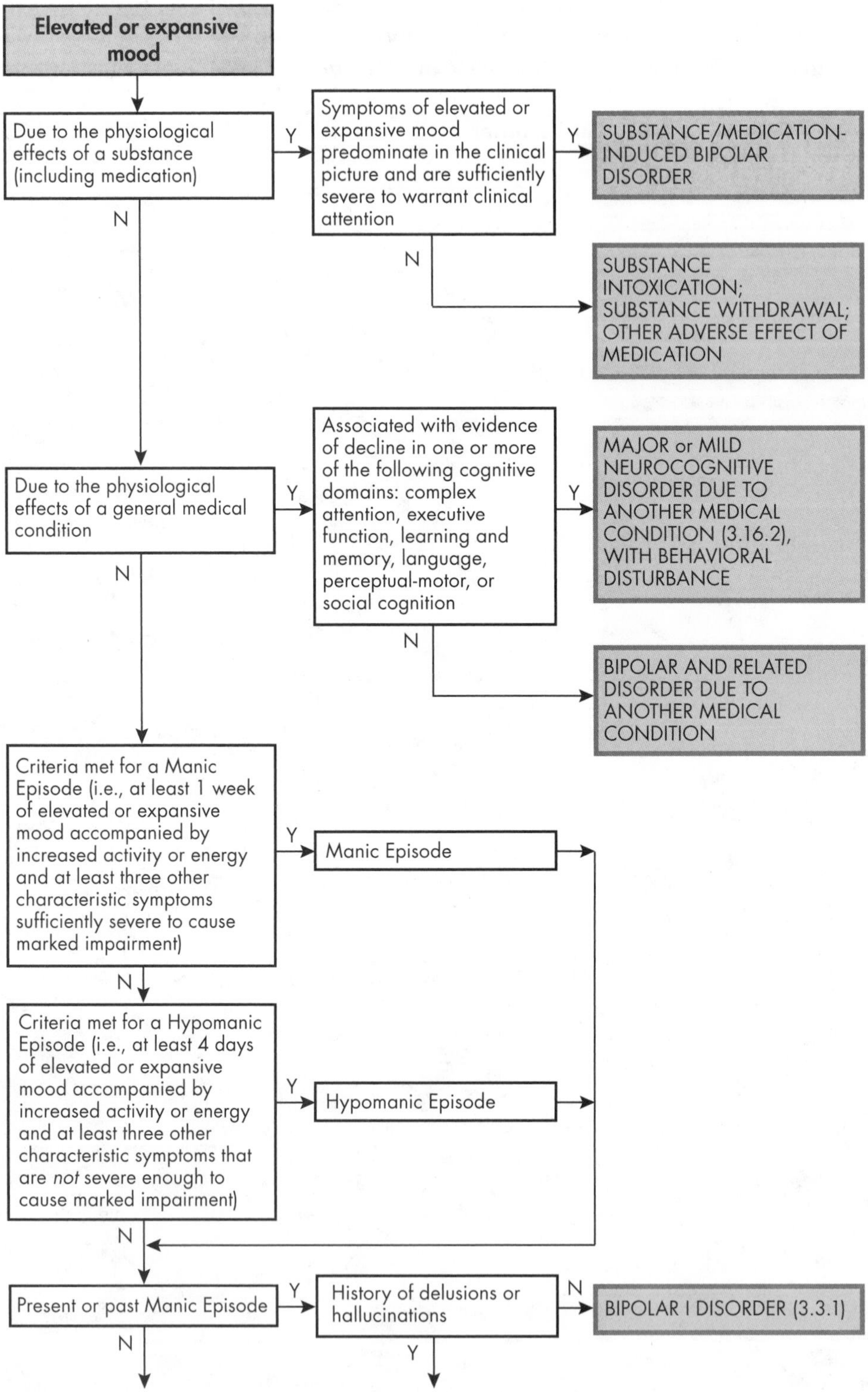
Elevated or expansive mood
Due to the physiological effects of a substance (including medication)
Y
Symptoms of elevated or expansive mood predominate in the clinical picture and are sufficiently severe to warrant clinical attention
Y
SUBSTANCE/MEDICATION-INDUCED BIPOLAR DISORDER
N
SUBSTANCE INTOXICATION; SUBSTANCE WITHDRAWAL; OTHER ADVERSE EFFECT OF MEDICATION
N
Due to the physiological effects of a general medical condition
Y
Associated with evidence of decline in one or more of the following cognitive domains: complex attention, executive function, learning and memory, language, perceptual-motor, or social cognition
Y
MAJOR or MILD NEUROCOGNITIVE DISORDER DUE TO ANOTHER MEDICAL CONDITION (3.16.2), WITH BEHAVIORAL DISTURBANCE
N
BIPOLAR AND RELATED DISORDER DUE TO ANOTHER MEDICAL CONDITION
N
Criteria met for a Manic Episode (i.e., at least 1 week of elevated or expansive mood accompanied by increased activity or energy and at least three other characteristic symptoms sufficiently severe to cause marked impairment)
Y
Manic Episode
N
Criteria met for a Hypomanic Episode (i.e., at least 4 days of elevated or expansive mood accompanied by increased activity or energy and at least three other characteristic symptoms that are *not* severe enough to cause marked impairment)
Y
Hypomanic Episode
N
Present or past Manic Episode
Y
History of delusions or hallucinations
N
BIPOLAR I DISORDER (3.3.1)
N
Y

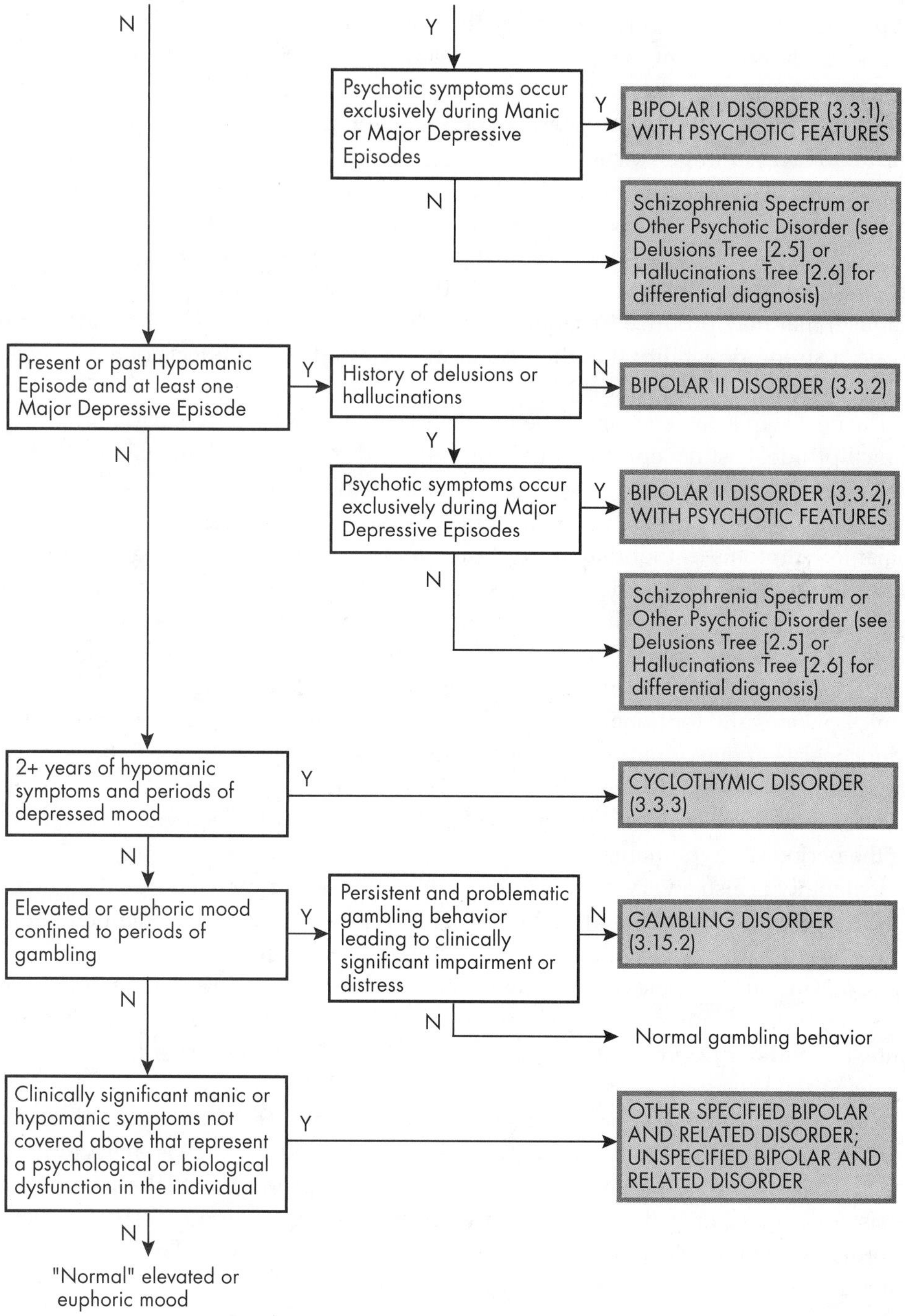
N
Y
Psychotic symptoms occur exclusively during Manic or Major Depressive Episodes
Y
BIPOLAR I DISORDER (3.3.1), WITH PSYCHOTIC FEATURES
N
Schizophrenia Spectrum or Other Psychotic Disorder (see Delusions Tree [2.5] or Hallucinations Tree [2.6] for differential diagnosis)
Present or past Hypomanic Episode and at least one Major Depressive Episode
Y
History of delusions or hallucinations
N
BIPOLAR II DISORDER (3.3.2)
Y
N
Psychotic symptoms occur exclusively during Major Depressive Episodes
Y
BIPOLAR II DISORDER (3.3.2), WITH PSYCHOTIC FEATURES
N
Schizophrenia Spectrum or Other Psychotic Disorder (see Delusions Tree [2.5] or Hallucinations Tree [2.6] for differential diagnosis)
2+ years of hypomanic symptoms and periods of depressed mood
Y
CYCLOTHYMIC DISORDER (3.3.3)
N
Elevated or euphoric mood confined to periods of gambling
Y
Persistent and problematic gambling behavior leading to clinically significant impairment or distress
N
GAMBLING DISORDER (3.15.2)
N
Normal gambling behavior
N
Clinically significant manic or hypomanic symptoms not covered above that represent a psychological or biological dysfunction in the individual
Y
OTHER SPECIFIED BIPOLAR AND RELATED DISORDER; UNSPECIFIED BIPOLAR AND RELATED DISORDER
N
"Normal" elevated or euphoric mood

2.9 Decision Tree for Irritable Mood

All people can become more or less irritable under the right set of circumstances (e.g., not enough sleep, caught in traffic, under deadline pressure). The decision tree for irritable mood is not meant to apply to everyday experiences of irritable mood but instead to periods of irritability that are either so persistent or so severe as to cause clinically significant distress or impairment.

The first step in the differential diagnosis is to ensure that the irritability is not caused by substance/medication use or a general medical condition. The clinician's first reflex, particularly for any late onset of these symptoms, should be to conduct a thorough medical workup and to evaluate whether the individual is using any medication (or drugs of abuse) that may produce irritability as a side effect. In younger individuals, there is always a strong possibility that the irritability is caused by the effects of Substance Intoxication or Substance Withdrawal.

The next step is to determine whether the irritable mood is part of a Manic or Hypomanic Episode. Distinct episodes of abnormally and persistently irritable mood accompanied by increased activity or energy and at least four other characteristic symptoms define a Manic Episode or Hypomanic Episode. Note that four associated manic or hypomanic symptoms (rather than the typical three) are required to make a diagnosis of a Manic or Hypomanic Episode in the absence of elevated or expansive mood so that the episode can more easily be differentiated from a Major Depressive Episode with associated irritability. These episodes are not coded separately in DSM-5 but instead form the building blocks for the bipolar disorders. Bipolar I Disorder consists of one or more Manic Episodes and (optionally) one or more Major Depressive Episodes. Bipolar II Disorder consists of one or more Major Depressive Episodes with intercurrent Hypomanic Episodes. In Cyclothymic Disorder, which is characterized by a persistent pattern of alternation between periods of hypomania and depression, irritable mood may occur during the periods of hypomania.

Irritability is also a very common associated feature of depressed mood. In fact, according to the original DSM-III definition, *major depressive episode* was defined in terms of a "dysphoric mood," which was characterized by symptoms such as feeling depressed, sad, blue, hopeless, low, down in the dumps, *or irritable*. Therefore, the next steps in the decision tree involve considering whether the irritable mood occurs in the context of a Major Depressive Episode, Persistent Depressive Disorder (Dysthymia), or Premenstrual Dysphoric Disorder.

Next in the differential are two disorders with prominent irritability that have their onset in childhood: Disruptive Mood Dysregulation Disorder, which is characterized by frequent severe temper outbursts that are grossly out of proportion to the situation with persistently angry or irritable mood between the outbursts, and Oppositional Defiant Disorder, which is also characterized by a pattern of persistent angry and irritable mood that is accompanied by argumentativeness, defiance, and vindictiveness. If the irritability is a fundamental part of the person's characteristic repertoire of mood states, then a diagnosis of a Personality Disorder may be most appropriate. Also, two of the DSM-5 personality disorders, Borderline Personality Disorder and Antisocial Personality Disorder, include chronic irritability among their characteristic features.

Finally, clinically significant irritability that is not covered so far could qualify for a diagnosis of Adjustment Disorder if it has occurred as a maladaptive response to a psychosocial stressor. Otherwise, clinically significant irritability that does not meet the criteria for any other mental disorder yet is judged to represent a psychological or biological dysfunction in the individual could qualify for a diagnosis of Other Specified Bipolar and Related Disorder or Unspecified Bipolar and Related Disorder.

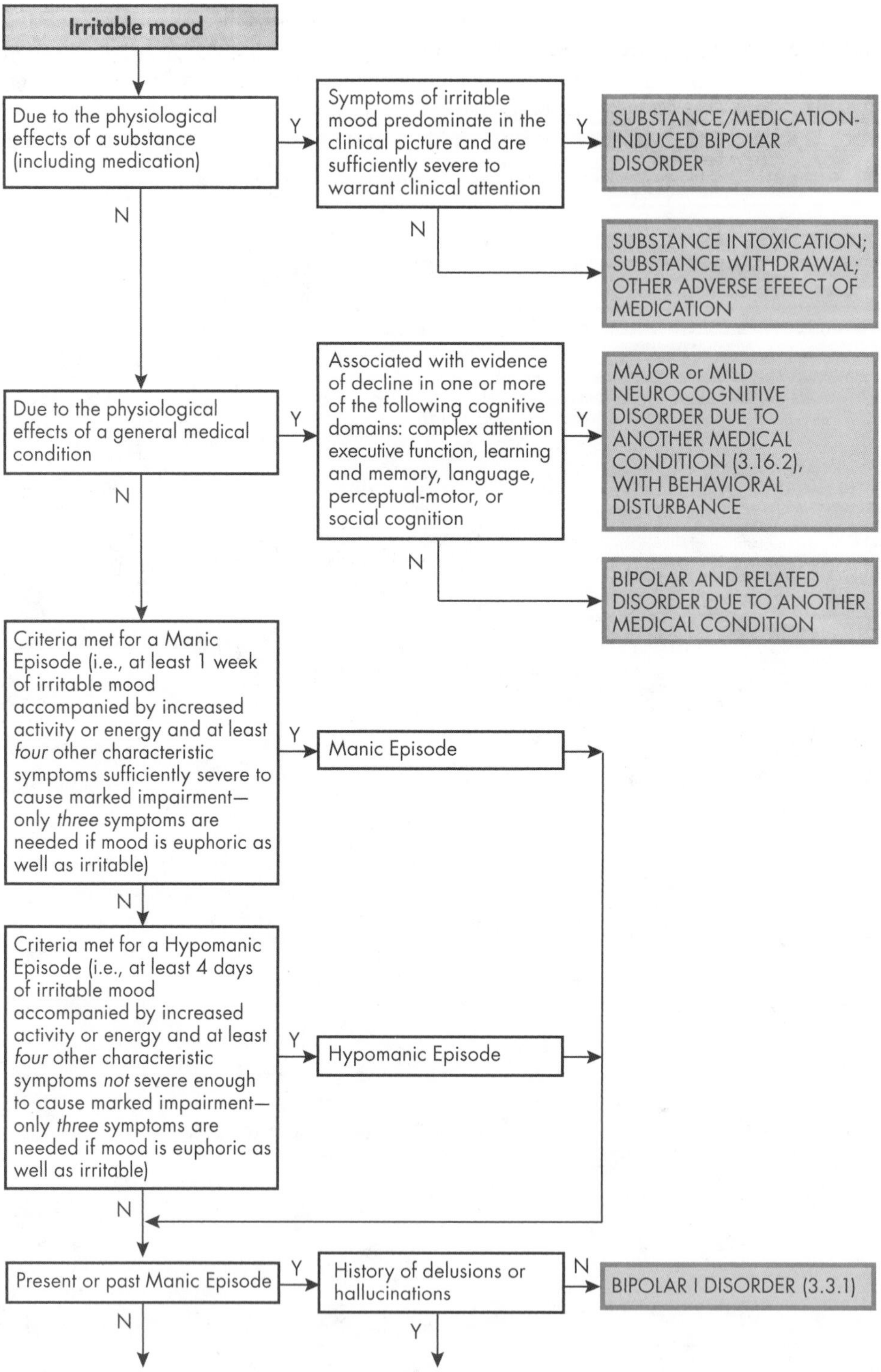
Irritable mood
Due to the physiological effects of a substance (including medication)
Symptoms of irritable mood predominate in the clinical picture and are sufficiently severe to warrant clinical attention
SUBSTANCE/MEDICATION-INDUCED BIPOLAR DISORDER
SUBSTANCE INTOXICATION; SUBSTANCE WITHDRAWAL; OTHER ADVERSE EFEECT OF MEDICATION
Due to the physiological effects of a general medical condition
Associated with evidence of decline in one or more of the following cognitive domains: complex attention executive function, learning and memory, language, perceptual-motor, or social cognition
MAJOR or MILD NEUROCOGNITIVE DISORDER DUE TO ANOTHER MEDICAL CONDITION (3.16.2), WITH BEHAVIORAL DISTURBANCE
BIPOLAR AND RELATED DISORDER DUE TO ANOTHER MEDICAL CONDITION
Criteria met for a Manic Episode (i.e., at least 1 week of irritable mood accompanied by increased activity or energy and at least *four* other characteristic symptoms sufficiently severe to cause marked impairment—only *three* symptoms are needed if mood is euphoric as well as irritable)
Manic Episode
Criteria met for a Hypomanic Episode (i.e., at least 4 days of irritable mood accompanied by increased activity or energy and at least *four* other characteristic symptoms *not* severe enough to cause marked impairment—only *three* symptoms are needed if mood is euphoric as well as irritable)
Hypomanic Episode
Present or past Manic Episode
History of delusions or hallucinations
BIPOLAR I DISORDER (3.3.1)
Y
N

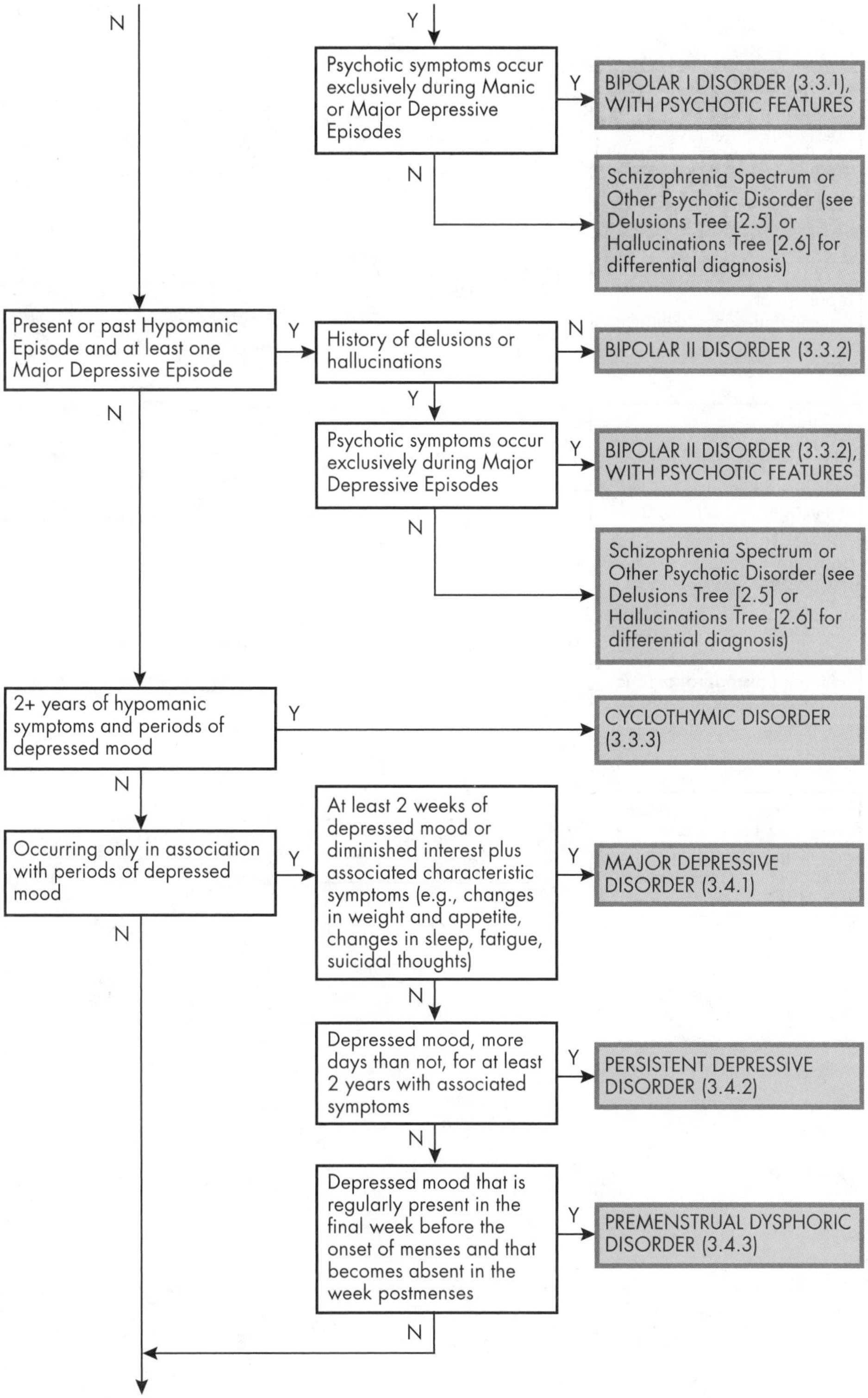
N
Y
Psychotic symptoms occur exclusively during Manic or Major Depressive Episodes
Y
BIPOLAR I DISORDER (3.3.1), WITH PSYCHOTIC FEATURES
N
Schizophrenia Spectrum or Other Psychotic Disorder (see Delusions Tree [2.5] or Hallucinations Tree [2.6] for differential diagnosis)
Present or past Hypomanic Episode and at least one Major Depressive Episode
Y
History of delusions or hallucinations
N
BIPOLAR II DISORDER (3.3.2)
N
Y
Psychotic symptoms occur exclusively during Major Depressive Episodes
Y
BIPOLAR II DISORDER (3.3.2), WITH PSYCHOTIC FEATURES
N
Schizophrenia Spectrum or Other Psychotic Disorder (see Delusions Tree [2.5] or Hallucinations Tree [2.6] for differential diagnosis)
2+ years of hypomanic symptoms and periods of depressed mood
Y
CYCLOTHYMIC DISORDER (3.3.3)
N
Occurring only in association with periods of depressed mood
Y
At least 2 weeks of depressed mood or diminished interest plus associated characteristic symptoms (e.g., changes in weight and appetite, changes in sleep, fatigue, suicidal thoughts)
Y
MAJOR DEPRESSIVE DISORDER (3.4.1)
N
N
Depressed mood, more days than not, for at least 2 years with associated symptoms
Y
PERSISTENT DEPRESSIVE DISORDER (3.4.2)
N
Depressed mood that is regularly present in the final week before the onset of menses and that becomes absent in the week postmenses
Y
PREMENSTRUAL DYSPHORIC DISORDER (3.4.3)
N

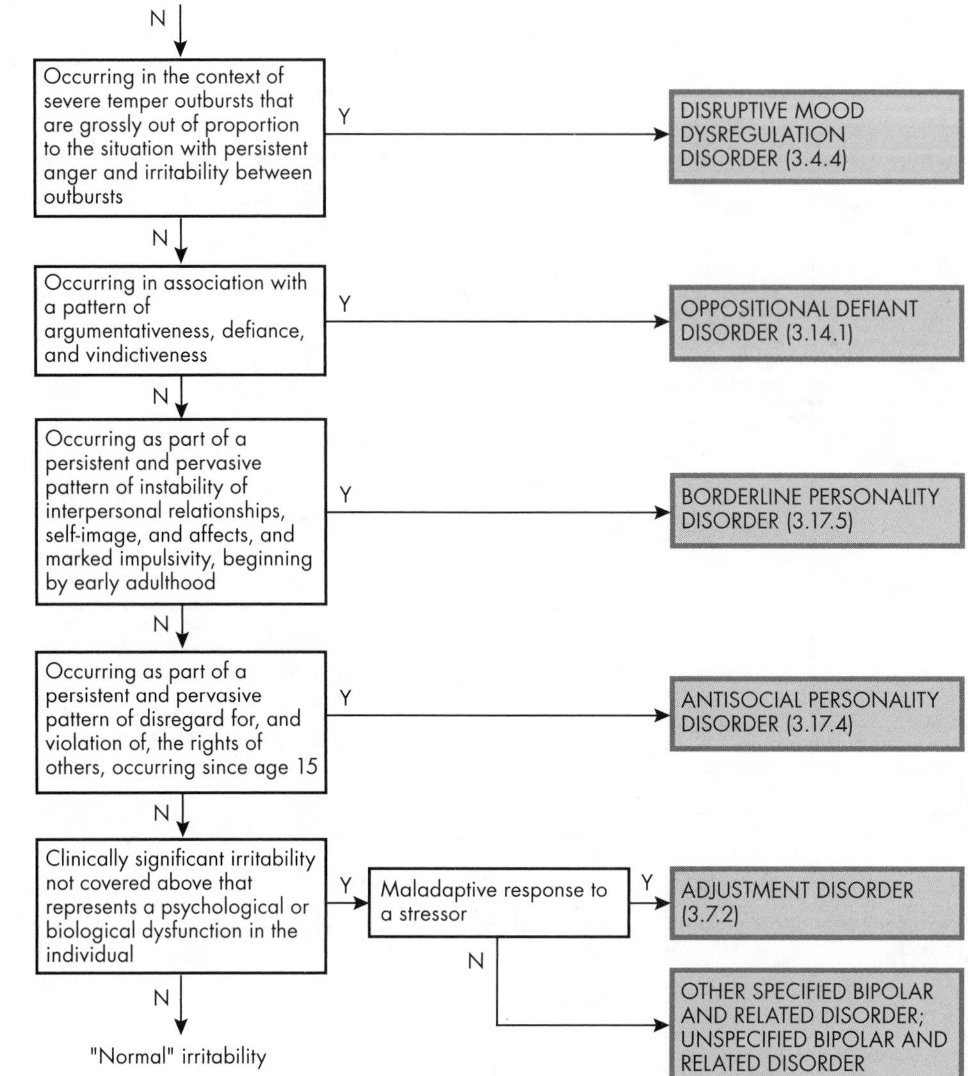
N
Occurring in the context of severe temper outbursts that are grossly out of proportion to the situation with persistent anger and irritability between outbursts
Y
DISRUPTIVE MOOD DYSREGULATION DISORDER (3.4.4)
N
Occurring in association with a pattern of argumentativeness, defiance, and vindictiveness
Y
OPPOSITIONAL DEFIANT DISORDER (3.14.1)
N
Occurring as part of a persistent and pervasive pattern of instability of interpersonal relationships, self-image, and affects, and marked impulsivity, beginning by early adulthood
Y
BORDERLINE PERSONALITY DISORDER (3.17.5)
N
Occurring as part of a persistent and pervasive pattern of disregard for, and violation of, the rights of others, occurring since age 15
Y
ANTISOCIAL PERSONALITY DISORDER (3.17.4)
N
Clinically significant irritability not covered above that represents a psychological or biological dysfunction in the individual
Y
Maladaptive response to a stressor
Y
ADJUSTMENT DISORDER (3.7.2)
N
OTHER SPECIFIED BIPOLAR AND RELATED DISORDER; UNSPECIFIED BIPOLAR AND RELATED DISORDER
N
"Normal" irritability

2.10 Decision Tree for Depressed Mood

Depressed or dysphoric mood is one of the most common presenting symptoms in mental health settings and is a component of many psychiatric conditions. The differential diagnosis of depressed mood requires a consideration of both the context in which the depression occurs and the clustering and duration of symptoms.

Substances (including both drugs of abuse and medication side effects) must first be ruled out. Depression can arise during intoxication with certain substances (e.g., cannabis), result from taking a medication, or be part of the withdrawal syndrome for a substance (e.g., cocaine). Because depressed mood is a frequent concomitant of intoxication and withdrawal, it usually does not require a separate diagnosis. However, if the depressive symptoms predominate in the clinical presentation and are sufficiently severe to warrant clinical attention, then a diagnosis of Substance/Medication-Induced Depressive Disorder may be more appropriate. The differential between Substance/Medication-Induced Depressive Disorder and a non-substance-induced depressive disorder can be made historically by documenting that the depressed mood occurs only in relation to substance/medication use. When such a history is not forthcoming, a period of abstinence is usually required to determine whether the depressed mood resolves once the effects of the substance wear off. DSM-5 suggests waiting for "about 1 month" after cessation of substance use to see whether the mood symptoms spontaneously resolve, although the actual time frame varies depending on the drug and the clinical situation. Other factors that should be considered include previous history of Major Depressive Episodes, family history, and the likelihood that this type of substance in the amount used could have caused the depressive symptoms. If the mood symptoms continue to persist after a reasonable waiting period, then a Substance/Medication-Induced Depressive Disorder is unlikely and the diagnosis should be a non-substance-induced depressive disorder.

One of the most difficult differential diagnostic determinations in psychiatry is to distinguish between primary depressive disorders and those that are the direct physiological consequences of a general medical condition. A very large number of general medical conditions are known to cause depression through their direct effect on the brain. If severe cognitive impairment is also present, Major Neurocognitive Disorder Due to Another Medical Condition, With Behavioral Disturbance, must be considered. However, it is important not to assume that the severity of the cognitive impairment necessarily indicates a diagnosis of Neurocognitive Disorder Due to Another Medical Condition. The cognitive impairment that can occur as part of a Major Depressive Episode can be so severe as to mimic a Major Neurocognitive Disorder. Often, only time, serial evaluations, and sequential antidepressant treatment trials will confirm whether a particular presentation is better explained by a Major Neurocognitive Disorder or a Major Depressive Episode with severe cognitive symptoms.

The next step of the differential diagnosis is to determine whether the depressed mood is part of a mood episode (e.g., Major Depressive Episode or a Manic Episode With Mixed Features). These episodes are not coded separately in DSM-5 but instead form the building blocks for the mood disorders (e.g., Major Depressive Disorder, Bipolar I Disorder, Bipolar II Disorder). A Major Depressive Episode requires a minimum duration of at least 2 weeks of depressed mood for most of the day, nearly every day. Furthermore, the depressed mood must be accompanied by at least four additional symptoms over the same time period (e.g., changes in appetite or weight, sleep, level of motor activity, and suicidal ideation). If the criteria are simultaneously met for a Manic Episode, then the combination of depressive and manic symptoms is considered in DSM-5 to be a Manic Episode, and the specifier "With Mixed Features" is used to indicate the concomitant depressive symptomatology.

The next three steps in the decision tree serve to identify those individuals whose current presentation is depressed but whose overall course is characteristic of one of the disorders in the Bipolar and Related Disorders diagnostic class in DSM-5. Depressive symptoms accompanied by a history of Manic Episodes indicate Bipolar I Disorder, Hypomanic Episodes with Major Depressive Episodes indicate Bipolar II Disorder, and persistent depressive symptoms alternating with periods of hypomanic symptoms warrant a diagnosis of Cyclothymic Disorder.

Once the presence of lifetime manic or hypomanic symptoms has been ruled out, the remaining decision points in the tree determine which depressive disorder best accounts for the symptomatic presentation. The specific diagnosis depends on the presence of Major Depressive Episodes, in which case the diagnosis is either Major Depressive Disorder or a Schizophrenia Spectrum or Other Psychotic Disorder (e.g., when psychotic symptoms persist in the absence of prominent depression). The persistence of the current Major Depressive Episode for at least 2 years warrants an additional diagnosis of Persistent Depressive Disorder (Dysthymia). A diagnosis of Persistent Depressive Disorder by itself is warranted for presentations characterized by chronic depression persisting for at least 2 years that is consistently below the symptom threshold for a Major Depressive Episode. Periods of depressed mood that are regularly present in the final week before the onset of menses and that become absent in the week postmenses are diagnosed as Premenstrual Dysphoric Disorder.

Finally, if the depression is not adequately explained by any of the decision points so far in the tree, it may still justify a DSM-5 diagnosis. If the depression is a symptomatic manifestation of a maladaptive response to a psychosocial stressor, a diagnosis of Adjustment Disorder With Depressed Mood might apply. If not, and the depression is clinically significant and represents a psychological or biological dysfunction in the individual (thus qualifying as a mental disorder), a residual category would apply, the choice depending on whether the clinician wishes to record the symptomatic presentation on the chart (in which case Other Specified Depressive Disorder would be used, followed by the specific reason) or not (in which case Unspecified Depressive Disorder would be used). Otherwise, the depression would be considered part of "normal" everyday blues and not indicative of a mental disorder.

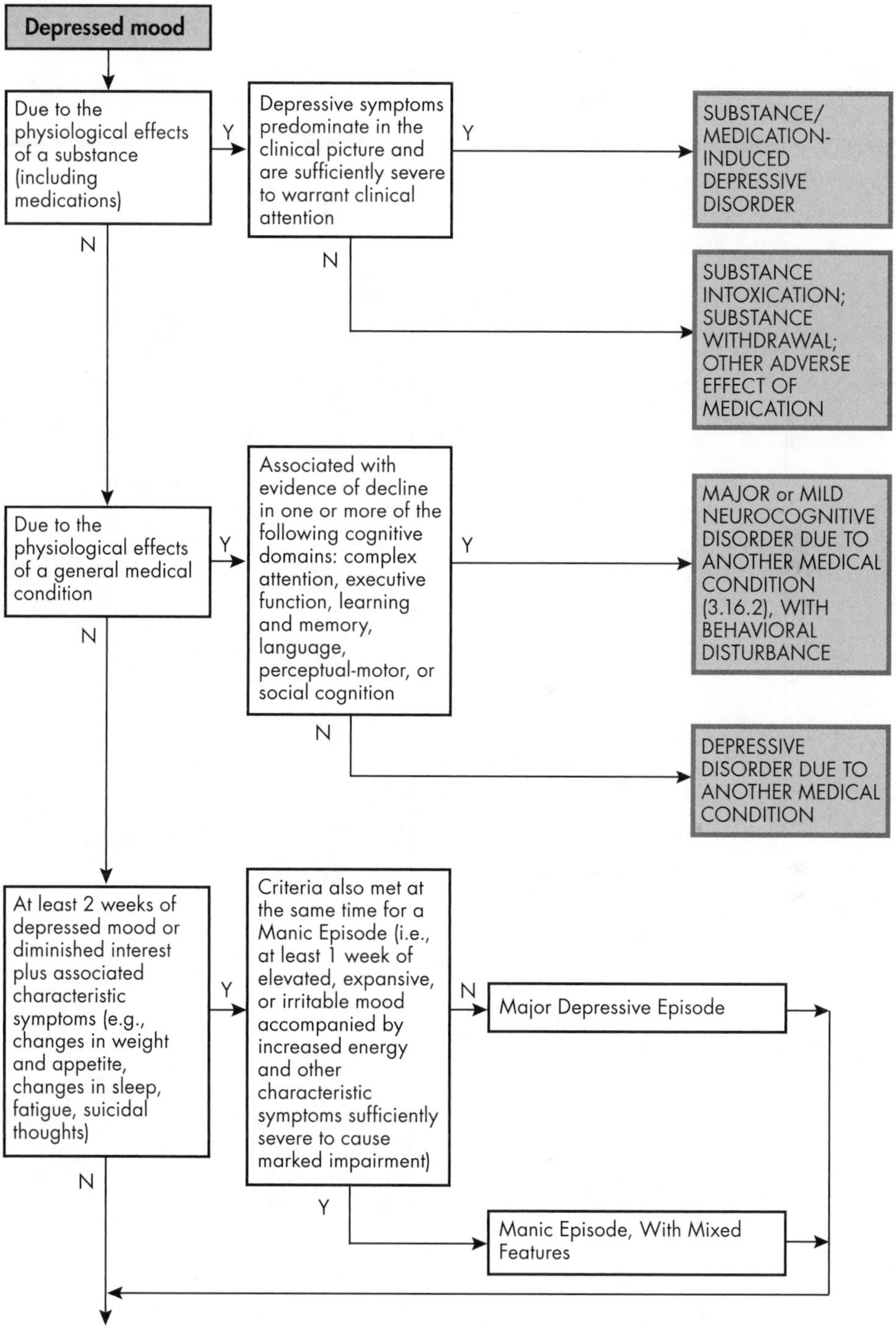
Depressed mood
Due to the physiological effects of a substance (including medications)
Y
N
Depressive symptoms predominate in the clinical picture and are sufficiently severe to warrant clinical attention
Y
N
SUBSTANCE/ MEDICATION-INDUCED DEPRESSIVE DISORDER
SUBSTANCE INTOXICATION; SUBSTANCE WITHDRAWAL; OTHER ADVERSE EFFECT OF MEDICATION
Due to the physiological effects of a general medical condition
Y
N
Associated with evidence of decline in one or more of the following cognitive domains: complex attention, executive function, learning and memory, language, perceptual-motor, or social cognition
Y
N
MAJOR or MILD NEUROCOGNITIVE DISORDER DUE TO ANOTHER MEDICAL CONDITION (3.16.2), WITH BEHAVIORAL DISTURBANCE
DEPRESSIVE DISORDER DUE TO ANOTHER MEDICAL CONDITION
At least 2 weeks of depressed mood or diminished interest plus associated characteristic symptoms (e.g., changes in weight and appetite, changes in sleep, fatigue, suicidal thoughts)
Y
N
Criteria also met at the same time for a Manic Episode (i.e., at least 1 week of elevated, expansive, or irritable mood accompanied by increased energy and other characteristic symptoms sufficiently severe to cause marked impairment)
N
Y
Major Depressive Episode
Manic Episode, With Mixed Features

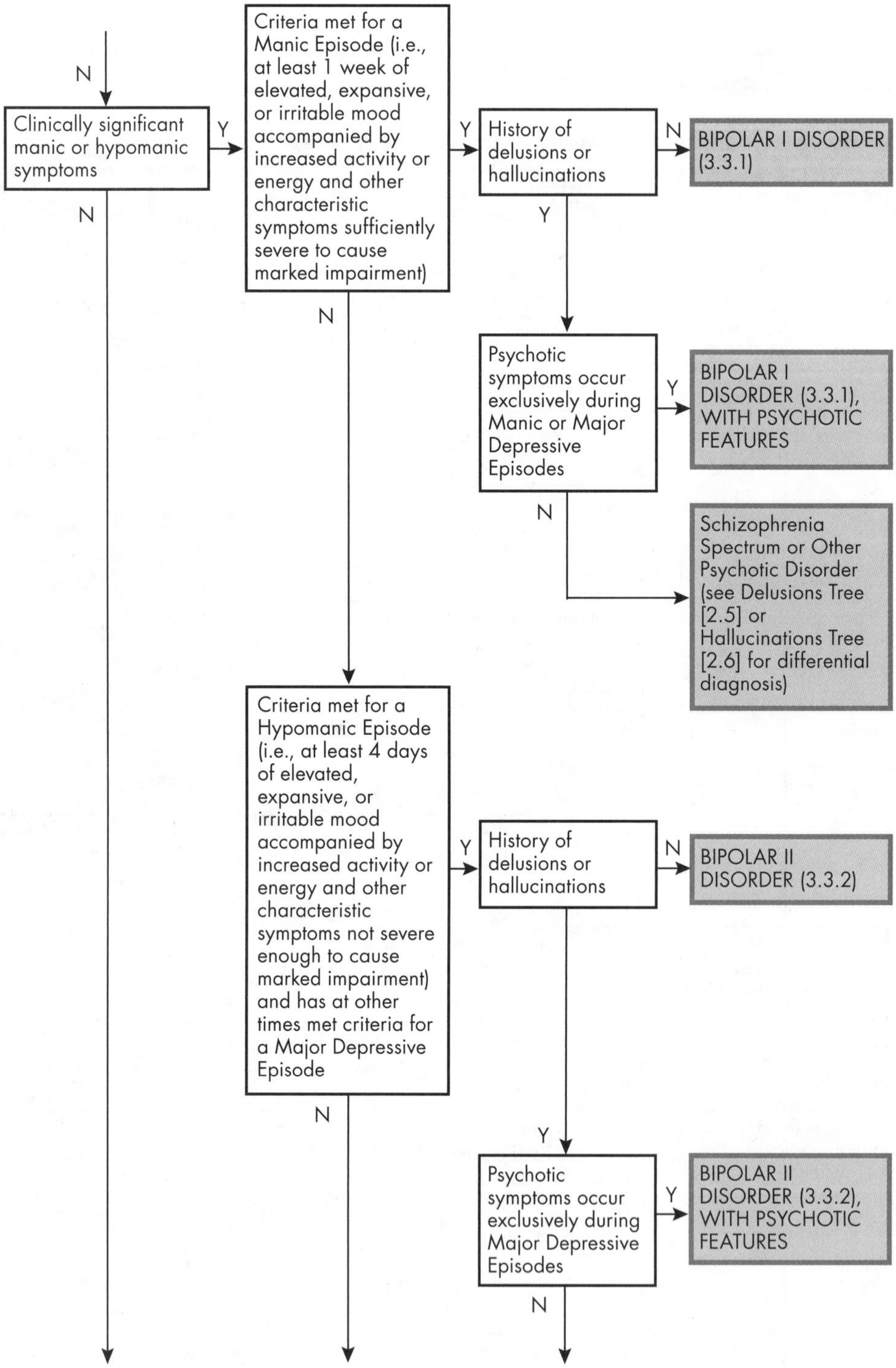
N
Clinically significant manic or hypomanic symptoms
Y
N
Criteria met for a Manic Episode (i.e., at least 1 week of elevated, expansive, or irritable mood accompanied by increased activity or energy and other characteristic symptoms sufficiently severe to cause marked impairment)
Y
N
History of delusions or hallucinations
N
BIPOLAR I DISORDER (3.3.1)
Y
Psychotic symptoms occur exclusively during Manic or Major Depressive Episodes
Y
BIPOLAR I DISORDER (3.3.1), WITH PSYCHOTIC FEATURES
N
Schizophrenia Spectrum or Other Psychotic Disorder (see Delusions Tree [2.5] or Hallucinations Tree [2.6] for differential diagnosis)
Criteria met for a Hypomanic Episode (i.e., at least 4 days of elevated, expansive, or irritable mood accompanied by increased activity or energy and other characteristic symptoms not severe enough to cause marked impairment) and has at other times met criteria for a Major Depressive Episode
Y
N
History of delusions or hallucinations
N
BIPOLAR II DISORDER (3.3.2)
Y
Psychotic symptoms occur exclusively during Major Depressive Episodes
Y
BIPOLAR II DISORDER (3.3.2), WITH PSYCHOTIC FEATURES
N

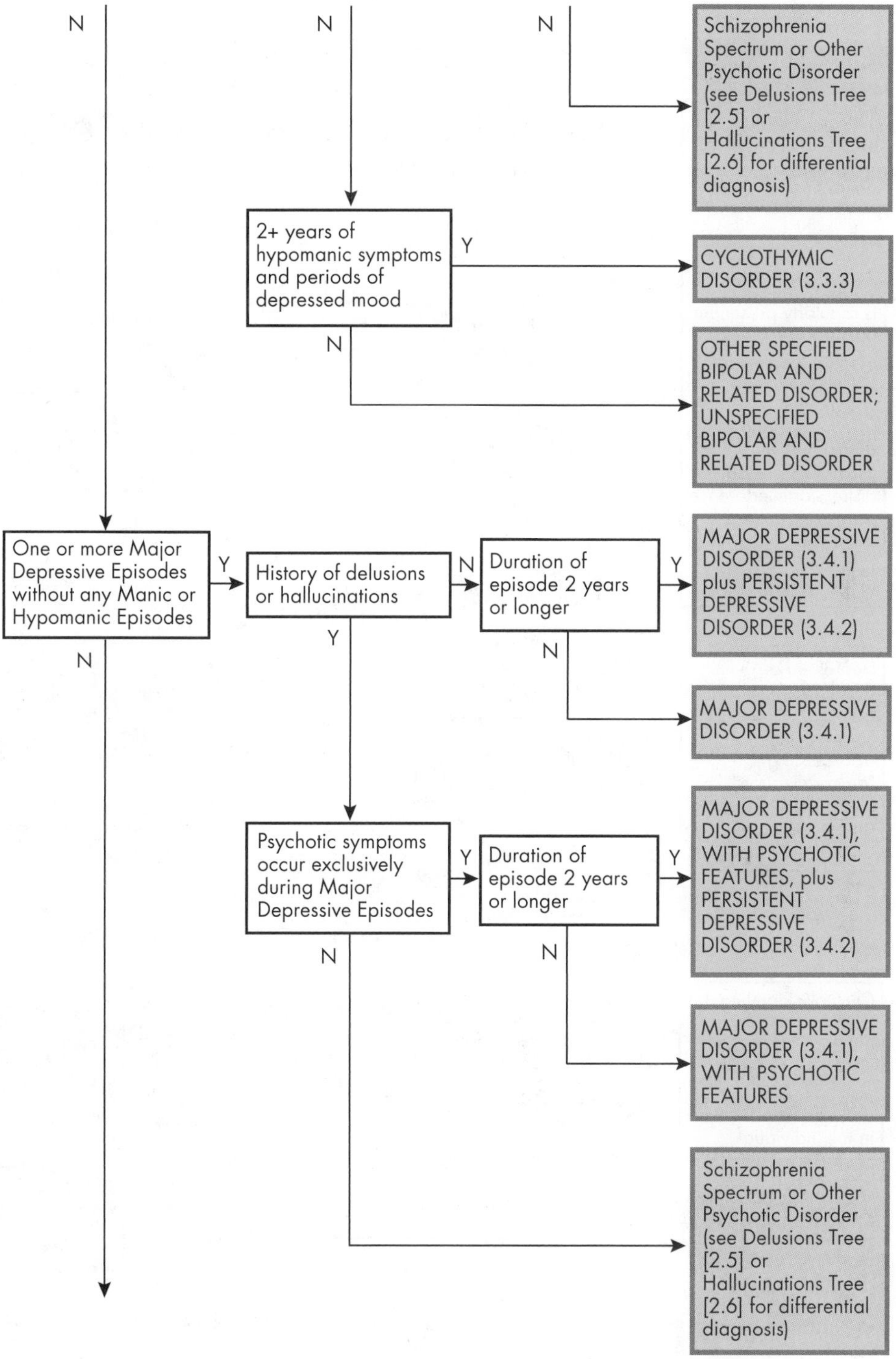
N
N
N
Schizophrenia Spectrum or Other Psychotic Disorder (see Delusions Tree [2.5] or Hallucinations Tree [2.6] for differential diagnosis)
2+ years of hypomanic symptoms and periods of depressed mood
Y
CYCLOTHYMIC DISORDER (3.3.3)
N
OTHER SPECIFIED BIPOLAR AND RELATED DISORDER; UNSPECIFIED BIPOLAR AND RELATED DISORDER
One or more Major Depressive Episodes without any Manic or Hypomanic Episodes
Y
History of delusions or hallucinations
N
Duration of episode 2 years or longer
Y
MAJOR DEPRESSIVE DISORDER (3.4.1) plus PERSISTENT DEPRESSIVE DISORDER (3.4.2)
N
MAJOR DEPRESSIVE DISORDER (3.4.1)
Y
N
Psychotic symptoms occur exclusively during Major Depressive Episodes
Y
Duration of episode 2 years or longer
Y
MAJOR DEPRESSIVE DISORDER (3.4.1), WITH PSYCHOTIC FEATURES, plus PERSISTENT DEPRESSIVE DISORDER (3.4.2)
N
MAJOR DEPRESSIVE DISORDER (3.4.1), WITH PSYCHOTIC FEATURES
N
Schizophrenia Spectrum or Other Psychotic Disorder (see Delusions Tree [2.5] or Hallucinations Tree [2.6] for differential diagnosis)

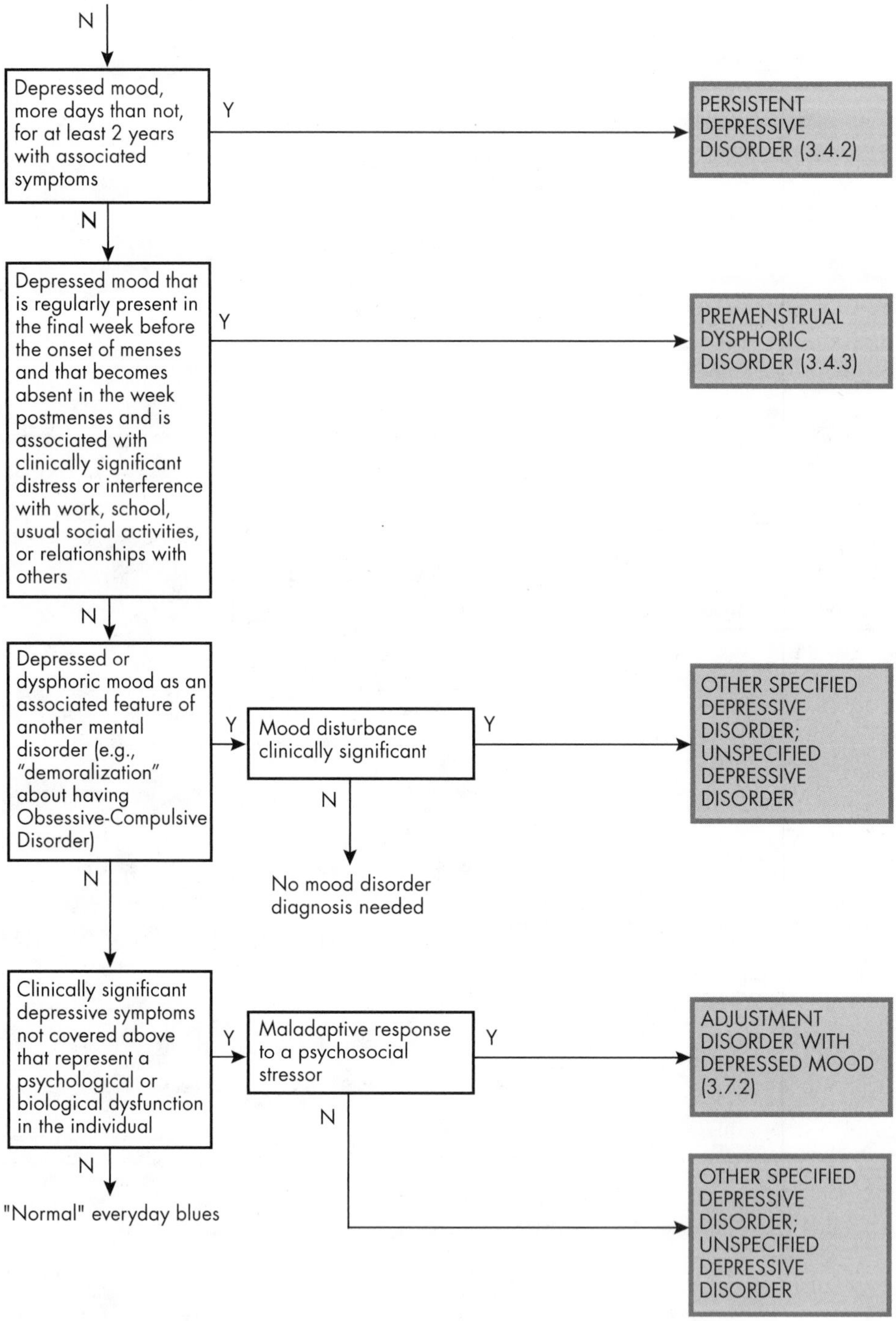
N
Depressed mood, more days than not, for at least 2 years with associated symptoms
Y
PERSISTENT DEPRESSIVE DISORDER (3.4.2)
N
Depressed mood that is regularly present in the final week before the onset of menses and that becomes absent in the week postmenses and is associated with clinically significant distress or interference with work, school, usual social activities, or relationships with others
Y
PREMENSTRUAL DYSPHORIC DISORDER (3.4.3)
N
Depressed or dysphoric mood as an associated feature of another mental disorder (e.g., "demoralization" about having Obsessive-Compulsive Disorder)
Y
Mood disturbance clinically significant
Y
OTHER SPECIFIED DEPRESSIVE DISORDER; UNSPECIFIED DEPRESSIVE DISORDER
N
No mood disorder diagnosis needed
N
Clinically significant depressive symptoms not covered above that represent a psychological or biological dysfunction in the individual
Y
Maladaptive response to a psychosocial stressor
Y
ADJUSTMENT DISORDER WITH DEPRESSED MOOD (3.7.2)
N
OTHER SPECIFIED DEPRESSIVE DISORDER; UNSPECIFIED DEPRESSIVE DISORDER
N
"Normal" everyday blues

2.11 Decision Tree for Suicidal Ideation or Behavior

When you are evaluating suicidality, it is important to determine the urgency of current suicidal thoughts, the degree to which definite plans have been formulated and acted on, the availability of a means of suicide, the lethality of the method, the urgency of the impulse, the presence of psychotic symptoms, the history of previous suicidal thoughts and attempts, family history of suicidal behavior, and current and past substance use. The degree of suicidality is on a continuum ranging from recurrent wishes to be dead, to feelings that others would be better off if one were dead ("passive suicidal thoughts"), to formulating suicidal plans, to overt suicidal behaviors.

Perhaps because suicidal behavior is a defining feature of a Major Depressive Episode, most people associate suicide most closely with mood disorders. For this reason, the third branch of the tree offers a "mini-differential diagnosis" of those DSM-5 conditions associated with depressed mood, and the fourth branch covers conditions with a concurrent mixture of depressive and manic symptoms (so-called mixed states). As this decision tree illustrates, although suicidal ideation is a characteristic feature of mood disorders, it must be considered in the management of a wide array of DSM-5 disorders. Moreover, the risk of suicide increases dramatically when the individual has more than one disorder because each disorder may independently contribute to the risk (e.g., a particularly common and dangerous combination includes Major Depressive Disorder, Alcohol Use Disorder, and Borderline Personality Disorder).

Suicidal behavior may result from symptoms other than depressed mood. For example, suicidal behavior may occur under the direction of delusions or command hallucinations (e.g., in Schizophrenia, Bipolar Disorder With Psychotic Features, or Major Depressive Disorder With Psychotic Features), may be related to confusion or other cognitive impairment (e.g., in Delirium, Major Neurocognitive Disorder, Substance Intoxication or Substance Withdrawal), or may result from disinhibition (e.g., in a Manic Episode or Substance Intoxication). Borderline Personality Disorder and Antisocial Personality Disorder have a 5%–10% risk of successful suicide, perhaps resulting from the impulsivity, labile moods, low frustration tolerance, and high rates of substance use characteristic of individuals with such disorders. Similarly, Conduct Disorder is an important predictor of suicide in adolescents, particularly when it is accompanied by substance use and mood symptoms.

The evaluation of suicidal ideation or behavior must take into account the fact that such symptoms are sometimes feigned as a way of gaining admission to the hospital or of "solving" other life problems. Patients quickly learn the power of saying the phrase, "I want to kill myself," as a way of influencing clinicians, family members, and other important individuals in their lives. In Malingering, the patient's motivation is some obvious external reward (e.g., getting transferred from prison to hospital, getting a place to spend the night). In contrast, in Factitious Disorder, the presumed motivation is a psychological need to assume the sick role, especially for individuals who are attempting to make the hospital their more or less permanent home. Adjustment Disorder applies to those individuals who develop suicidal ideation or behavior in response to psychosocial stressors and in the absence of other symptoms that would meet the criteria for a specific DSM-5 disorder. This diagnosis is most commonly used to describe suicidal behavior in adolescents.

Another possibility is that in certain extreme circumstances (e.g., an intractable terminal illness), the desire to kill oneself may not necessarily represent a mental disorder. However, before a clinician can arrive at this conclusion, a thorough evaluation is necessary to rule out all other more treatable causes of suicidal ideation (e.g., depression, pain, insomnia, psychosis, Delirium).

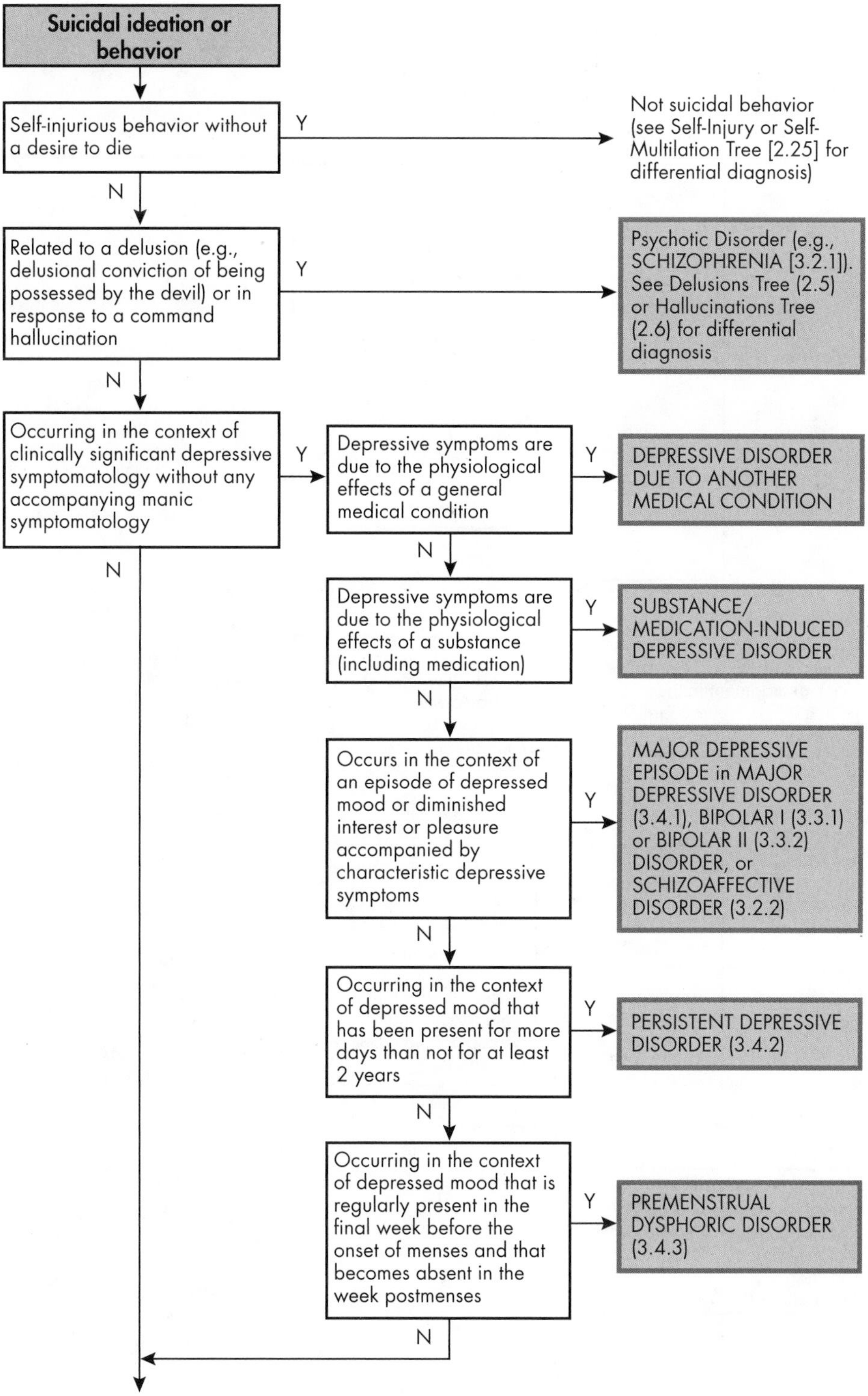
Suicidal ideation or behavior
Self-injurious behavior without a desire to die
Y
Not suicidal behavior (see Self-Injury or Self-Multilation Tree [2.25] for differential diagnosis)
N
Related to a delusion (e.g., delusional conviction of being possessed by the devil) or in response to a command hallucination
Y
Psychotic Disorder (e.g., SCHIZOPHRENIA [3.2.1]). See Delusions Tree (2.5) or Hallucinations Tree (2.6) for differential diagnosis
N
Occurring in the context of clinically significant depressive symptomatology without any accompanying manic symptomatology
Y
Depressive symptoms are due to the physiological effects of a general medical condition
Y
DEPRESSIVE DISORDER DUE TO ANOTHER MEDICAL CONDITION
N
Depressive symptoms are due to the physiological effects of a substance (including medication)
Y
SUBSTANCE/MEDICATION-INDUCED DEPRESSIVE DISORDER
N
Occurs in the context of an episode of depressed mood or diminished interest or pleasure accompanied by characteristic depressive symptoms
Y
MAJOR DEPRESSIVE EPISODE in MAJOR DEPRESSIVE DISORDER (3.4.1), BIPOLAR I (3.3.1) or BIPOLAR II (3.3.2) DISORDER, or SCHIZOAFFECTIVE DISORDER (3.2.2)
N
Occurring in the context of depressed mood that has been present for more days than not for at least 2 years
Y
PERSISTENT DEPRESSIVE DISORDER (3.4.2)
N
Occurring in the context of depressed mood that is regularly present in the final week before the onset of menses and that becomes absent in the week postmenses
Y
PREMENSTRUAL DYSPHORIC DISORDER (3.4.3)
N
N

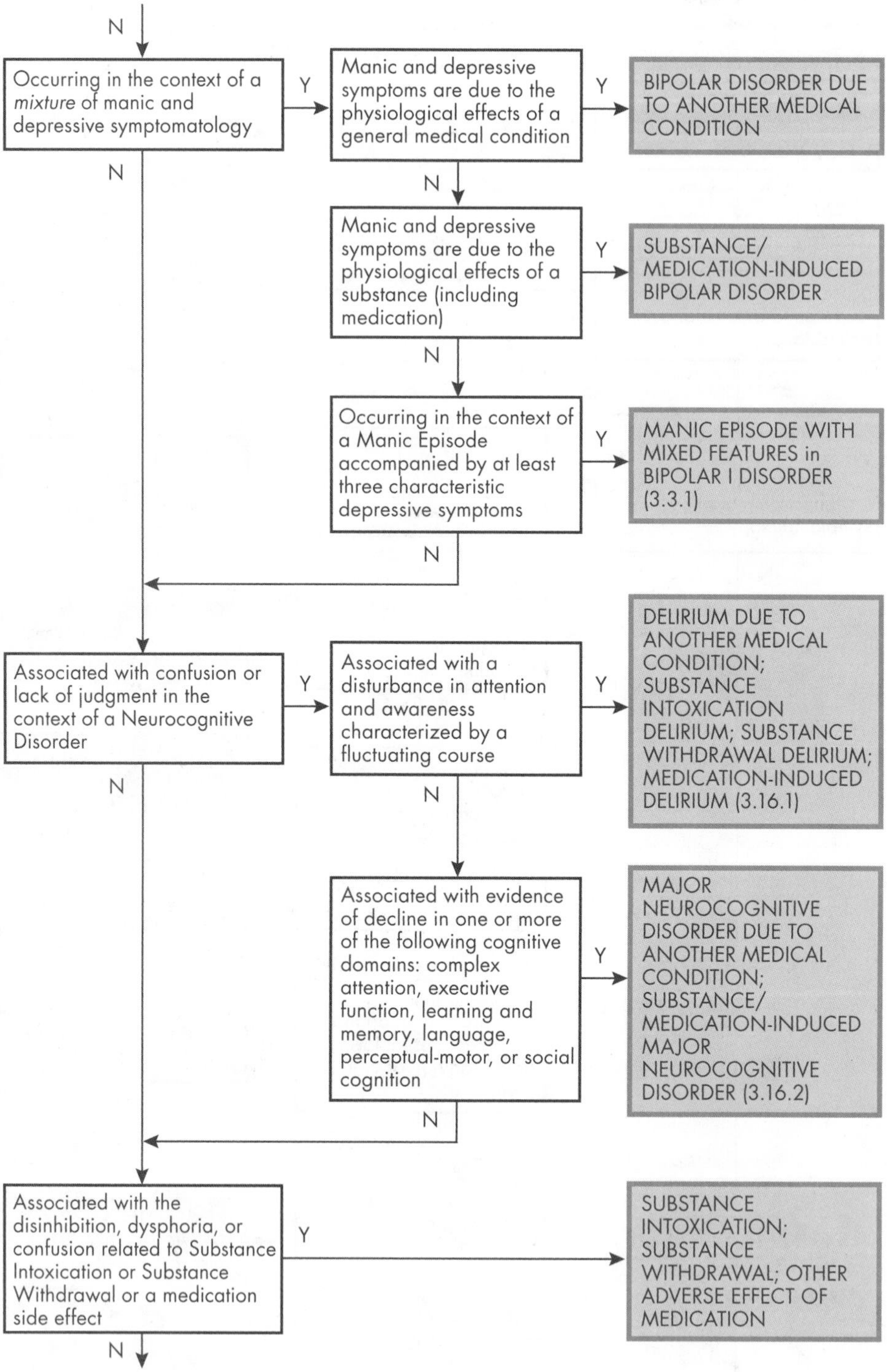
N
Occurring in the context of a *mixture* of manic and depressive symptomatology
Y
Manic and depressive symptoms are due to the physiological effects of a general medical condition
Y
BIPOLAR DISORDER DUE TO ANOTHER MEDICAL CONDITION
N
N
Manic and depressive symptoms are due to the physiological effects of a substance (including medication)
Y
SUBSTANCE/ MEDICATION-INDUCED BIPOLAR DISORDER
N
Occurring in the context of a Manic Episode accompanied by at least three characteristic depressive symptoms
Y
MANIC EPISODE WITH MIXED FEATURES in BIPOLAR I DISORDER (3.3.1)
N
Associated with confusion or lack of judgment in the context of a Neurocognitive Disorder
Y
Associated with a disturbance in attention and awareness characterized by a fluctuating course
Y
DELIRIUM DUE TO ANOTHER MEDICAL CONDITION; SUBSTANCE INTOXICATION DELIRIUM; SUBSTANCE WITHDRAWAL DELIRIUM; MEDICATION-INDUCED DELIRIUM (3.16.1)
N
N
Associated with evidence of decline in one or more of the following cognitive domains: complex attention, executive function, learning and memory, language, perceptual-motor, or social cognition
Y
MAJOR NEUROCOGNITIVE DISORDER DUE TO ANOTHER MEDICAL CONDITION; SUBSTANCE/ MEDICATION-INDUCED MAJOR NEUROCOGNITIVE DISORDER (3.16.2)
N
Associated with the disinhibition, dysphoria, or confusion related to Substance Intoxication or Substance Withdrawal or a medication side effect
Y
SUBSTANCE INTOXICATION; SUBSTANCE WITHDRAWAL; OTHER ADVERSE EFFECT OF MEDICATION
N

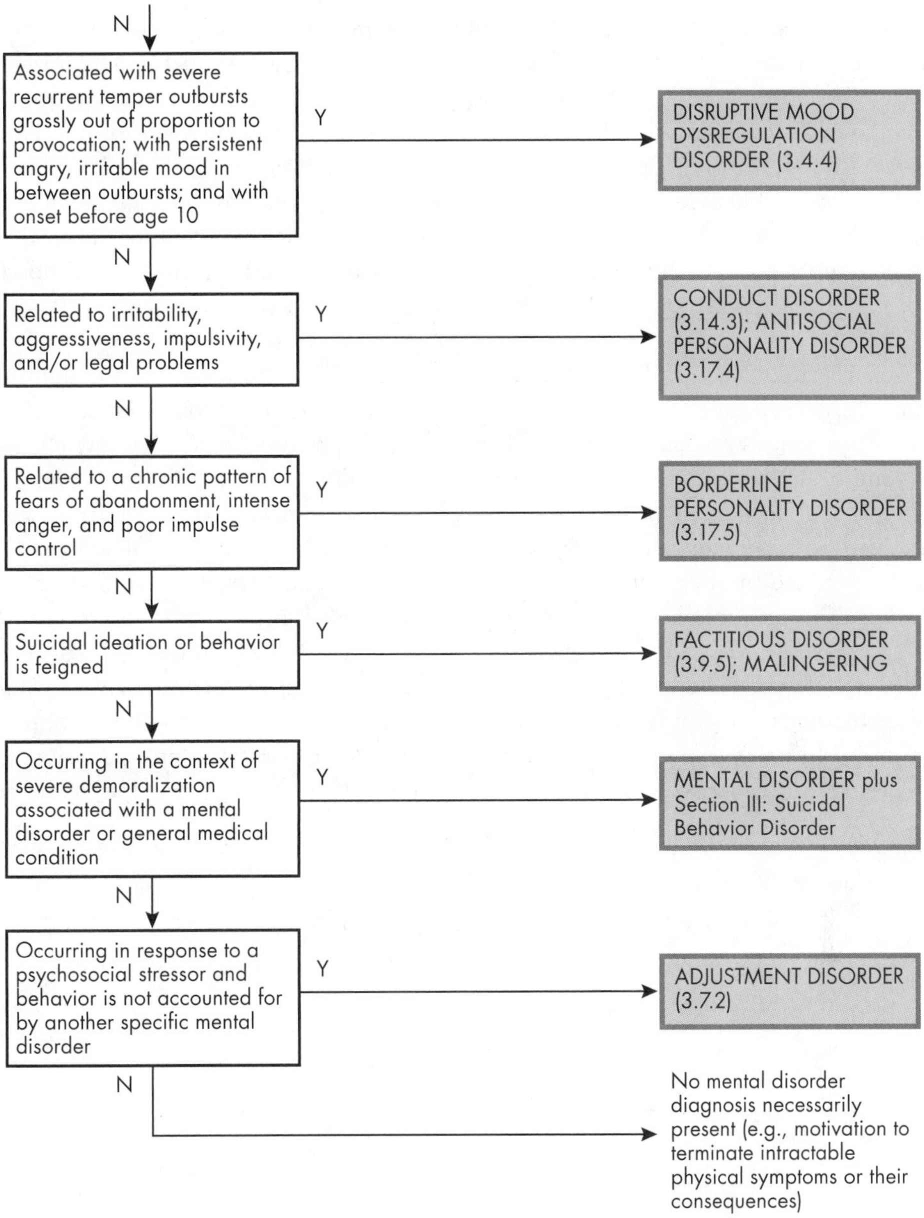
N
Associated with severe recurrent temper outbursts grossly out of proportion to provocation; with persistent angry, irritable mood in between outbursts; and with onset before age 10
Y
DISRUPTIVE MOOD DYSREGULATION DISORDER (3.4.4)
N
Related to irritability, aggressiveness, impulsivity, and/or legal problems
Y
CONDUCT DISORDER (3.14.3); ANTISOCIAL PERSONALITY DISORDER (3.17.4)
N
Related to a chronic pattern of fears of abandonment, intense anger, and poor impulse control
Y
BORDERLINE PERSONALITY DISORDER (3.17.5)
N
Suicidal ideation or behavior is feigned
Y
FACTITIOUS DISORDER (3.9.5); MALINGERING
N
Occurring in the context of severe demoralization associated with a mental disorder or general medical condition
Y
MENTAL DISORDER plus Section III: Suicidal Behavior Disorder
N
Occurring in response to a psychosocial stressor and behavior is not accounted for by another specific mental disorder
Y
ADJUSTMENT DISORDER (3.7.2)
N
No mental disorder diagnosis necessarily present (e.g., motivation to terminate intractable physical symptoms or their consequences)

2.12 Decision Tree for Psychomotor Retardation

Psychomotor retardation is defined as visible generalized slowing of movements and speech. In its extreme form, psychomotor retardation may be characterized by unresponsiveness and mutism that is indistinguishable from catatonic stupor. The symptom of psychomotor retardation should be distinguished from other similar symptoms. Fatigue is a subjective sense of having decreased energy or being tired all the time but is not characterized by visible evidence of slowed movements. Leaden paralysis is the subjective sense that one's arms and legs are as "heavy as lead" and is a part of the "atypical" pattern of symptoms in a Major Depressive Episode With Atypical Features. Avolition (one of the negative symptoms of Schizophrenia) is characterized by a lack of motivation to carry out behaviors rather than being physically slowed down.

General medical conditions may cause psychomotor retardation that usually does not warrant a separate mental disorder diagnosis. It is important to remember that psychomotor changes associated with Delirium go in both directions. Very few clinicians miss the dramatic presentations of Delirium associated with psychomotor agitation (e.g., the patient pulling out an intravenous line). The "quiet" cases of Delirium associated with psychomotor retardation are much more likely to go unrecognized. Such scenarios are noted by specifying the psychomotor level of activity as being "hypoactive." Another common "missed" cause of slowed movements is Neuroleptic-Induced Parkinsonism. This differentiation is complicated by the fact that a number of disorders for which neuroleptics are given can themselves present with psychomotor retardation (e.g., Schizophrenia, Bipolar Disorder or Major Depressive Disorder With Psychotic Features, Delirium). A change in medication (e.g., reducing the neuroleptic dosage or administering anticholinergic medication) can often be helpful in making the distinction.

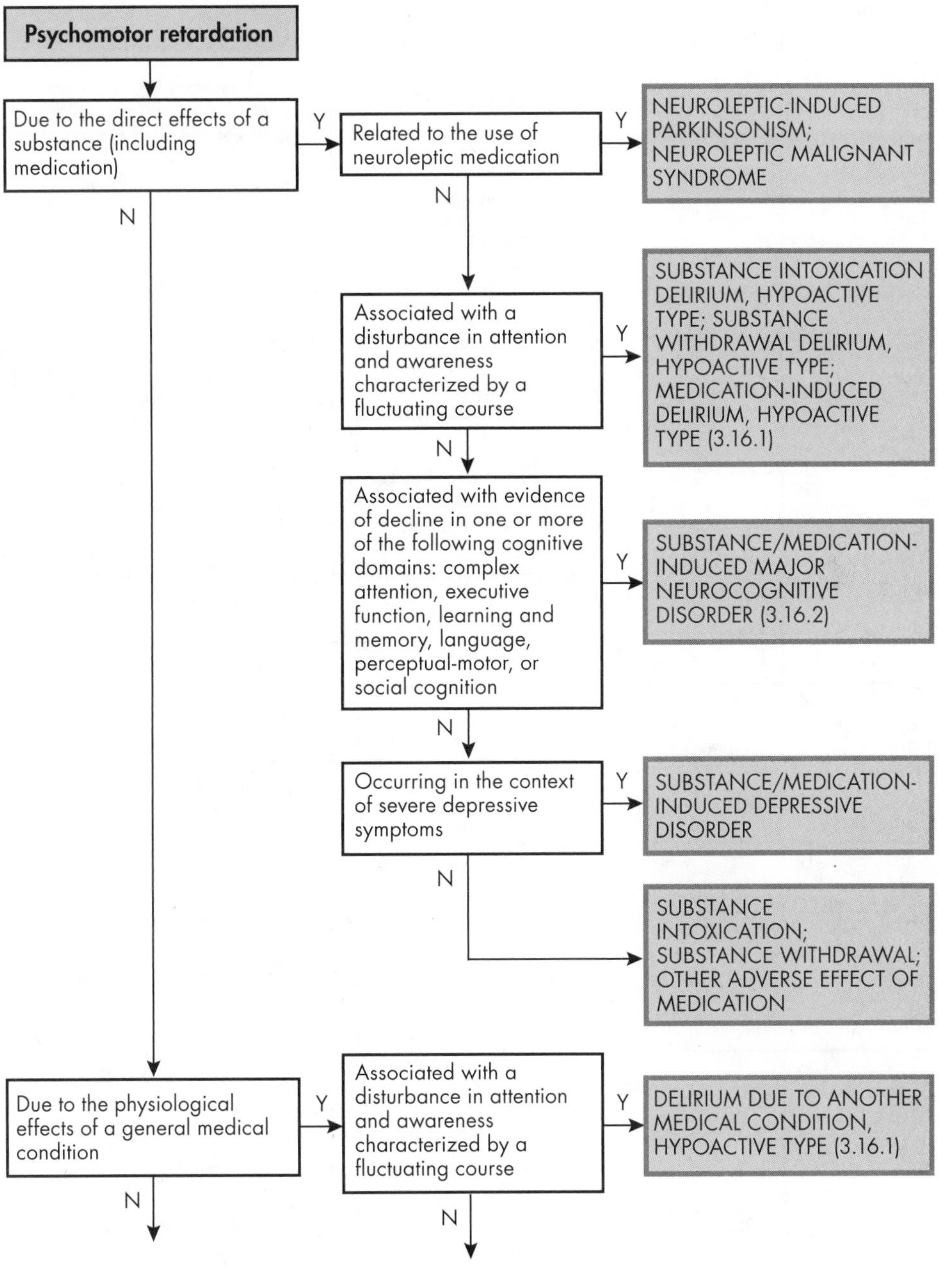
Psychomotor retardation
Due to the direct effects of a substance (including medication)
Y
Related to the use of neuroleptic medication
Y
NEUROLEPTIC-INDUCED PARKINSONISM; NEUROLEPTIC MALIGNANT SYNDROME
N
Associated with a disturbance in attention and awareness characterized by a fluctuating course
Y
SUBSTANCE INTOXICATION DELIRIUM, HYPOACTIVE TYPE; SUBSTANCE WITHDRAWAL DELIRIUM, HYPOACTIVE TYPE; MEDICATION-INDUCED DELIRIUM, HYPOACTIVE TYPE (3.16.1)
N
Associated with evidence of decline in one or more of the following cognitive domains: complex attention, executive function, learning and memory, language, perceptual-motor, or social cognition
Y
SUBSTANCE/MEDICATION-INDUCED MAJOR NEUROCOGNITIVE DISORDER (3.16.2)
N
Occurring in the context of severe depressive symptoms
Y
SUBSTANCE/MEDICATION-INDUCED DEPRESSIVE DISORDER
N
SUBSTANCE INTOXICATION; SUBSTANCE WITHDRAWAL; OTHER ADVERSE EFFECT OF MEDICATION
N
Due to the physiological effects of a general medical condition
Y
Associated with a disturbance in attention and awareness characterized by a fluctuating course
Y
DELIRIUM DUE TO ANOTHER MEDICAL CONDITION, HYPOACTIVE TYPE (3.16.1)
N
N

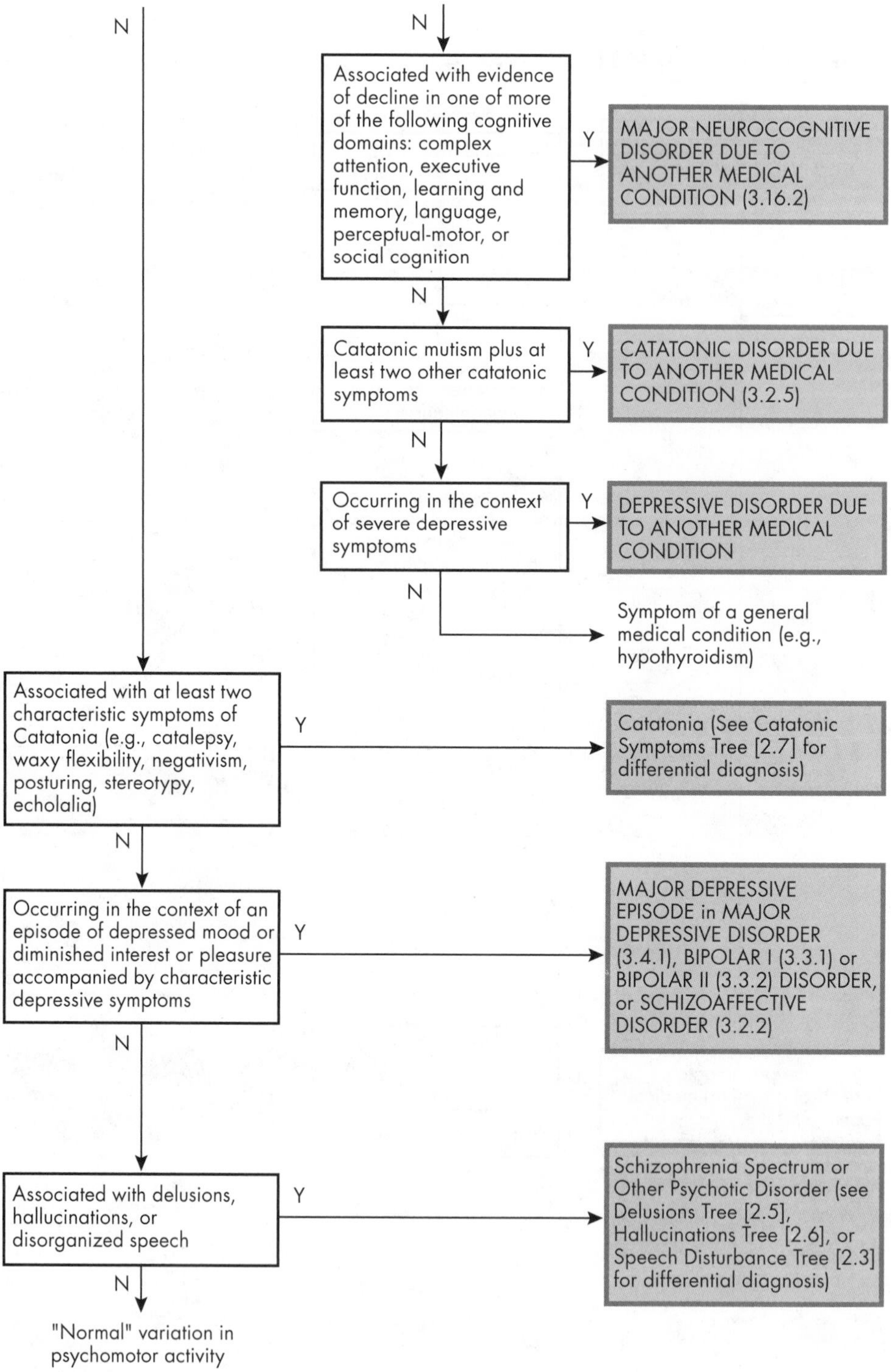
N
N
Associated with evidence of decline in one of more of the following cognitive domains: complex attention, executive function, learning and memory, language, perceptual-motor, or social cognition
Y
MAJOR NEUROCOGNITIVE DISORDER DUE TO ANOTHER MEDICAL CONDITION (3.16.2)
N
Catatonic mutism plus at least two other catatonic symptoms
Y
CATATONIC DISORDER DUE TO ANOTHER MEDICAL CONDITION (3.2.5)
N
Occurring in the context of severe depressive symptoms
Y
DEPRESSIVE DISORDER DUE TO ANOTHER MEDICAL CONDITION
N
Symptom of a general medical condition (e.g., hypothyroidism)
Associated with at least two characteristic symptoms of Catatonia (e.g., catalepsy, waxy flexibility, negativism, posturing, stereotypy, echolalia)
Y
Catatonia (See Catatonic Symptoms Tree [2.7] for differential diagnosis)
N
Occurring in the context of an episode of depressed mood or diminished interest or pleasure accompanied by characteristic depressive symptoms
Y
MAJOR DEPRESSIVE EPISODE in MAJOR DEPRESSIVE DISORDER (3.4.1), BIPOLAR I (3.3.1) or BIPOLAR II (3.3.2) DISORDER, or SCHIZOAFFECTIVE DISORDER (3.2.2)
N
Associated with delusions, hallucinations, or disorganized speech
Y
Schizophrenia Spectrum or Other Psychotic Disorder (see Delusions Tree [2.5], Hallucinations Tree [2.6], or Speech Disturbance Tree [2.3] for differential diagnosis)
N
"Normal" variation in psychomotor activity

2.13 Decision Tree for Anxiety

As is always the case, the first step in the differential diagnosis is to rule out substance/medication use or a general medical condition as the direct physiological cause of a patient's anxiety. Because anxiety can be an associated feature of Delirium and Major or Mild Neurocognitive Disorder, these more specific conditions are also considered within this section of the decision tree.

When the anxiety occurs in discrete episodes with a sudden onset and is accompanied by a number of somatic symptoms (e.g., palpitations, shortness of breath, dizziness) and cognitive symptoms (e.g., fear of going crazy or having a heart attack), it is considered to be a Panic Attack (or, if the number of characteristic symptoms falls short of the minimum threshold of four, a "limited-symptom attack"). Because of the specific treatment implications of panic attacks, a separate decision tree (2.14) is provided for them.

The remaining decision points in the anxiety tree differentiate among the Anxiety Disorders by determining what the individual is afraid of, what situations are avoided, and whether the anxiety is in response to a stressor. In Panic Disorder, the anxiety is related to the fear of having additional panic attacks and the possible consequences of these attacks. Agoraphobia is similar in that the person is afraid of places or situations that would be difficult or embarrassing to get out of in the event of a Panic Attack or panic-like symptoms, but the focus is on the fear and avoidance of the places and situations rather than on the Panic Attack itself. Reflecting the more generalized nature of the avoidance in Agoraphobia (compared with the more limited nature of avoided situations in conditions such as Specific Phobia), a diagnosis of Agoraphobia requires that the individual must be fearful of situations from at least two "agoraphobic clusters": public transportation, open spaces, enclosed spaces, standing in a line or being in a crowd, and being outside the home alone. Separation Anxiety Disorder, Social Anxiety Disorder (Social Phobia), Specific Phobia, and Illness Anxiety Disorder each has a specific focus of fear and avoidance (i.e., about separation from major attachment figures, situations in which the person may be exposed to scrutiny of others, exposure to a feared object [e.g., spider] or situation [e.g., flying in an airplane], and having or acquiring a serious illness, respectively). Disorders from the Obsessive-Compulsive and Related Disorders grouping may also be associated with anxiety (e.g., anxiety associated with the preoccupation with an imagined bodily defect in Body Dysmorphic Disorder, being contaminated in Obsessive-Compulsive Disorder, being forced to discard personal items by an individual with Hoarding Disorder). Although not included in the Obsessive-Compulsive and Related Disorders diagnostic class, Generalized Anxiety Disorder is phenomenologically similar in that it is characterized by excessive ruminations and worries about untoward events that go along with the chronic anxiety.

Anxiety that develops in response to exposure to a traumatic stressor may be indicative of Posttraumatic Stress Disorder or Acute Stress Disorder if the other characteristic features are also present (i.e., intrusion and avoidance symptoms related to the traumatic stressor or its circumstances, negative alterations in cognitions and mood, and alterations in arousal and activity); the differentiation is based on duration (i.e., 1 month or less for Acute Stress Disorder, greater than 1 month for Posttraumatic Stress Disorder).

Anxiety occurs so commonly with Major Depressive Episodes, Manic Episodes, and Hypomanic Episodes that its co-occurrence is more the rule than the exception. To indicate the comorbid presence of anxiety, DSM-5 has introduced the specifier With Anxious Distress that allows the clinician to indicate the severity of comorbid anxiety (ranging from mild to severe). Finally, if the anxiety is not adequately explained by any of the decision points so far in the tree, a DSM-5 diagnosis may still be justified. If the anxiety is a symptomatic manifestation of a maladaptive response to a psychosocial stressor, the diagnosis is Adjustment Disorder With Anxiety. If not, and it is clinically significant and represents a psychological or biological dysfunction in the individual (thus qualifying as a mental disorder), a residual category would apply, the choice depending on whether the clinician wishes to record the symptomatic presentation on the chart (in which case Other Specified Anxiety Disorder would be used, followed by the specific reason) or not (in which case Unspecified Anxiety Disorder would be used). Otherwise, the anxiety would be considered part of the normal repertoire of emotional expression and not indicative of a mental disorder.

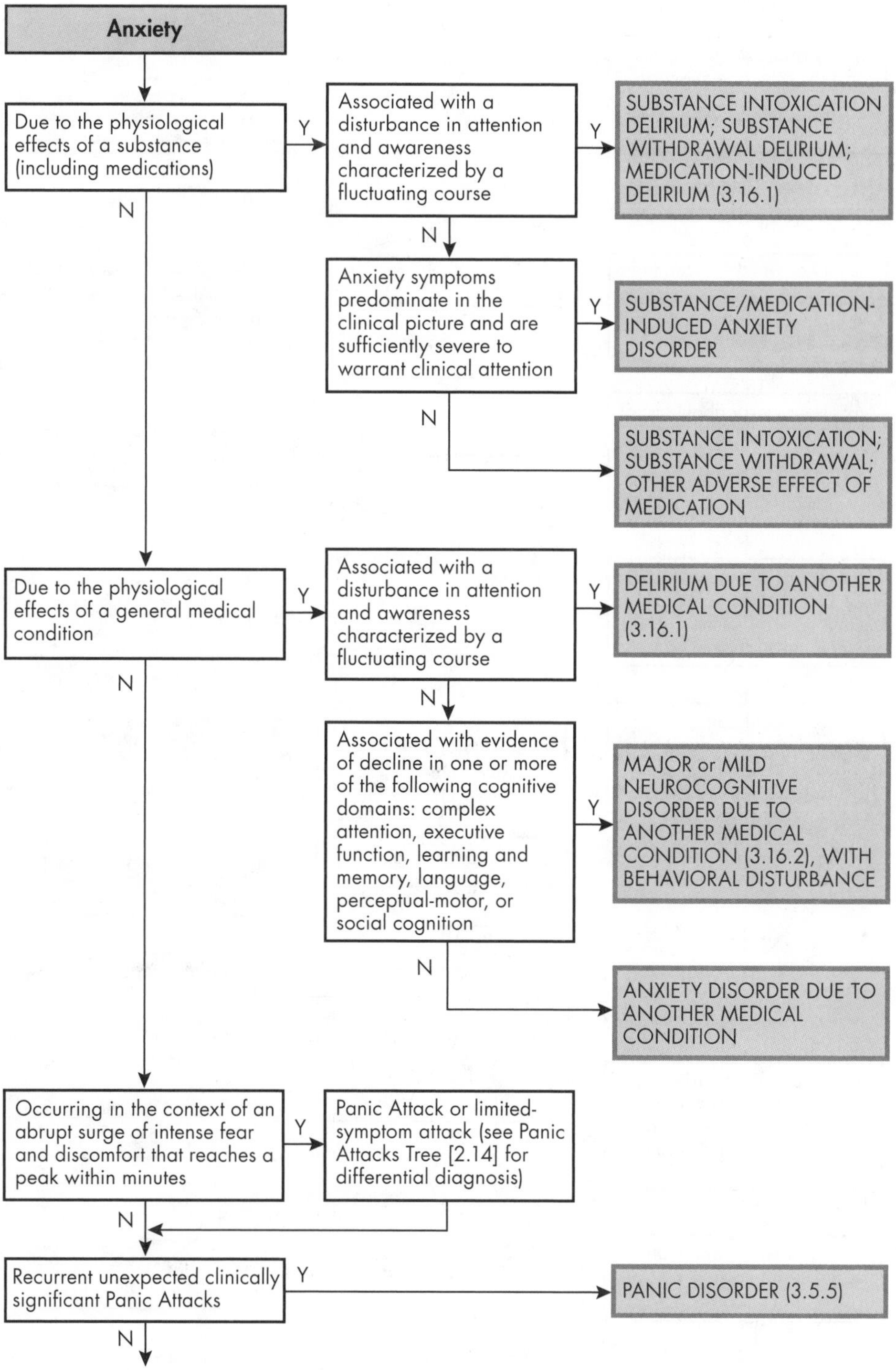
Anxiety
Due to the physiological effects of a substance (including medications)
Y
Associated with a disturbance in attention and awareness characterized by a fluctuating course
Y
SUBSTANCE INTOXICATION DELIRIUM; SUBSTANCE WITHDRAWAL DELIRIUM; MEDICATION-INDUCED DELIRIUM (3.16.1)
N
Anxiety symptoms predominate in the clinical picture and are sufficiently severe to warrant clinical attention
Y
SUBSTANCE/MEDICATION-INDUCED ANXIETY DISORDER
N
SUBSTANCE INTOXICATION; SUBSTANCE WITHDRAWAL; OTHER ADVERSE EFFECT OF MEDICATION
N
Due to the physiological effects of a general medical condition
Y
Associated with a disturbance in attention and awareness characterized by a fluctuating course
Y
DELIRIUM DUE TO ANOTHER MEDICAL CONDITION (3.16.1)
N
Associated with evidence of decline in one or more of the following cognitive domains: complex attention, executive function, learning and memory, language, perceptual-motor, or social cognition
Y
MAJOR or MILD NEUROCOGNITIVE DISORDER DUE TO ANOTHER MEDICAL CONDITION (3.16.2), WITH BEHAVIORAL DISTURBANCE
N
ANXIETY DISORDER DUE TO ANOTHER MEDICAL CONDITION
N
Occurring in the context of an abrupt surge of intense fear and discomfort that reaches a peak within minutes
Y
Panic Attack or limited-symptom attack (see Panic Attacks Tree [2.14] for differential diagnosis)
N
Recurrent unexpected clinically significant Panic Attacks
Y
PANIC DISORDER (3.5.5)
N

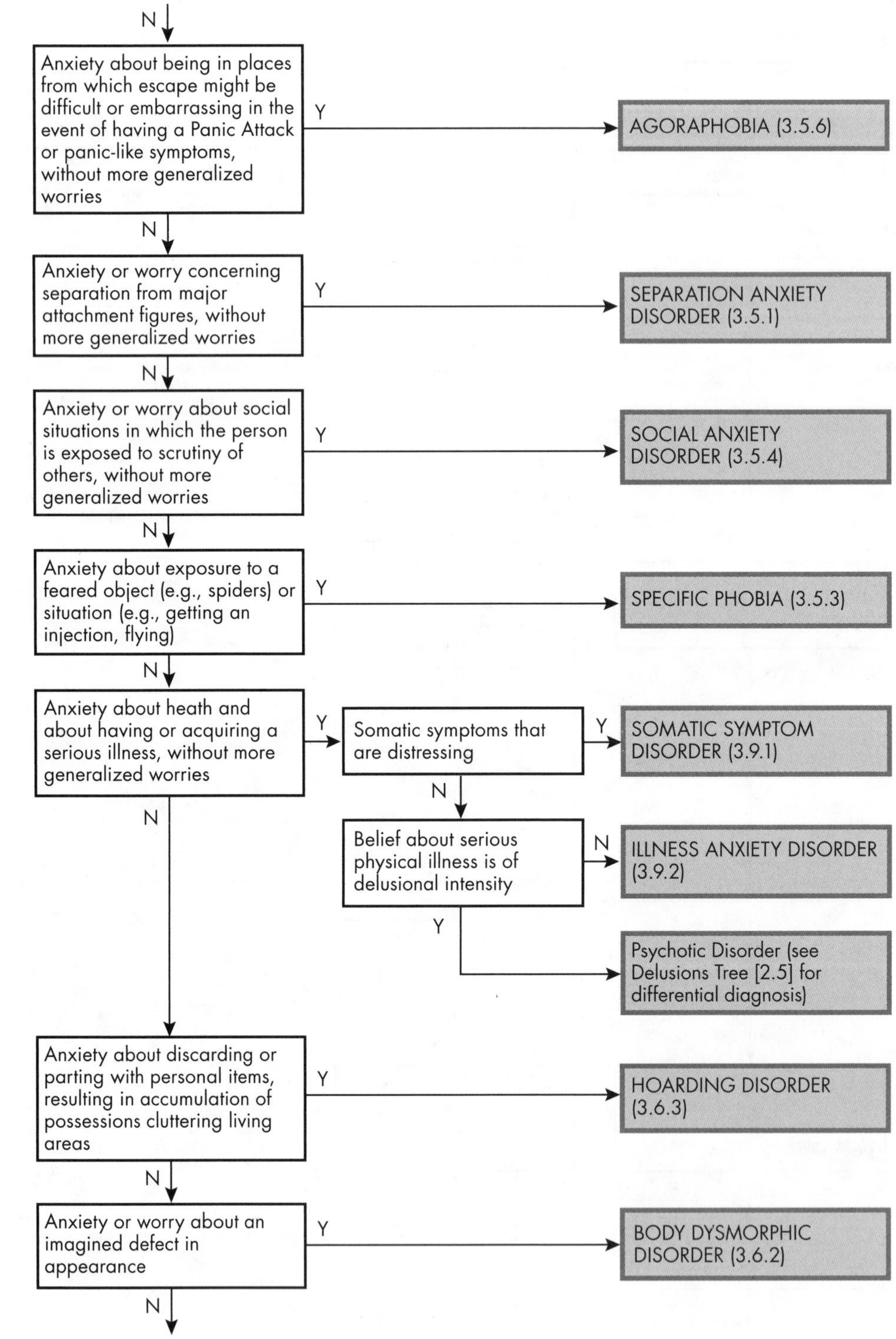
N
Anxiety about being in places from which escape might be difficult or embarrassing in the event of having a Panic Attack or panic-like symptoms, without more generalized worries
Y
AGORAPHOBIA (3.5.6)
N
Anxiety or worry concerning separation from major attachment figures, without more generalized worries
Y
SEPARATION ANXIETY DISORDER (3.5.1)
N
Anxiety or worry about social situations in which the person is exposed to scrutiny of others, without more generalized worries
Y
SOCIAL ANXIETY DISORDER (3.5.4)
N
Anxiety about exposure to a feared object (e.g., spiders) or situation (e.g., getting an injection, flying)
Y
SPECIFIC PHOBIA (3.5.3)
N
Anxiety about heath and about having or acquiring a serious illness, without more generalized worries
Y
Somatic symptoms that are distressing
Y
SOMATIC SYMPTOM DISORDER (3.9.1)
N
Belief about serious physical illness is of delusional intensity
N
ILLNESS ANXIETY DISORDER (3.9.2)
Y
Psychotic Disorder (see Delusions Tree [2.5] for differential diagnosis)
N
Anxiety about discarding or parting with personal items, resulting in accumulation of possessions cluttering living areas
Y
HOARDING DISORDER (3.6.3)
N
Anxiety or worry about an imagined defect in appearance
Y
BODY DYSMORPHIC DISORDER (3.6.2)
N

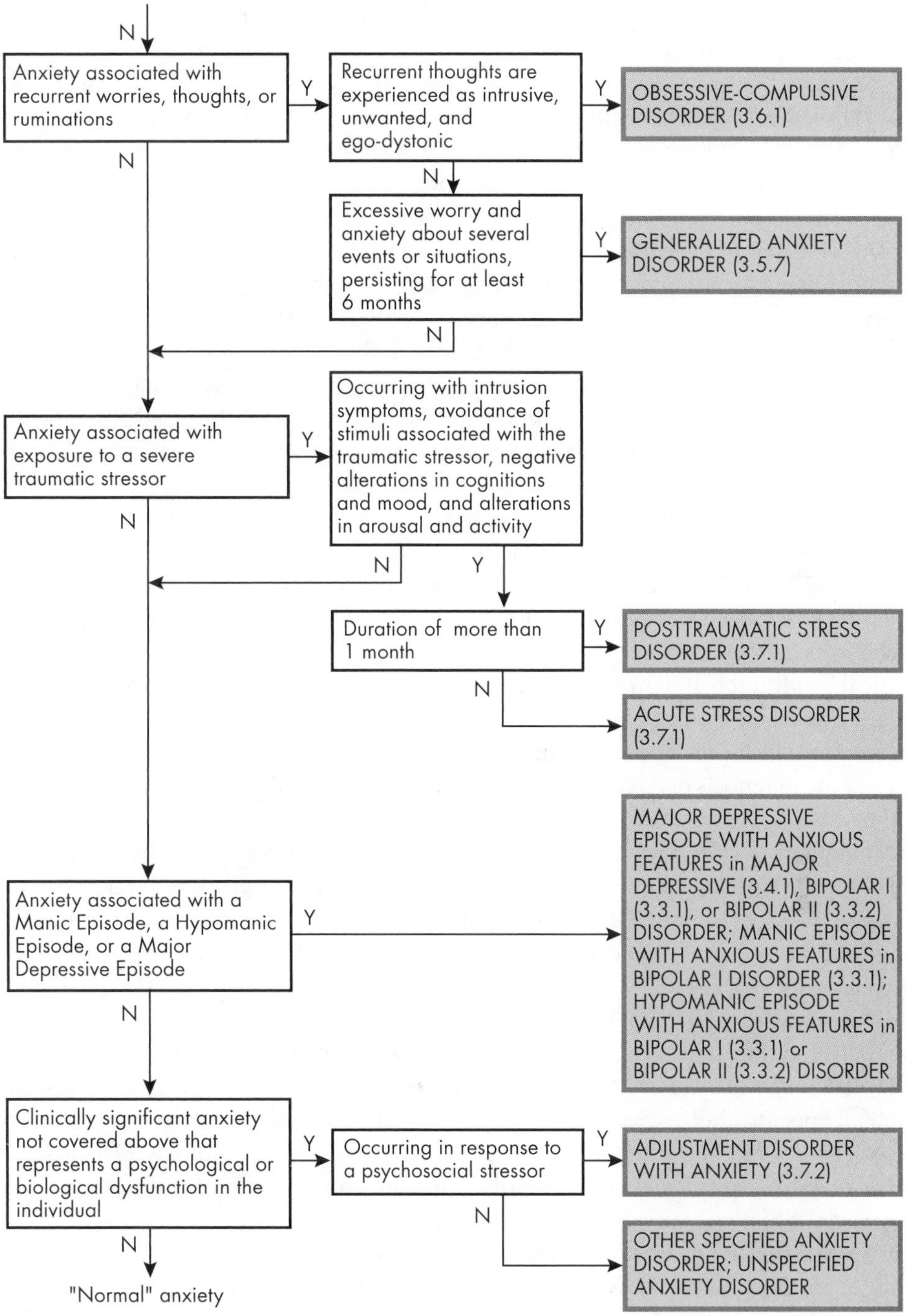
N
Anxiety associated with recurrent worries, thoughts, or ruminations
Y
Recurrent thoughts are experienced as intrusive, unwanted, and ego-dystonic
Y
OBSESSIVE-COMPULSIVE DISORDER (3.6.1)
N
Excessive worry and anxiety about several events or situations, persisting for at least 6 months
Y
GENERALIZED ANXIETY DISORDER (3.5.7)
N
N
Anxiety associated with exposure to a severe traumatic stressor
Y
Occurring with intrusion symptoms, avoidance of stimuli associated with the traumatic stressor, negative alterations in cognitions and mood, and alterations in arousal and activity
N
N
Y
Duration of more than 1 month
Y
POSTTRAUMATIC STRESS DISORDER (3.7.1)
N
ACUTE STRESS DISORDER (3.7.1)
Anxiety associated with a Manic Episode, a Hypomanic Episode, or a Major Depressive Episode
Y
MAJOR DEPRESSIVE EPISODE WITH ANXIOUS FEATURES in MAJOR DEPRESSIVE (3.4.1), BIPOLAR I (3.3.1), or BIPOLAR II (3.3.2) DISORDER; MANIC EPISODE WITH ANXIOUS FEATURES in BIPOLAR I DISORDER (3.3.1); HYPOMANIC EPISODE WITH ANXIOUS FEATURES in BIPOLAR I (3.3.1) or BIPOLAR II (3.3.2) DISORDER
N
Clinically significant anxiety not covered above that represents a psychological or biological dysfunction in the individual
Y
Occurring in response to a psychosocial stressor
Y
ADJUSTMENT DISORDER WITH ANXIETY (3.7.2)
N
OTHER SPECIFIED ANXIETY DISORDER; UNSPECIFIED ANXIETY DISORDER
N
"Normal" anxiety

2.14 Decision Tree for Panic Attacks

Panic attacks are discrete episodes of intense fear or discomfort accompanied by symptoms such as palpitations, shortness of breath, sweating, trembling, derealization, and a fear of losing control or dying. Although panic attacks are required for a diagnosis of Panic Disorder, they also occur in association with a number of other DSM-5 disorders listed in the tree. For example, if a patient with a snake phobia goes on a hike and steps on a snake, that experience could easily result in a Panic Attack that would be indicative of a Specific Phobia rather than Panic Disorder.

The first step in the differential for a Panic Attack is to rule out the presence of etiological substance/medication use. When taken in high enough doses or during Substance Withdrawal, a number of substances and medications can lead to a Panic Attack. Because caffeine is a common but covert culprit in this regard, taking a careful history of the consumption of caffeine-containing substances is important. If substance-related Panic Attacks warrant clinical attention, Substance/Medication-Induced Anxiety Disorder should be diagnosed; otherwise, a diagnosis of Substance Intoxication or Substance Withdrawal will suffice. Sometimes, individuals have their first Panic Attack while taking a substance and then go on to have additional attacks even when they are not taking any substances. Such subsequent attacks should not be considered substance-induced Panic Attacks but instead might warrant a diagnosis of Panic Disorder.

Next, possible etiological general medical conditions, such as hyperthyroidism or a pheochromocytoma, should be considered. If evidence indicates that such a general medical condition is the direct cause of the Panic Attack (e.g., the onset of the Panic Attacks paralleled the onset of the general medical condition, and the Panic Attacks remitted after initiation of successful treatment for the general medical condition), that would suggest the diagnosis of Anxiety Disorder Due to Another Medical Condition. Although mitral valve prolapse appears to be more frequent in individuals with Panic Attacks, a direct etiological connection has not been established; therefore, an individual with mitral valve prolapse and Panic Attacks is considered to have a primary Panic Disorder.

Once it is clear that the Panic Attacks are not the direct physiological consequence of a substance or general medical condition, the next step is to determine the relationship between the Panic Attacks and a possible situational trigger. By definition, at least two of the panic attacks in Panic Disorder must be unexpected—that is, there is no relationship between the attacks and a situational cue (i.e., they arise "out of the blue"). In contrast, the panic attacks that occur in patients with Social Anxiety Disorder (Social Phobia), Specific Phobia, Separation Anxiety Disorder, Posttraumatic Stress Disorder or Acute Stress Disorder, Illness Anxiety Disorder, Obsessive-Compulsive Disorder, and Generalized Anxiety Disorder are closely related to the pertinent situational trigger (e.g., social situations such as public speaking, a specific situation such as closed places, being separated from major attachment figures, being exposed to reminders of the trauma, the possibility of having a serious illness, obsessive concerns such as contamination fears, and worry about a number of events or situations, respectively). If the Panic Attacks are not an associated feature of a specific DSM-5 disorder but nonetheless are judged to be clinically significant, either a diagnosis of Adjustment Disorder (if the Panic Attacks are a response to a psychosocial stressor) or a diagnosis of a residual category

(Other Specified Anxiety Disorder or Unspecified Anxiety Disorder) may be appropriate. Finally, Panic Attacks triggered by a realistic threat (e.g., being held up at gunpoint) or the experience of a single isolated Panic Attack (or very occasional Panic Attacks) does not warrant a diagnosis of a mental disorder.

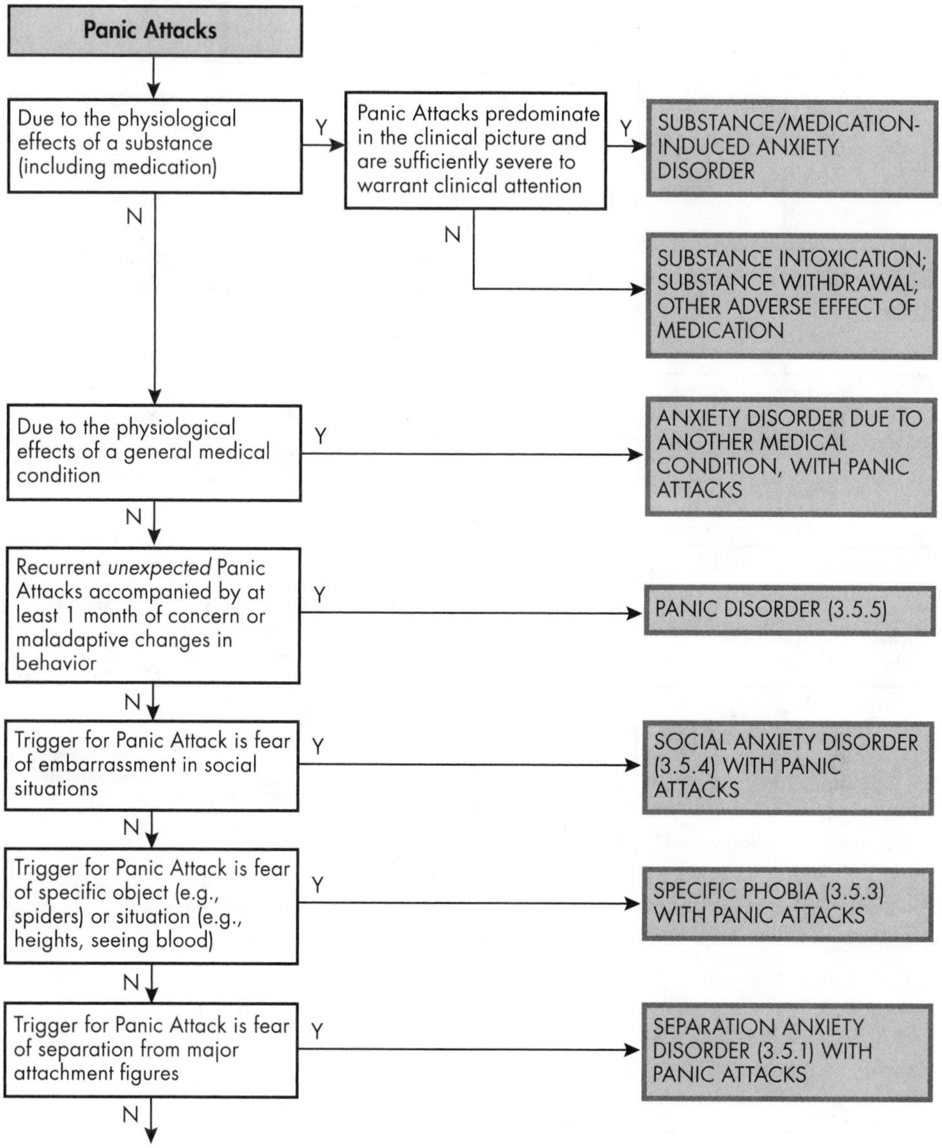

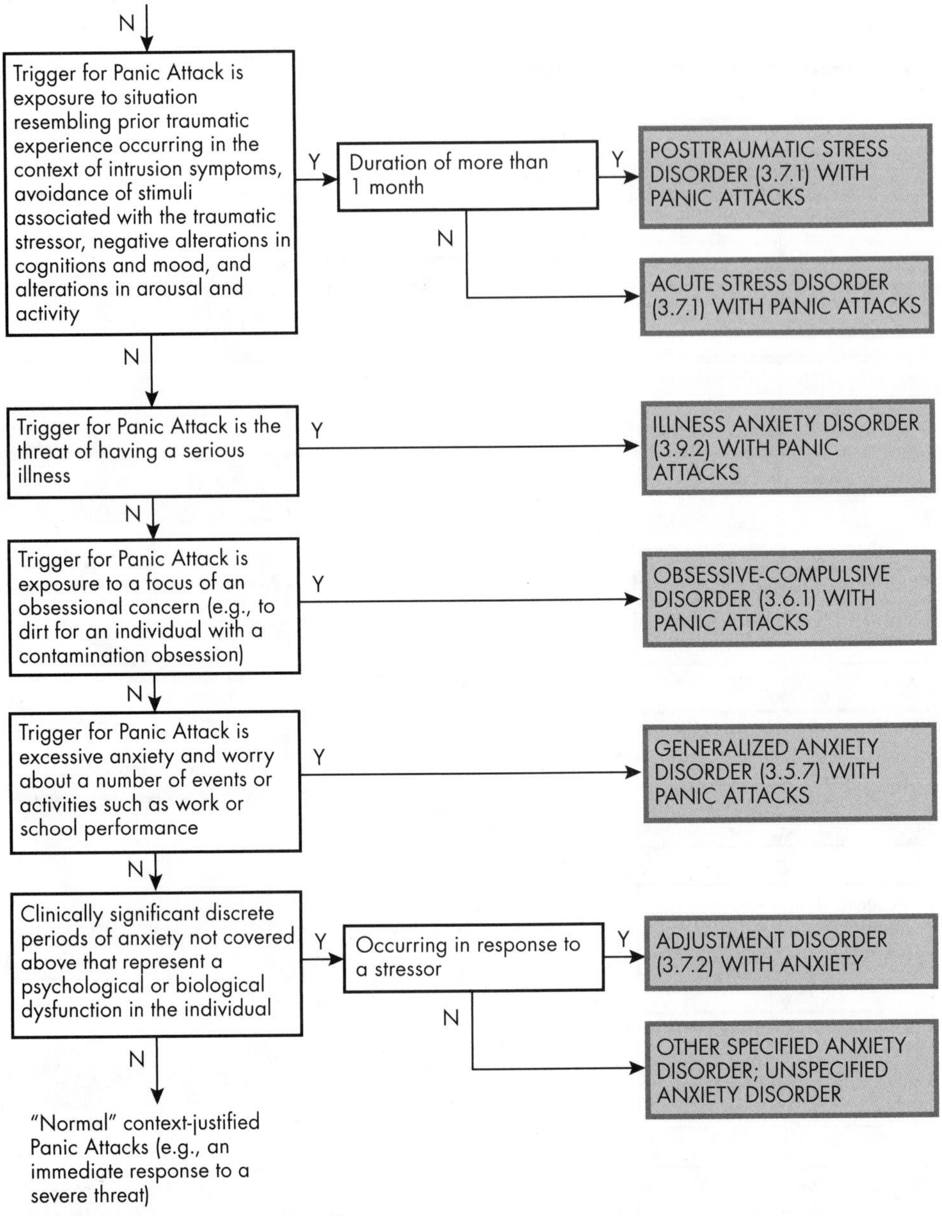
N
Trigger for Panic Attack is exposure to situation resembling prior traumatic experience occurring in the context of intrusion symptoms, avoidance of stimuli associated with the traumatic stressor, negative alterations in cognitions and mood, and alterations in arousal and activity
Y
Duration of more than 1 month
Y
POSTTRAUMATIC STRESS DISORDER (3.7.1) WITH PANIC ATTACKS
N
ACUTE STRESS DISORDER (3.7.1) WITH PANIC ATTACKS
N
Trigger for Panic Attack is the threat of having a serious illness
Y
ILLNESS ANXIETY DISORDER (3.9.2) WITH PANIC ATTACKS
N
Trigger for Panic Attack is exposure to a focus of an obsessional concern (e.g., to dirt for an individual with a contamination obsession)
Y
OBSESSIVE-COMPULSIVE DISORDER (3.6.1) WITH PANIC ATTACKS
N
Trigger for Panic Attack is excessive anxiety and worry about a number of events or activities such as work or school performance
Y
GENERALIZED ANXIETY DISORDER (3.5.7) WITH PANIC ATTACKS
N
Clinically significant discrete periods of anxiety not covered above that represent a psychological or biological dysfunction in the individual
Y
Occurring in response to a stressor
Y
ADJUSTMENT DISORDER (3.7.2) WITH ANXIETY
N
OTHER SPECIFIED ANXIETY DISORDER; UNSPECIFIED ANXIETY DISORDER
N
"Normal" context-justified Panic Attacks (e.g., an immediate response to a severe threat)

2.15 Decision Tree for Avoidance Behavior

Avoidance behavior (particularly of realistically harmful situations) is often adaptive. This decision tree applies only when the avoidance is based on unrealistic or excessive fears and leads to clinically significant distress or impairment. Avoidance is a fairly ubiquitous and nonspecific symptom and is an associated feature of many disorders. The evaluation of this symptom requires determining the specific circumstances triggering the avoidance. This is one of the few decision trees included in this handbook that does not include a decision point for ruling out substance/medication use or a general medical condition as an etiological factor. This is because avoidance behavior is almost invariably a psychological reaction to an underlying anxiety or fear. Although substance/medication use or a general medical condition can cause anxiety, the lack of contextual associations makes the development of avoidance behavior related to Substance/Medication-Induced Anxiety Disorder or Anxiety Disorder Due to Another Medical Condition unlikely.

The first order of business is determining whether the avoidance behavior involves multiple situations and places. If so, and if the situations are avoided due to thoughts that escape might be difficult or help might not be available in the event of developing panic-like symptoms, the diagnosis of Agoraphobia might apply. Individuals associate the risk of having a Panic Attack or panic-like symptoms with particular locations or situations that then become conditioned stimuli particularly likely to trigger additional attacks. The individuals then avoid what appear to be "triggering" situations in an effort to minimize the chance of having panic attacks or panic-like symptoms.

The avoidance in Social Anxiety Disorder (Social Phobia) is related to the fear of social embarrassment. This avoidance comes in two forms: the performance anxiety form of Social Anxiety Disorder concerns the avoidance of public activities (e.g., speaking, playing music, acting, eating, urinating, writing) that can easily be performed by the individual in the privacy of his or her own home, and can be indicated by the "Performance Only" specifier; the generalized form includes virtually any situation that involves social interaction and in many cases may be virtually identical to Avoidant Personality Disorder. The Specific Phobias probably involve some interaction between evolutionarily predetermined inborn fears and the occurrence of aversive early-life experiences that reinforce them. In Separation Anxiety Disorder, which can occur in both childhood and in adulthood, situations in which the person is apart from major attachment figures are avoided. In Posttraumatic Stress Disorder and Acute Stress Disorder, the individual avoids situations that are reminiscent of the traumatic stressor (e.g., someone who resembles the assailant, loud sounds that recall wartime, tremors that recall a major earthquake). Some individuals with Obsessive-Compulsive Disorder learn that avoiding certain triggering situations will prevent the onset of obsessions (e.g., avoidance of handshakes will help reduce contamination obsessions). Similarly, some individuals with Illness Anxiety Disorder will avoid situations that they feel might jeopardize their health (e.g., visiting sick family members) lest they trigger ruminations about having contracted a serious illness.

Many other psychiatric disorders can have avoidance as an associated feature. For example, in psychotic disorders avoidance behavior can occur in the context of a particular delusional system, such as when a delusional patient avoids going outside for fear that the FBI is after him or her. Low motivation, which may be due to the anhedonia in a Major

Depressive Episode or as part of the negative symptoms in Schizophrenia, may lead to a generalized avoidance of going out of the house. Because of a sexual dysfunction, sexual situations may be avoided because of anxiety about poor sexual performance. Individuals with Anorexia Nervosa and Avoidant/Restrictive Food Intake Disorder avoid certain foods (e.g., high-calorie foods in Anorexia Nervosa, aversive foods in Avoidant/Restrictive Food Intake Disorder), leading to clinically significant weight loss and potential malnutrition. A generalized pattern of avoidance characterizes Avoidant Personality Disorder, which by definition has its onset by early adulthood and tends to be relatively persistent and stable over the course of the person's lifetime.

Finally, if the avoidance behavior is not adequately explained by any of the decision points so far in the tree, it may still justify a DSM-5 diagnosis. If the avoidance behavior is a symptomatic manifestation of a maladaptive response to a psychosocial stressor, a diagnosis of Adjustment Disorder might apply. If not, and it is clinically significant and represents a psychological or biological dysfunction in the individual (thus qualifying as a mental disorder), a residual category would apply. DSM-5 does not include a residual category for avoidance behavior per se. The closest residual category would be Other Specified Anxiety Disorder or Unspecified Anxiety Disorder because most likely the avoidance is serving to prevent some sort of anxiety. The choice of category depends on whether the clinician wishes to record the symptomatic presentation on the chart (in which case Other Specified Anxiety Disorder would be used, followed by the specific reason) or not (in which case Unspecified Anxiety Disorder would be used). Otherwise, the avoidance would be considered part of the normal repertoire of human behavior and not indicative of a mental disorder.

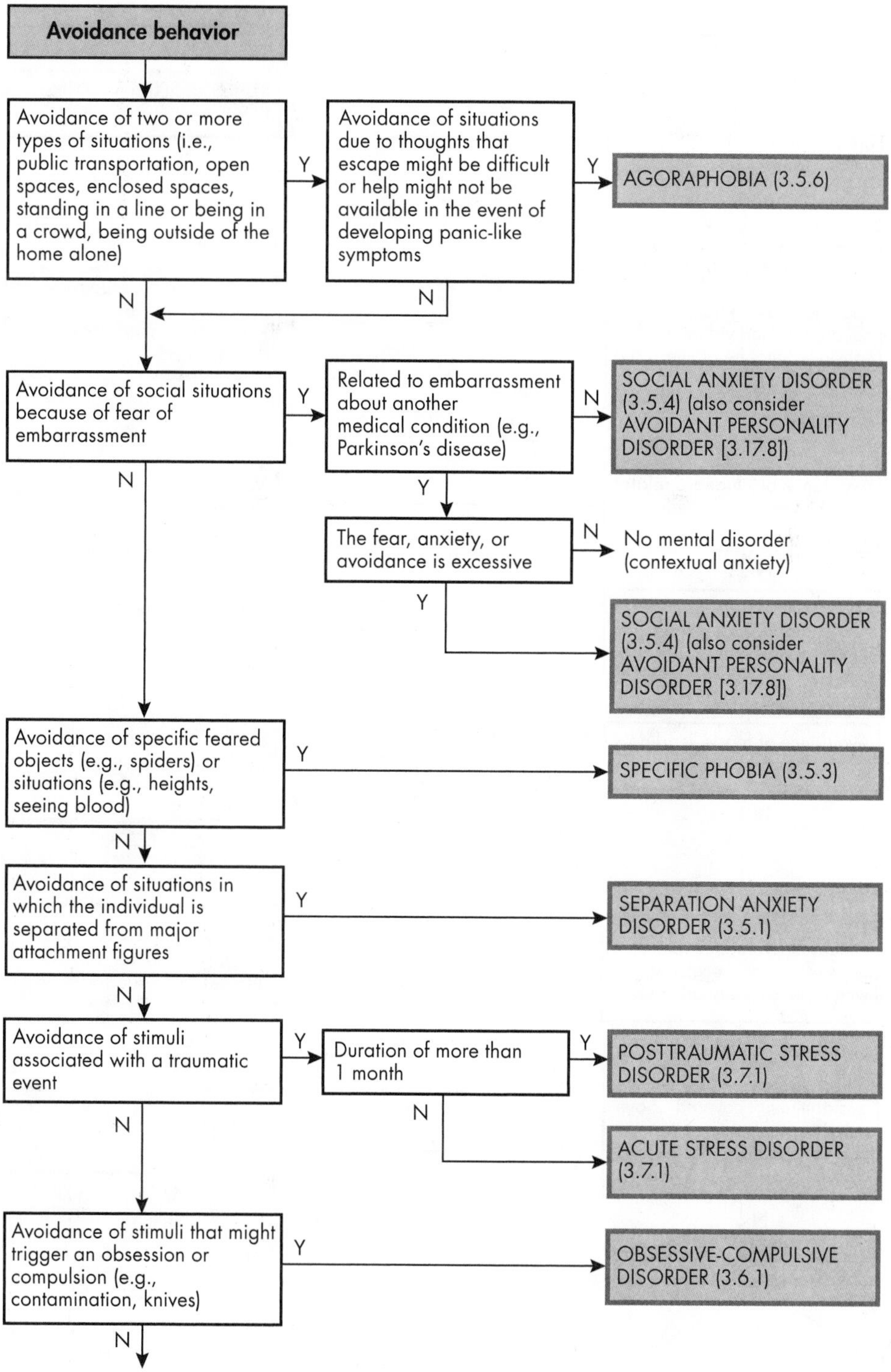
Avoidance behavior
Avoidance of two or more types of situations (i.e., public transportation, open spaces, enclosed spaces, standing in a line or being in a crowd, being outside of the home alone)
Y
Avoidance of situations due to thoughts that escape might be difficult or help might not be available in the event of developing panic-like symptoms
Y
AGORAPHOBIA (3.5.6)
N
N
Avoidance of social situations because of fear of embarrassment
Y
Related to embarrassment about another medical condition (e.g., Parkinson's disease)
N
SOCIAL ANXIETY DISORDER (3.5.4) (also consider AVOIDANT PERSONALITY DISORDER [3.17.8])
Y
The fear, anxiety, or avoidance is excessive
N
No mental disorder (contextual anxiety)
Y
SOCIAL ANXIETY DISORDER (3.5.4) (also consider AVOIDANT PERSONALITY DISORDER [3.17.8])
N
Avoidance of specific feared objects (e.g., spiders) or situations (e.g., heights, seeing blood)
Y
SPECIFIC PHOBIA (3.5.3)
N
Avoidance of situations in which the individual is separated from major attachment figures
Y
SEPARATION ANXIETY DISORDER (3.5.1)
N
Avoidance of stimuli associated with a traumatic event
Y
Duration of more than 1 month
Y
POSTTRAUMATIC STRESS DISORDER (3.7.1)
N
ACUTE STRESS DISORDER (3.7.1)
N
Avoidance of stimuli that might trigger an obsession or compulsion (e.g., contamination, knives)
Y
OBSESSIVE-COMPULSIVE DISORDER (3.6.1)
N

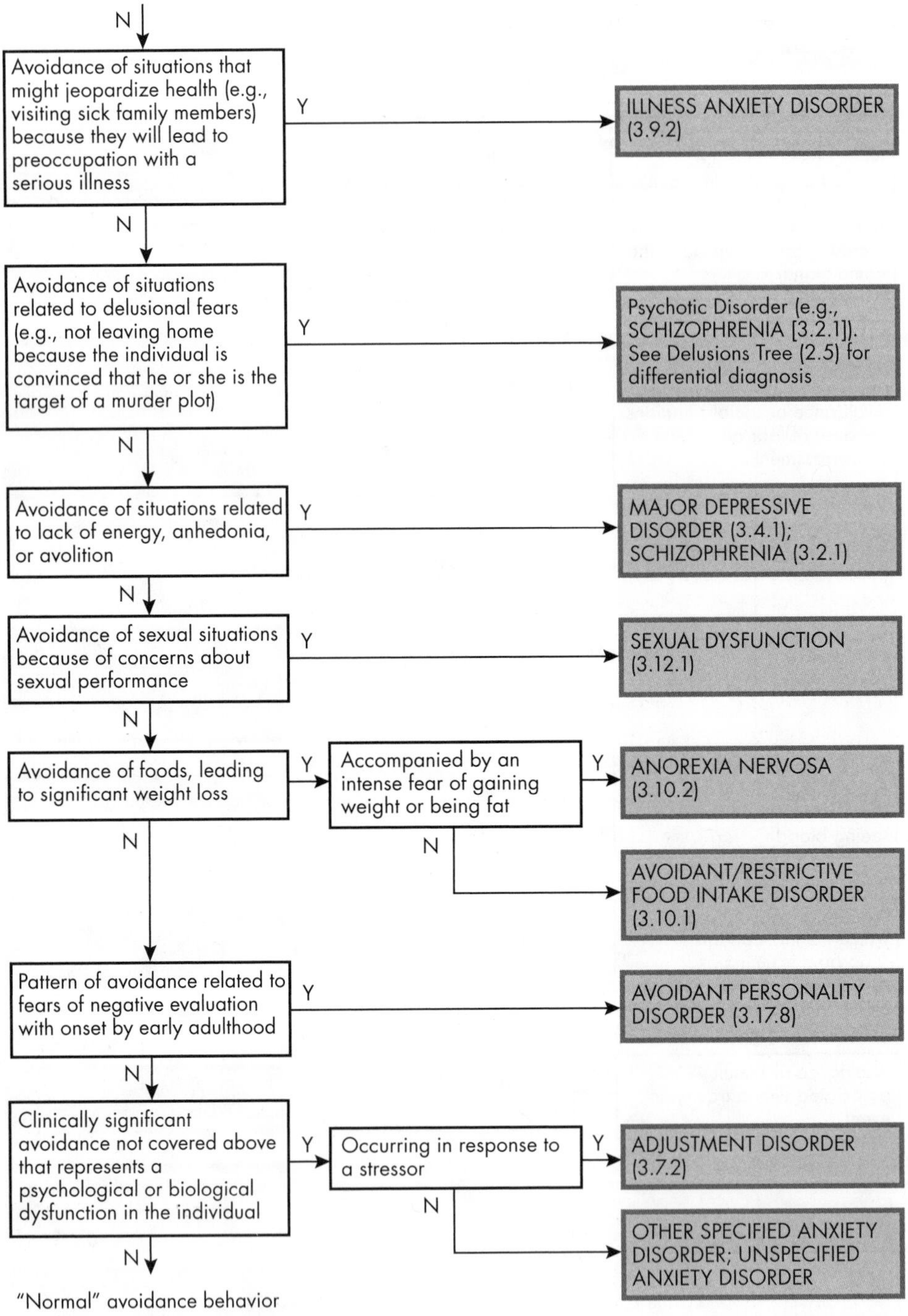
N
Avoidance of situations that might jeopardize health (e.g., visiting sick family members) because they will lead to preoccupation with a serious illness
Y
ILLNESS ANXIETY DISORDER (3.9.2)
N
Avoidance of situations related to delusional fears (e.g., not leaving home because the individual is convinced that he or she is the target of a murder plot)
Y
Psychotic Disorder (e.g., SCHIZOPHRENIA [3.2.1]). See Delusions Tree (2.5) for differential diagnosis
N
Avoidance of situations related to lack of energy, anhedonia, or avolition
Y
MAJOR DEPRESSIVE DISORDER (3.4.1); SCHIZOPHRENIA (3.2.1)
N
Avoidance of sexual situations because of concerns about sexual performance
Y
SEXUAL DYSFUNCTION (3.12.1)
N
Avoidance of foods, leading to significant weight loss
Y
Accompanied by an intense fear of gaining weight or being fat
Y
ANOREXIA NERVOSA (3.10.2)
N
AVOIDANT/RESTRICTIVE FOOD INTAKE DISORDER (3.10.1)
N
Pattern of avoidance related to fears of negative evaluation with onset by early adulthood
Y
AVOIDANT PERSONALITY DISORDER (3.17.8)
N
Clinically significant avoidance not covered above that represents a psychological or biological dysfunction in the individual
Y
Occurring in response to a stressor
Y
ADJUSTMENT DISORDER (3.7.2)
N
OTHER SPECIFIED ANXIETY DISORDER; UNSPECIFIED ANXIETY DISORDER
N
"Normal" avoidance behavior

2.16 Decision Tree for Trauma or Psychosocial Stressors Involved in the Etiology

Psychosocial stressors are important in the pathogenesis of all of the DSM-5 disorders, but their specific etiological role serves as a defining feature for only a few. Four disorders in DSM-5 can be diagnosed only when the individual has been exposed to an extreme stressor: Posttraumatic Stress Disorder, Acute Stress Disorder, Reactive Attachment Disorder, and Disinhibited Social Engagement Disorder. Posttraumatic Stress Disorder requires exposure to an event that involved actual or threatened death, serious injury, or sexual violation, and is characterized by persistent intrusion symptoms associated with the traumatic event (e.g., intrusive memories of the event, distressing dreams, flashbacks, distress upon exposure to cues reminiscent of the event), avoidance of stimuli associated with the event, negative alterations in cognitions and moods associated with the event (e.g., negative beliefs about oneself and the world, distorted blame of self or others, feelings of detachment, persistent negative state, inability to experience positive emotions), and marked alterations in reactivity and arousal. The symptom profile of Acute Stress Disorder closely resembles that of Posttraumatic Stress Disorder except that the symptoms have lasted for less than 1 month. Reactive Attachment Disorder and Disinhibited Social Engagement Disorder both require extended exposure to extremes of insufficient care as a young child, such as frequent changes in primary caregivers or being raised in poorly staffed institutional settings.

Although not required as part of the disorder definition, Brief Psychotic Disorder, Dissociative Amnesia, and Conversion Disorder (Functional Neurological Symptom Disorder) often develop in response to a severe psychosocial stressor. A diagnosis of Brief Psychotic Disorder applies if the reaction to an extreme stressor involves the development of psychotic symptoms lasting for less than 1 month. If the individual is unable to recall important autobiographical information related to a traumatic experience, then the diagnosis of Dissociative Amnesia might apply. If the person develops symptoms of altered voluntary motor or sensory function that are incompatible with any recognized neurological condition in response to a psychosocial stressor, then a diagnosis of Conversion Disorder would apply. Although the development of each of these disorders is often related to exposure to a traumatic stressor, any of these conditions can develop without exposure to a stressor.

Many clinicians are confused about the relationship between the Adjustment Disorders and the other conditions in DSM-5 that are often precipitated by the presence of a psychosocial stressor. Adjustment Disorder is diagnosed for those presentations in which the maladaptive response to the stressor causes clinically significant distress or impairment but does not meet the threshold requirements for any specific DSM-5 disorder. In contrast, when the criteria are met for a specific DSM-5 disorder, that disorder is diagnosed regardless of the presence or absence of associated stressors. For example, if a depressive reaction occurs in response to a job loss or learning that one has a serious illness, the diagnosis is Major Depressive Disorder if the reaction meets the full criteria for a Major Depressive Episode. A less severe, but nonetheless clinically significant, depressive reaction might instead be diagnosed as Adjustment Disorder With Depressed Mood.

Finally, some individuals, in response to the loss of a loved one, develop a persistent, prolonged, and abnormal grief response that has been given the name Persistent Complex Bereavement Disorder (see "Conditions for Further Study" in DSM-5 Section III). It involves the persistence for at least 12 months of symptoms such as longing or yearning for the deceased, intense sorrow and pain, and preoccupation with the deceased and the circumstances of the death. Although there are undoubtedly individuals suffering from this syndrome who would benefit from treatment, the developers of DSM-5 felt that insufficient data exist regarding the specifics of the definition to warrant its inclusion in the main body of DSM-5. Clinicians wishing to make this diagnosis must use Other Specified Trauma- and Stressor-Related Disorder, and specify Persistent Complex Bereavement Disorder.

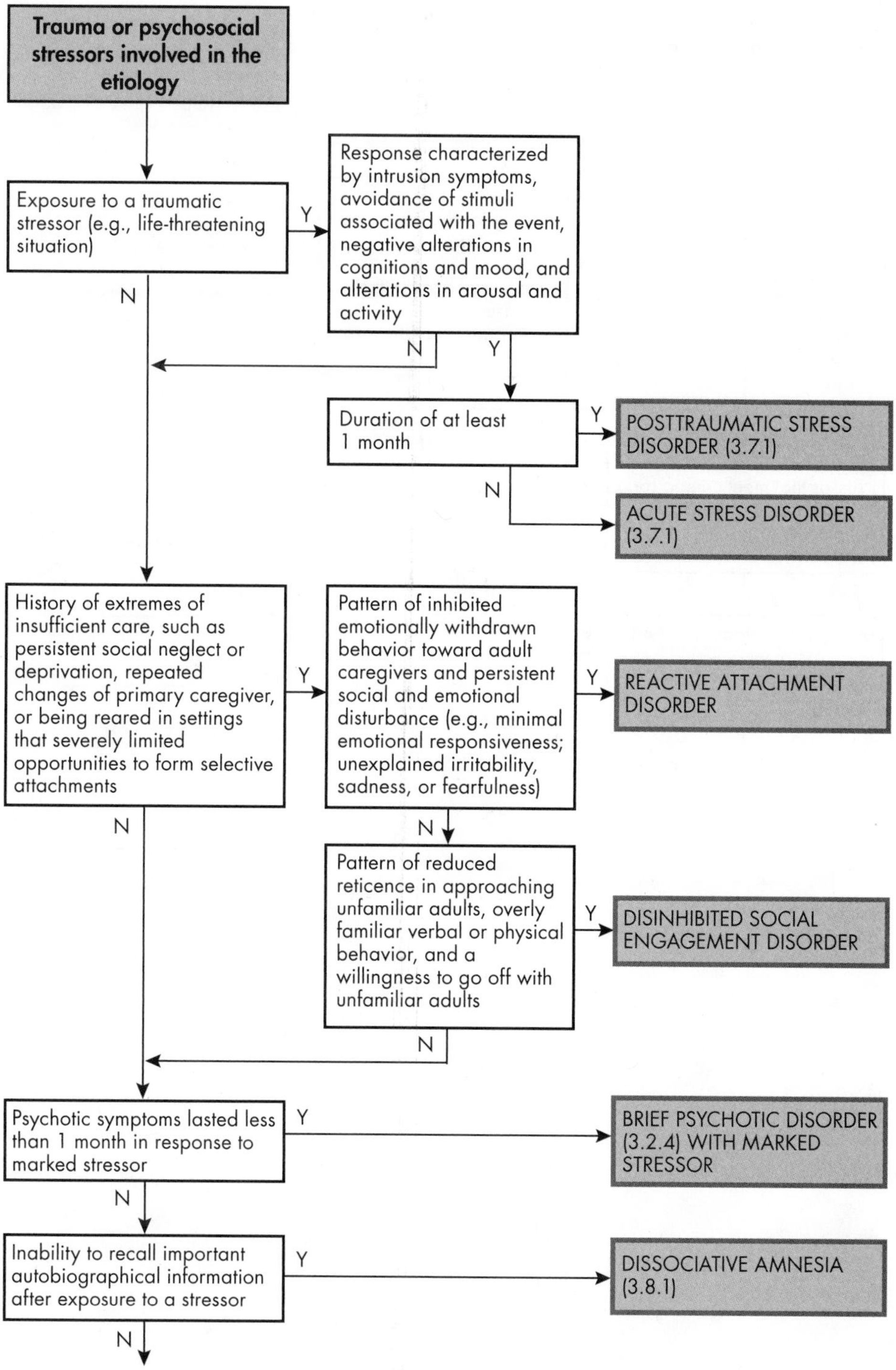
Trauma or psychosocial stressors involved in the etiology
Exposure to a traumatic stressor (e.g., life-threatening situation)
Y
N
Response characterized by intrusion symptoms, avoidance of stimuli associated with the event, negative alterations in cognitions and mood, and alterations in arousal and activity
N
Y
Duration of at least 1 month
Y
POSTTRAUMATIC STRESS DISORDER (3.7.1)
N
ACUTE STRESS DISORDER (3.7.1)
History of extremes of insufficient care, such as persistent social neglect or deprivation, repeated changes of primary caregiver, or being reared in settings that severely limited opportunities to form selective attachments
Y
N
Pattern of inhibited emotionally withdrawn behavior toward adult caregivers and persistent social and emotional disturbance (e.g., minimal emotional responsiveness; unexplained irritability, sadness, or fearfulness)
Y
REACTIVE ATTACHMENT DISORDER
N
Pattern of reduced reticence in approaching unfamiliar adults, overly familiar verbal or physical behavior, and a willingness to go off with unfamiliar adults
Y
DISINHIBITED SOCIAL ENGAGEMENT DISORDER
N
Psychotic symptoms lasted less than 1 month in response to marked stressor
Y
BRIEF PSYCHOTIC DISORDER (3.2.4) WITH MARKED STRESSOR
N
Inability to recall important autobiographical information after exposure to a stressor
Y
DISSOCIATIVE AMNESIA (3.8.1)
N

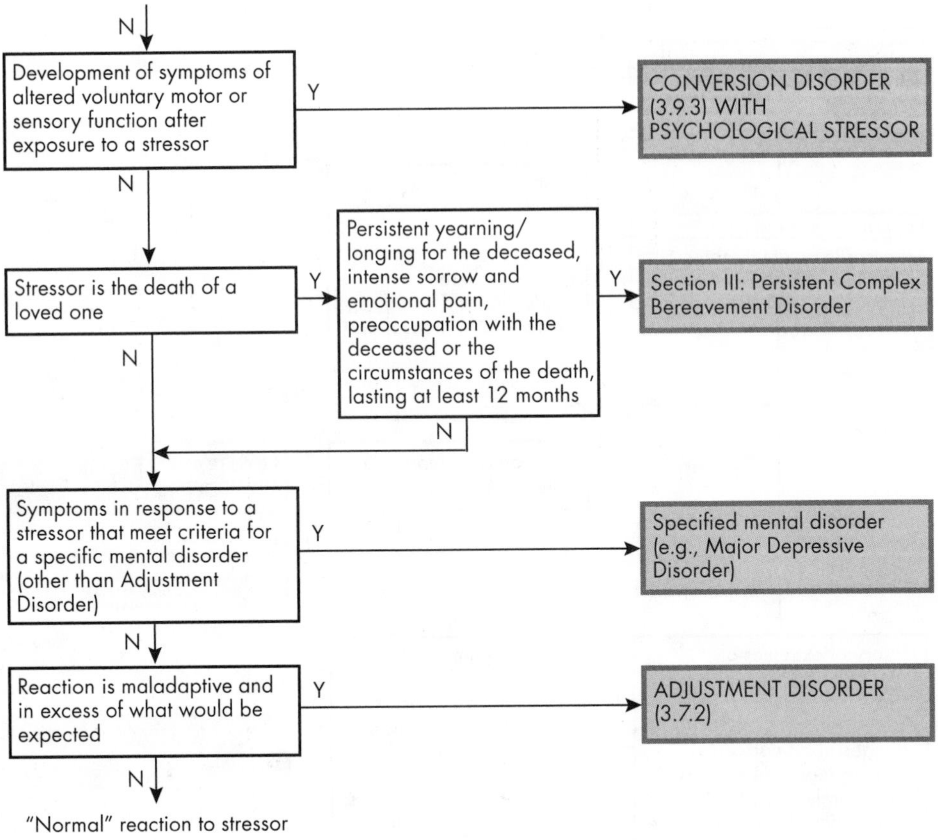
N
Development of symptoms of altered voluntary motor or sensory function after exposure to a stressor
Y
CONVERSION DISORDER (3.9.3) WITH PSYCHOLOGICAL STRESSOR
N
Stressor is the death of a loved one
Y
Persistent yearning/ longing for the deceased, intense sorrow and emotional pain, preoccupation with the deceased or the circumstances of the death, lasting at least 12 months
Y
Section III: Persistent Complex Bereavement Disorder
N
N
Symptoms in response to a stressor that meet criteria for a specific mental disorder (other than Adjustment Disorder)
Y
Specified mental disorder (e.g., Major Depressive Disorder)
N
Reaction is maladaptive and in excess of what would be expected
Y
ADJUSTMENT DISORDER (3.7.2)
N
"Normal" reaction to stressor

2.17 Decision Tree for Somatic Complaints or Illness/Appearance Anxiety

When a patient presents with distressing somatic complaints, the focus of the differential diagnosis is usually on which general medical condition best explains the somatic complaints. However, when the somatic complaints are accompanied by abnormal thoughts, feelings, and behaviors, the presence of a Somatic Symptom Disorder or other mental disorder should be considered.

Physical complaints that are feigned by the patient warrant either the mental disorder diagnosis Factitious Disorder or the nondisordered condition known as Malingering. The differentiation between these two conditions depends on a consideration of the context in which the somatic symptoms developed. If the feigning of the symptoms occurs in the absence of obvious external rewards, the diagnosis is Factitious Disorder, whereas feigning in settings in which the presence of the somatic symptoms provides an obvious financial or other benefit to the patient suggests Malingering.

Somatic complaints can occur as a manifestation of a wide variety of psychiatric conditions. Substance Intoxication or Substance Withdrawal is typically manifested as a characteristic syndrome of somatic and behavioral symptoms. States of high anxiety are typically associated with a variety of somatic complaints. Consequently, somatic complaints are commonly associated with many of the Anxiety Disorders. For some Anxiety Disorders, such as Panic Disorder and Generalized Anxiety Disorder, the distressing somatic complaints characteristic of these disorders may be the reason for the patient to seek treatment. In other cases, the somatic complaints are related to the manifestations of a psychotic disorder (e.g., somatic delusions) or an Obsessive-Compulsive and Related Disorder, such as the preoccupation with an imagined physical defect in Body Dysmorphic Disorder.

When the somatic complaints themselves are the patient's central focus, a diagnosis of one of the DSM-5 Somatic Symptom and Related Disorders might be most appropriate. Patients presenting with neurological symptoms such as paralysis or seizures which, upon examination and laboratory investigation, do not conform to a pattern characteristic of a known neurological or other medical condition, can be diagnosed with Conversion Disorder (Functional Neurological Symptom Disorder). Other types of somatic complaints, when accompanied by disproportionate thoughts about the seriousness of the illness, persistently high levels of anxiety about health or about symptoms, or the devotion of excessive time and energy to symptoms or health concerns, may warrant a diagnosis of Somatic Symptom Disorder. In contrast to the DSM-IV Somatoform Disorder diagnoses in which the somatic complaints were by definition medically unexplained, a diagnosis of Somatic Symptom Disorder in DSM-5 can be given to patients with a bona fide medical illness. The DSM-5 diagnosis depends on the presence of cognitions, feelings, and behaviors that are, in the clinician's judgment, "excessive" given the nature of the general medical condition. To avoid pathologizing appropriate reactions to serious or disabling general medical conditions, this diagnosis should be used very cautiously in medically ill individuals, being reserved only for cases in which the person's reactions to having the medical illness are clearly extreme and maladaptive.

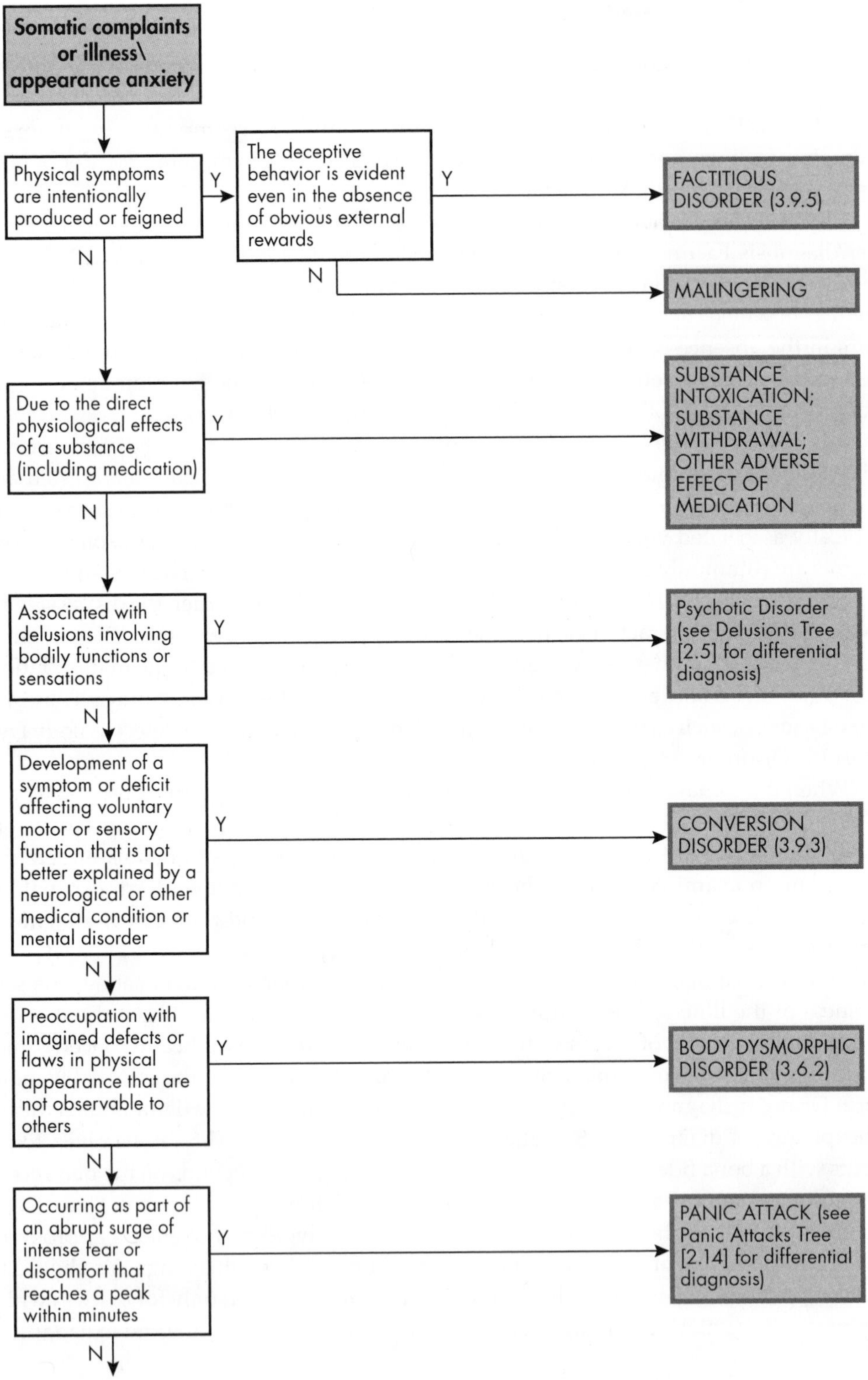
Somatic complaints or illness\ appearance anxiety
Physical symptoms are intentionally produced or feigned
Y
The deceptive behavior is evident even in the absence of obvious external rewards
Y
FACTITIOUS DISORDER (3.9.5)
N
MALINGERING
N
Due to the direct physiological effects of a substance (including medication)
Y
SUBSTANCE INTOXICATION; SUBSTANCE WITHDRAWAL; OTHER ADVERSE EFFECT OF MEDICATION
N
Associated with delusions involving bodily functions or sensations
Y
Psychotic Disorder (see Delusions Tree [2.5] for differential diagnosis)
N
Development of a symptom or deficit affecting voluntary motor or sensory function that is not better explained by a neurological or other medical condition or mental disorder
Y
CONVERSION DISORDER (3.9.3)
N
Preoccupation with imagined defects or flaws in physical appearance that are not observable to others
Y
BODY DYSMORPHIC DISORDER (3.6.2)
N
Occurring as part of an abrupt surge of intense fear or discomfort that reaches a peak within minutes
Y
PANIC ATTACK (see Panic Attacks Tree [2.14] for differential diagnosis)
N

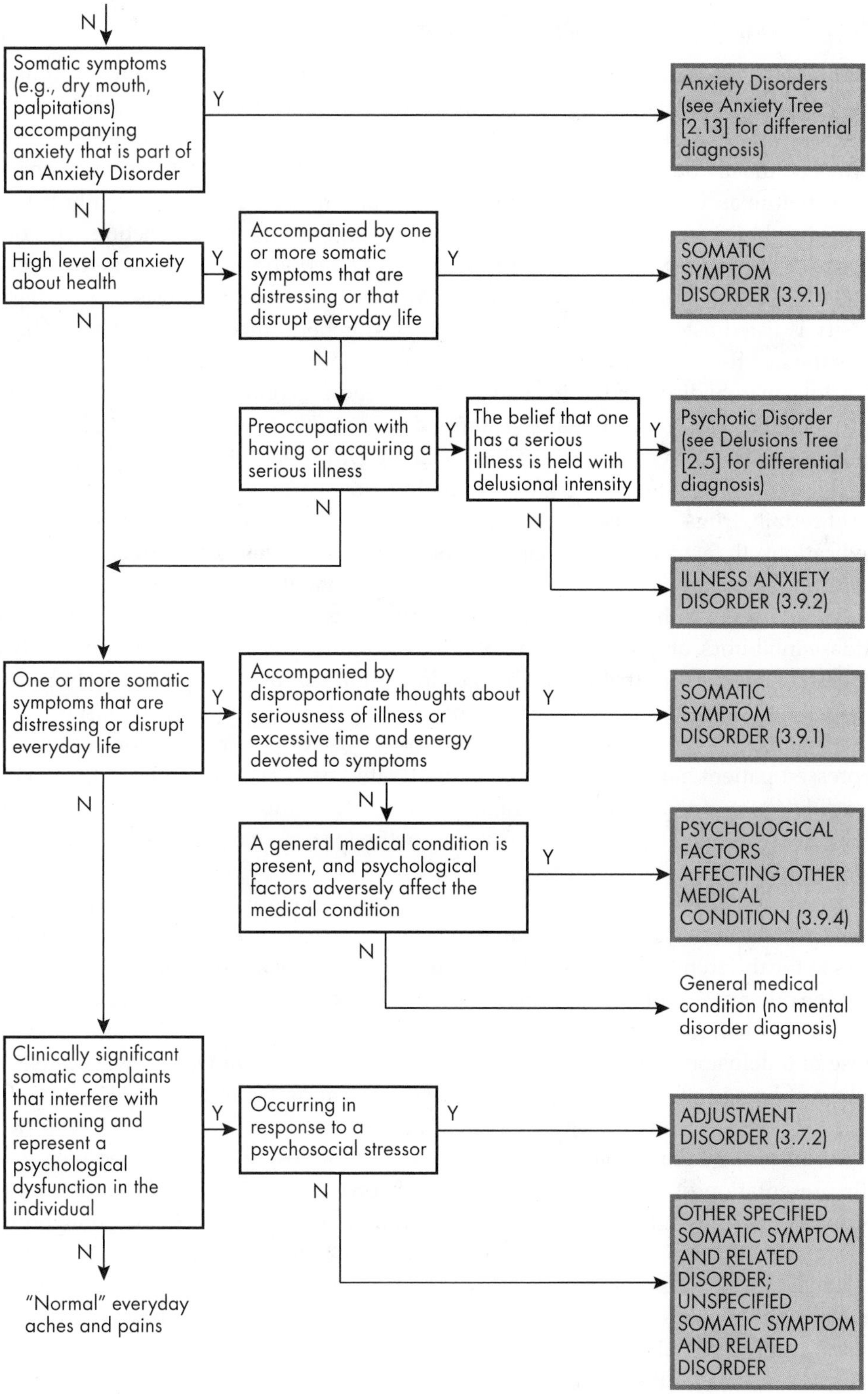
N
Somatic symptoms (e.g., dry mouth, palpitations) accompanying anxiety that is part of an Anxiety Disorder
Y
Anxiety Disorders (see Anxiety Tree [2.13] for differential diagnosis)
N
High level of anxiety about health
Y
Accompanied by one or more somatic symptoms that are distressing or that disrupt everyday life
Y
SOMATIC SYMPTOM DISORDER (3.9.1)
N
N
Preoccupation with having or acquiring a serious illness
Y
The belief that one has a serious illness is held with delusional intensity
Y
Psychotic Disorder (see Delusions Tree [2.5] for differential diagnosis)
N
N
ILLNESS ANXIETY DISORDER (3.9.2)
One or more somatic symptoms that are distressing or disrupt everyday life
Y
Accompanied by disproportionate thoughts about seriousness of illness or excessive time and energy devoted to symptoms
Y
SOMATIC SYMPTOM DISORDER (3.9.1)
N
N
A general medical condition is present, and psychological factors adversely affect the medical condition
Y
PSYCHOLOGICAL FACTORS AFFECTING OTHER MEDICAL CONDITION (3.9.4)
N
General medical condition (no mental disorder diagnosis)
Clinically significant somatic complaints that interfere with functioning and represent a psychological dysfunction in the individual
Y
Occurring in response to a psychosocial stressor
Y
ADJUSTMENT DISORDER (3.7.2)
N
OTHER SPECIFIED SOMATIC SYMPTOM AND RELATED DISORDER; UNSPECIFIED SOMATIC SYMPTOM AND RELATED DISORDER
N
"Normal" everyday aches and pains

2.18 Decision Tree for Appetite Changes or Unusual Eating Behavior

This decision tree covers several disparate symptoms associated with eating: weight and appetite changes, binge eating, rumination, and pica. Because changes in appetite and weight are commonly caused by general medical conditions, your first thought should always be to rule out cancer, endocrine disturbances, chronic infections, and other illnesses before assuming that the symptoms are psychiatric. This is especially the case when weight loss or gain is of major proportion and occurs in conjunction with other physical symptoms. Note that in the assessment of an etiological general medical condition in the branch of the decision tree covering the differential diagnosis of weight gain, obesity is listed as one of the possible etiological general medical conditions. This reflects the fact that obesity (defined as a body mass index [BMI] ≥30) by itself is considered not a mental disorder but instead a general medical condition. A BMI of ≥30 would be considered a component of a psychiatric disorder only when it is a consequence of a disturbed eating pattern (such as in Binge-Eating Disorder).

Changes in appetite and weight (in both directions) are also frequently caused by the use of certain drugs of abuse (especially stimulants and cannabis) and certain prescribed medications. In fact, one of the major reasons for noncompliance with many of the psychotropic medications (e.g., selective serotonin reuptake inhibitors, serotonin-norepinephrine reuptake inhibitors, tricyclic antidepressants, lithium, divalproex, monoamine oxidase inhibitors, atypical antipsychotics) is the fear of weight gain that commonly accompanies their use. Attributing changes in weight can be difficult precisely because many of the conditions treated by these psychotropic medications are themselves associated with changes in weight independent of the use of medication. For example, if a depressed patient gains weight while being treated with an antidepressant, this could be a side effect of the antidepressant, a characteristic symptom of the depression, or a desirable treatment effect (e.g., improved appetite in someone previously experiencing loss of appetite).

Because changes in appetite and gains or losses in weight are common in many different psychiatric disorders, they are relatively nonspecific on their own in providing clues to the differential diagnosis. Therefore, you must rely on the temporal relationship with the other presenting symptoms in deciding which is the most appropriate explanation for the change in appetite or weight. For example, is the individual not eating because of a delusion that the food is poisoned (as in Delusional Disorder), because of a feeling of being unworthy or a loss of pleasure in eating (as in Major Depressive Episode), or because of a diminished appetite or being "too busy" (as in Manic Episode)?

In some individuals, weight loss or weight gain is most often associated with a specific presentation of severe body image distortions and/or binge eating. In Anorexia Nervosa, the pathological fear of being (or becoming) fat results in an often dangerously low weight. Some individuals with Anorexia Nervosa engage in binge eating and purging behavior, whereas others achieve low weight exclusively through fasting and excessive exercise. In contrast to those with Anorexia Nervosa, individuals with Bulimia Nervosa have normal or above normal weight. They engage in cycles of binge eating compensated for by the use of inappropriate methods of counteracting the effects of their excessive caloric intake (e.g., self-induced vomiting, misuse of laxatives, fasting, excessive exercise). Individuals with Binge-Eating Disorder, however, engage in regular binge eating (i.e., at least once per week for at least 3 months) without employing any inappropriate compensatory mechanisms to keep from gaining weight. Thus, these individuals are typically overweight. Some individuals have a significant weight loss (or a failure to make expected weight gain) in the absence of a fear of gaining weight or being fat. Instead, their weight loss occurs as a result of lack of interest in eating, avoidance of food based on extreme sensitivity to its sensory characteristics (e.g., appearance, color, texture, temperature, taste), or anticipation of aversive consequences to eating such as choking. Such individuals may be diagnosed with Avoidant/Restrictive Food Intake Disorder.

The decision tree also contains several eating disturbances that occur primarily in infants, young children, or individuals with Intellectual Disability (Intellectual Developmental Disorder). Pica is the developmentally inappropriate and persistent eating of nonnutritive substances (e.g., paint chips, string, dirt, animal droppings). Rumination Disorder is the repeated regurgitation and rechewing of food. The previously discussed category Avoidant/Restrictive Food Intake Disorder is also applicable to infants or children with severe weight loss (or failure of weight gain) that usually results from a combination of a difficult-to-feed child and an inexperienced caretaker.

Clinically significant changes in weight and pathological eating behavior that are not covered so far in the decision tree could occur as a response to a psychosocial stressor, in which case a diagnosis of Adjustment Disorder may be appropriate. Other clinically significant Eating Disorders that do not meet criteria for one of the specific DSM-5 Eating Disorder categories (e.g., recurrent purging without binge eating) would be diagnosed using a residual category, the choice depending on whether the clinician wishes to record the symptomatic presentation on the chart (in which case Other Specified Feeding or Eating Disorder would be used, followed by the specific reason) or not (in which case Unspecified Feeding or Eating Disorder would be used). Finally, it is important to remember that concerns about body appearance, gaining and losing weight, and fad dieting are fairly ubiquitous aspects of life. A diagnosis of Other Specified or Unspecified Feeding or Eating Disorder should be given only if the eating disturbance represents a psychological or biological dysfunction in the individual.

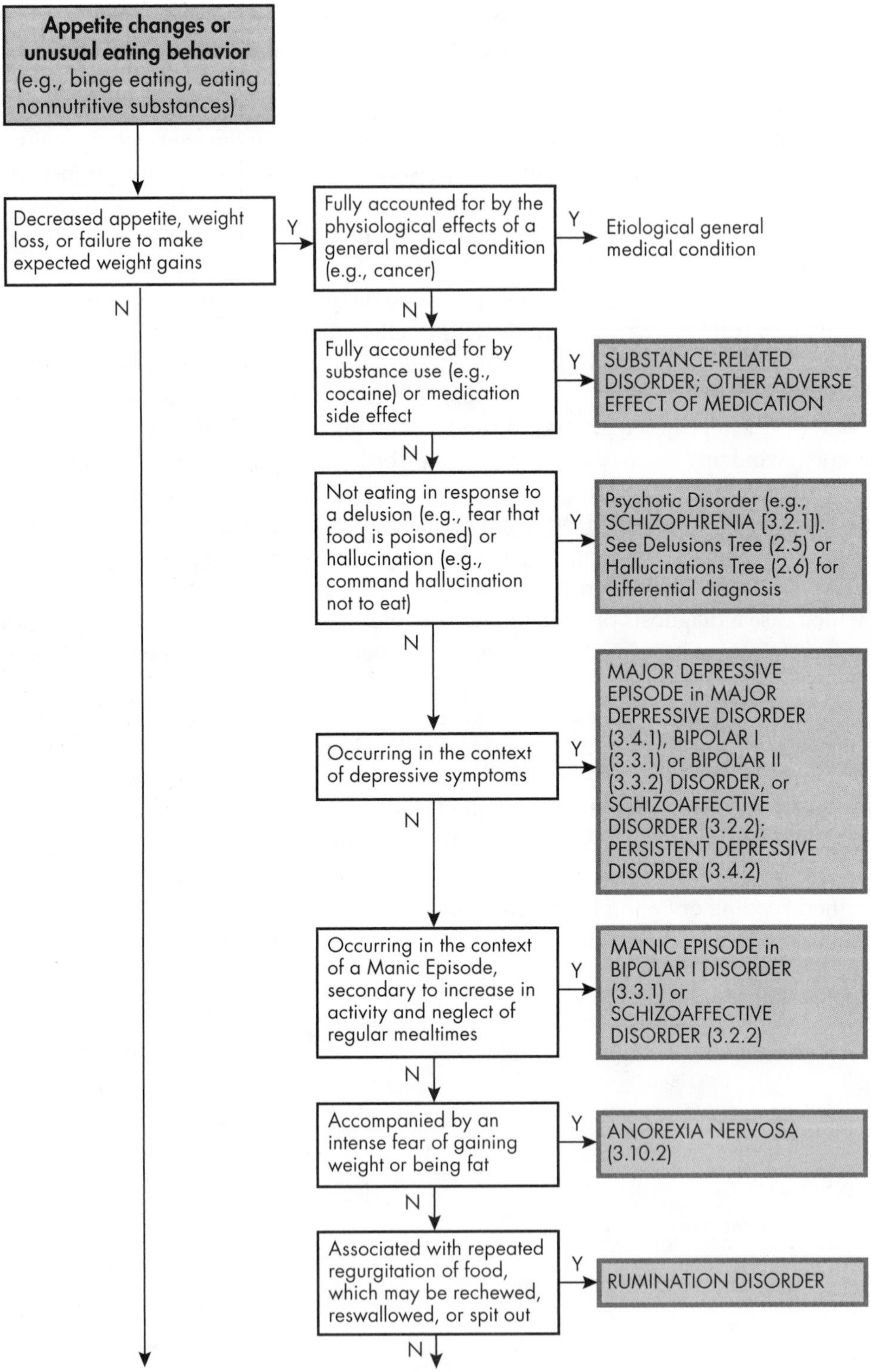
Appetite changes or unusual eating behavior (e.g., binge eating, eating nonnutritive substances)
Decreased appetite, weight loss, or failure to make expected weight gains
Y
Fully accounted for by the physiological effects of a general medical condition (e.g., cancer)
Y
Etiological general medical condition
N
N
Fully accounted for by substance use (e.g., cocaine) or medication side effect
Y
SUBSTANCE-RELATED DISORDER; OTHER ADVERSE EFFECT OF MEDICATION
N
Not eating in response to a delusion (e.g., fear that food is poisoned) or hallucination (e.g., command hallucination not to eat)
Y
Psychotic Disorder (e.g., SCHIZOPHRENIA [3.2.1]). See Delusions Tree (2.5) or Hallucinations Tree (2.6) for differential diagnosis
N
Occurring in the context of depressive symptoms
Y
MAJOR DEPRESSIVE EPISODE in MAJOR DEPRESSIVE DISORDER (3.4.1), BIPOLAR I (3.3.1) or BIPOLAR II (3.3.2) DISORDER, or SCHIZOAFFECTIVE DISORDER (3.2.2); PERSISTENT DEPRESSIVE DISORDER (3.4.2)
N
Occurring in the context of a Manic Episode, secondary to increase in activity and neglect of regular mealtimes
Y
MANIC EPISODE in BIPOLAR I DISORDER (3.3.1) or SCHIZOAFFECTIVE DISORDER (3.2.2)
N
Accompanied by an intense fear of gaining weight or being fat
Y
ANOREXIA NERVOSA (3.10.2)
N
Associated with repeated regurgitation of food, which may be rechewed, reswallowed, or spit out
Y
RUMINATION DISORDER
N

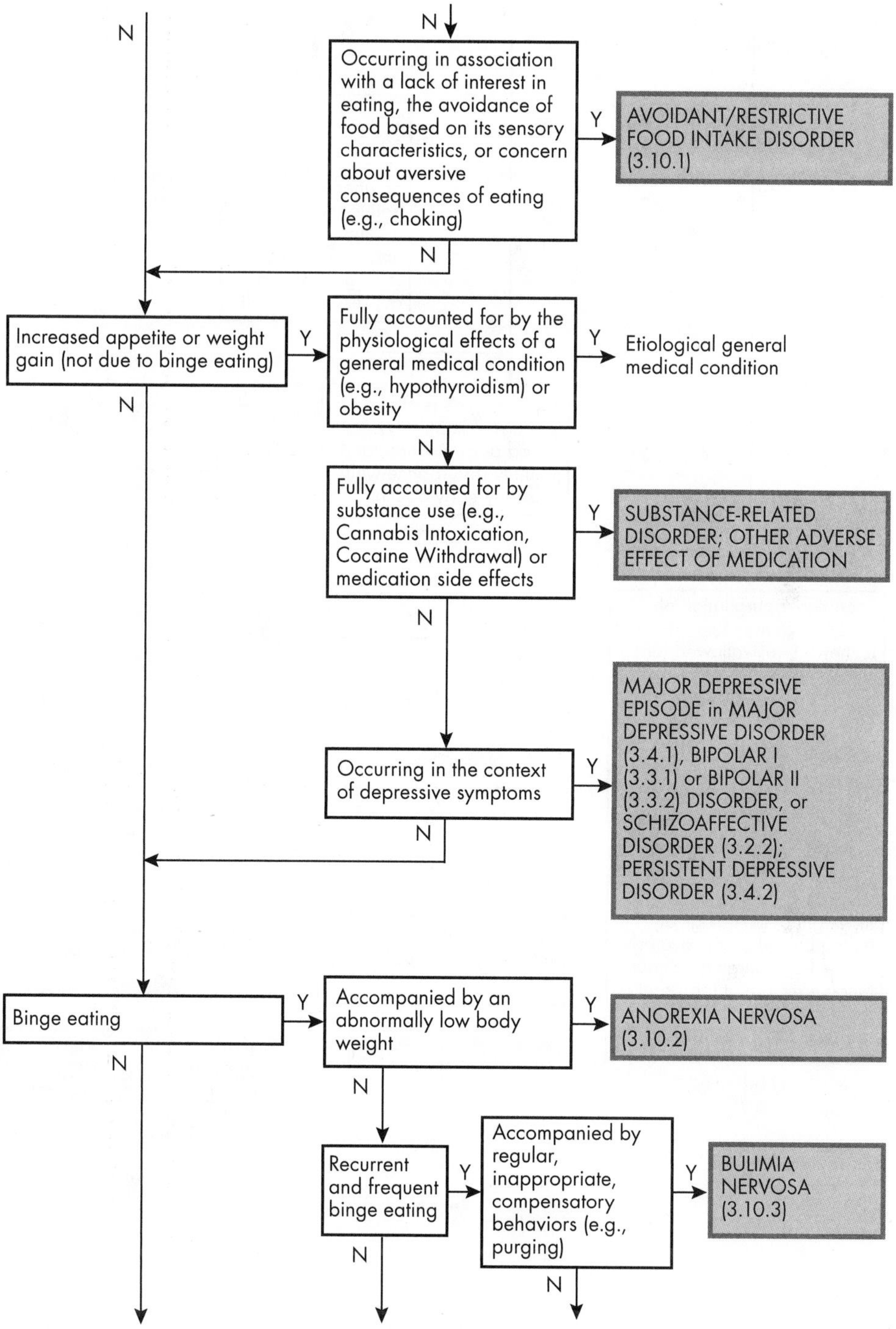
N
N
Occurring in association with a lack of interest in eating, the avoidance of food based on its sensory characteristics, or concern about aversive consequences of eating (e.g., choking)
Y
AVOIDANT/RESTRICTIVE FOOD INTAKE DISORDER (3.10.1)
N
Increased appetite or weight gain (not due to binge eating)
Y
Fully accounted for by the physiological effects of a general medical condition (e.g., hypothyroidism) or obesity
Y
Etiological general medical condition
N
N
Fully accounted for by substance use (e.g., Cannabis Intoxication, Cocaine Withdrawal) or medication side effects
Y
SUBSTANCE-RELATED DISORDER; OTHER ADVERSE EFFECT OF MEDICATION
N
Occurring in the context of depressive symptoms
Y
MAJOR DEPRESSIVE EPISODE in MAJOR DEPRESSIVE DISORDER (3.4.1), BIPOLAR I (3.3.1) or BIPOLAR II (3.3.2) DISORDER, or SCHIZOAFFECTIVE DISORDER (3.2.2); PERSISTENT DEPRESSIVE DISORDER (3.4.2)
N
Binge eating
Y
Accompanied by an abnormally low body weight
Y
ANOREXIA NERVOSA (3.10.2)
N
N
Recurrent and frequent binge eating
Y
Accompanied by regular, inappropriate, compensatory behaviors (e.g., purging)
Y
BULIMIA NERVOSA (3.10.3)
N
N

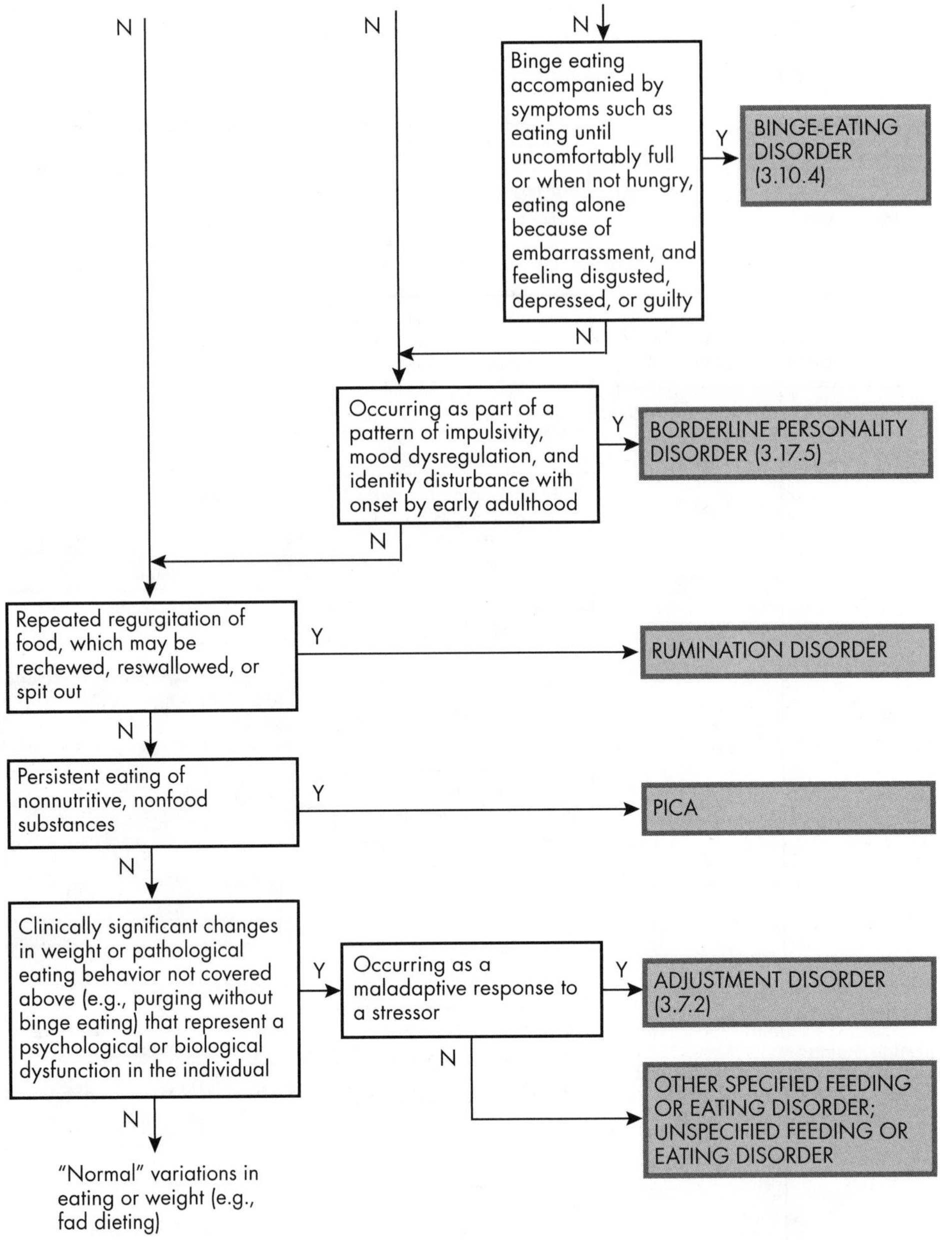
N
N
N
Binge eating accompanied by symptoms such as eating until uncomfortably full or when not hungry, eating alone because of embarrassment, and feeling disgusted, depressed, or guilty
Y
BINGE-EATING DISORDER (3.10.4)
N
Occurring as part of a pattern of impulsivity, mood dysregulation, and identity disturbance with onset by early adulthood
Y
BORDERLINE PERSONALITY DISORDER (3.17.5)
N
Repeated regurgitation of food, which may be rechewed, reswallowed, or spit out
Y
RUMINATION DISORDER
N
Persistent eating of nonnutritive, nonfood substances
Y
PICA
N
Clinically significant changes in weight or pathological eating behavior not covered above (e.g., purging without binge eating) that represent a psychological or biological dysfunction in the individual
Y
Occurring as a maladaptive response to a stressor
Y
ADJUSTMENT DISORDER (3.7.2)
N
OTHER SPECIFIED FEEDING OR EATING DISORDER; UNSPECIFIED FEEDING OR EATING DISORDER
N
"Normal" variations in eating or weight (e.g., fad dieting)

2.19 Decision Tree for Insomnia

Insomnia is defined in DSM-5 as dissatisfaction with sleep quantity or quality with complaints of difficulty initiating or maintaining sleep. Drugs of abuse and many prescribed and over-the-counter medications have insomnia as a significant side effect. For drugs of abuse, typically a diagnosis of Substance Intoxication or Substance Withdrawal will suffice to cover the symptoms of insomnia. A diagnosis of Substance/Medication-Induced Sleep Disorder, Insomnia Type, should be considered only if the insomnia predominates in the clinical picture and is sufficiently severe to warrant clinical attention. A diagnosis of Substance/Medication-Induced Sleep Disorder can also be given for clinically notable insomnia related to medications.

You must then rule out other more specific sleep disorders as the cause of the insomnia because the manifestations of the other sleep disorders can interrupt nighttime sleep. Narcolepsy is characterized by recurrent periods of an irrepressible need for sleep accompanied by cataplexy (i.e., brief periods of sudden bilateral loss of muscle tone precipitated by laughter), hypocretin deficiency (as measured in cerebrospinal fluid), or characteristic polysomnographic findings (i.e., rapid eye movement [REM] sleep latency of 15 minutes or less, or multiple sleep latency test with mean sleep latency of 8 minutes or less and two or more sleep-onset REM periods). DSM-5 includes three distinct disorders under the general rubric of Breathing-Related Sleep Disorders, each of which can cause insomnia because of middle-of-the-night awakenings. Obstructive Sleep Apnea Hypopnea, which is the most common form of Breathing-Related Sleep Disorder, is characterized by repeated episodes of upper airway obstruction during sleep. Central Sleep Apnea is characterized by repeated episodes of apneas and hypopneas during sleep caused by variability in respiratory effort. Sleep-Related Hypoventilation is characterized by episodes of decreased ventilation during sleep associated with elevated CO_2 levels. Non–Rapid Eye Movement Sleep Arousal Disorder is characterized by recurrent episodes of incomplete awakening from sleep, usually during the first third of the night, which can take the form of Sleep Terrors or Sleepwalking. Nightmare Disorder and REM Sleep Behavior Disorder describe problematic phenomena occurring during REM sleep: extended, extremely dysphoric, and well-remembered dreams in the case of Nightmare Disorder, and repeated arousals during REM sleep with vocalizations or complex motor behavior in the case of REM Sleep Behavior Disorder. Restless Legs Syndrome is characterized by recurrent or persistent urges to move the legs in response to unpleasant sensations. Circadian Rhythm Sleep-Wake Disorder is characterized by a mismatch between the individual's schedule and natural sleep-wake patterns. Insomnia that occurs exclusively during, and is better explained by, any of these sleep disorders does not warrant a separate diagnosis of Insomnia Disorder. If the severity of the insomnia exceeds what would be expected from another sleep disorder or occurs at times other than when that sleep disorder is present, a comorbid diagnosis of Insomnia Disorder may be appropriate.

The next step in the assessment is to consider whether the insomnia is actually a symptom of another mental disorder. A number of mental disorders, such as Major Depressive Disorder, may include prominent symptoms of insomnia. If the insomnia is adequately explained by the mental disorder, only the mental disorder is diagnosed and an additional diagnosis of Insomnia Disorder is not made. If, however, the insomnia predominates in the clinical picture and warrants clinical attention, then a comorbid diagnosis of Insomnia Disorder may be appropriate. Similarly, a number of general medical conditions, such as back pain, may significantly disrupt sleep. An additional diagnosis of Insomnia Disorder may also be appropriate in such cases if the insomnia is not adequately explained by the general medical condition.

Some difficulty falling asleep (or maintaining sleep) is to be expected in everyone's life, especially in association with psychosocial stressors and as part of advancing age. Insomnia should be considered as evidence of a mental disorder only if the insomnia is severe, is prolonged, and results in clinically significant distress or impairment.

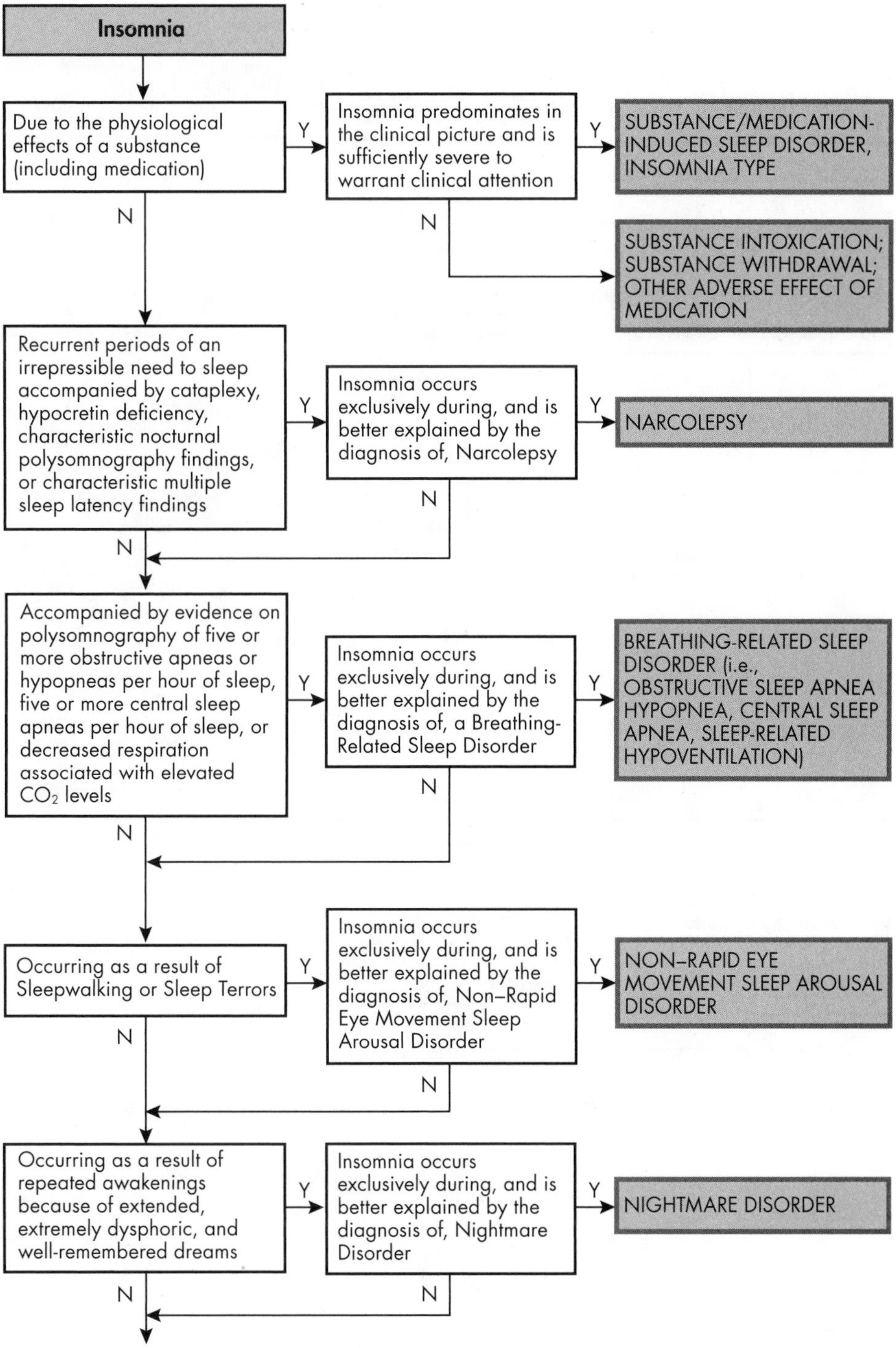
Insomnia
Due to the physiological effects of a substance (including medication)
Y
Insomnia predominates in the clinical picture and is sufficiently severe to warrant clinical attention
Y
SUBSTANCE/MEDICATION-INDUCED SLEEP DISORDER, INSOMNIA TYPE
N
SUBSTANCE INTOXICATION; SUBSTANCE WITHDRAWAL; OTHER ADVERSE EFFECT OF MEDICATION
N
Recurrent periods of an irrepressible need to sleep accompanied by cataplexy, hypocretin deficiency, characteristic nocturnal polysomnography findings, or characteristic multiple sleep latency findings
Y
Insomnia occurs exclusively during, and is better explained by the diagnosis of, Narcolepsy
Y
NARCOLEPSY
N
N
Accompanied by evidence on polysomnography of five or more obstructive apneas or hypopneas per hour of sleep, five or more central sleep apneas per hour of sleep, or decreased respiration associated with elevated CO2 levels
Y
Insomnia occurs exclusively during, and is better explained by the diagnosis of, a Breathing-Related Sleep Disorder
Y
BREATHING-RELATED SLEEP DISORDER (i.e., OBSTRUCTIVE SLEEP APNEA HYPOPNEA, CENTRAL SLEEP APNEA, SLEEP-RELATED HYPOVENTILATION)
N
N
Occurring as a result of Sleepwalking or Sleep Terrors
Y
Insomnia occurs exclusively during, and is better explained by the diagnosis of, Non–Rapid Eye Movement Sleep Arousal Disorder
Y
NON–RAPID EYE MOVEMENT SLEEP AROUSAL DISORDER
N
N
Occurring as a result of repeated awakenings because of extended, extremely dysphoric, and well-remembered dreams
Y
Insomnia occurs exclusively during, and is better explained by the diagnosis of, Nightmare Disorder
Y
NIGHTMARE DISORDER
N
N

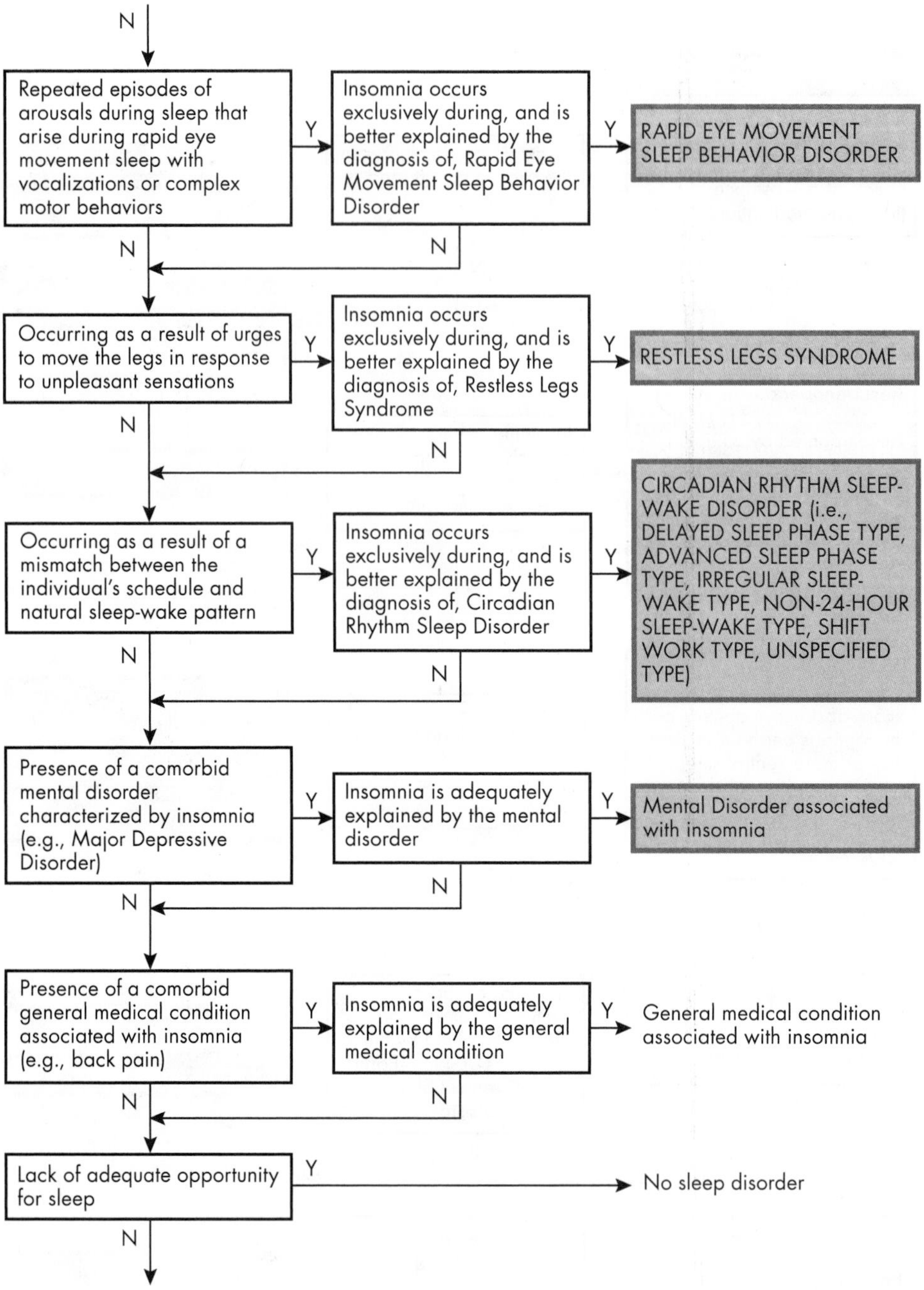
N
Repeated episodes of arousals during sleep that arise during rapid eye movement sleep with vocalizations or complex motor behaviors
Y
Insomnia occurs exclusively during, and is better explained by the diagnosis of, Rapid Eye Movement Sleep Behavior Disorder
Y
RAPID EYE MOVEMENT SLEEP BEHAVIOR DISORDER
N
N
Occurring as a result of urges to move the legs in response to unpleasant sensations
Y
Insomnia occurs exclusively during, and is better explained by the diagnosis of, Restless Legs Syndrome
Y
RESTLESS LEGS SYNDROME
N
N
Occurring as a result of a mismatch between the individual's schedule and natural sleep-wake pattern
Y
Insomnia occurs exclusively during, and is better explained by the diagnosis of, Circadian Rhythm Sleep Disorder
Y
CIRCADIAN RHYTHM SLEEP-WAKE DISORDER (i.e., DELAYED SLEEP PHASE TYPE, ADVANCED SLEEP PHASE TYPE, IRREGULAR SLEEP-WAKE TYPE, NON-24-HOUR SLEEP-WAKE TYPE, SHIFT WORK TYPE, UNSPECIFIED TYPE)
N
N
Presence of a comorbid mental disorder characterized by insomnia (e.g., Major Depressive Disorder)
Y
Insomnia is adequately explained by the mental disorder
Y
Mental Disorder associated with insomnia
N
N
Presence of a comorbid general medical condition associated with insomnia (e.g., back pain)
Y
Insomnia is adequately explained by the general medical condition
Y
General medical condition associated with insomnia
N
N
Lack of adequate opportunity for sleep
Y
No sleep disorder
N

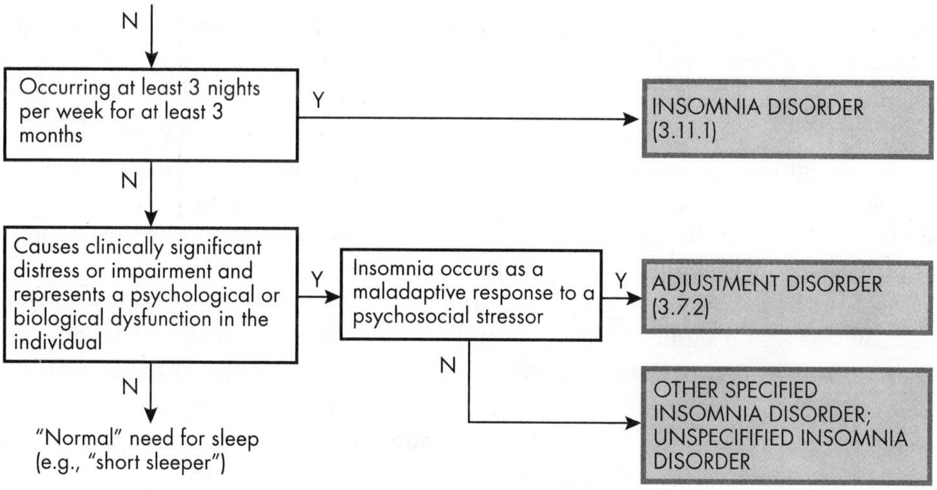
N
Occurring at least 3 nights per week for at least 3 months
Y
INSOMNIA DISORDER (3.11.1)
N
Causes clinically significant distress or impairment and represents a psychological or biological dysfunction in the individual
Y
Insomnia occurs as a maladaptive response to a psychosocial stressor
Y
ADJUSTMENT DISORDER (3.7.2)
N
OTHER SPECIFIED INSOMNIA DISORDER; UNSPECIFIED INSOMNIA DISORDER
N
"Normal" need for sleep (e.g., "short sleeper")

2.20 Decision Tree for Hypersomnolence

Hypersomnolence is a broad diagnostic term and includes symptoms of excessive quantity of sleep (e.g., extended nighttime sleep or involuntary daytime naps), deteriorated quality of wakefulness (e.g., difficulty awakening or inability to remain awake when required), and sleep inertia (i.e., a period of impaired performance and reduced vigilance upon awakening). A diagnosis of Hypersomnolence Disorder should be considered only if the person has been regularly getting adequate amounts of sleep—individuals would not qualify for this diagnosis if they are sleep deprived either because of insomnia or to accommodate their overscheduled lives.

Drugs of abuse and many prescribed and over-the-counter medications have daytime drowsiness as a significant side effect. For drugs of abuse, typically a diagnosis of Substance Intoxication or Substance Withdrawal will suffice to cover the hypersomnolence. A diagnosis of Substance-Induced Sleep Disorder, Daytime Sleepiness Type, should be considered only if the hypersomnolence predominates in the clinical picture and is sufficiently severe to warrant clinical attention. A diagnosis of Medication-Induced Sleep Disorder can also be given for clinically notable hypersomnolence related to medications.

You must then rule out other specific sleep disorders as the cause of the hypersomnolence, given that daytime sleepiness is a characteristic feature of some specific sleep disorders (e.g., Narcolepsy) or might be a consequence of the disturbance in nighttime sleep caused by the other sleep disorder (e.g., Nightmare Disorder). Narcolepsy is characterized by recurrent periods of an irrepressible need for sleep accompanied by cataplexy (i.e., brief periods of sudden bilateral loss of muscle tone precipitated by laughter), hypocretin deficiency (as measured in cerebrospinal fluid), or characteristic polysomnographic findings (i.e., rapid eye movement [REM] sleep latency of 15 minutes or less, or multiple sleep latency test with mean sleep latency of 8 minutes or less and two or more sleep-onset REM periods). DSM-5 includes three distinct disorders under the general rubric of Breathing-Related Sleep Disorders, each of which can cause daytime fatigue. Obstructive Sleep Apnea Hypopnea, which is the most common form of Breathing-Related Sleep Disorder, is characterized by repeated episodes of upper airway obstruction during sleep. Central Sleep Apnea is characterized by repeated episodes of apneas and hypopneas during sleep caused by variability in respiratory effort. Sleep-Related Hypoventilation is characterized by episodes of decreased ventilation during sleep associated with elevated CO_2 levels. Non–Rapid Eye Movement Sleep Arousal Disorder is characterized by recurrent episodes of incomplete awakening from sleep, usually during the first third of the night, which can take the form of Sleep Terrors or Sleepwalking. Nightmare Disorder and REM Sleep Behavior Disorder describe problematic phenomena occurring during REM sleep: extended extremely dysphoric and well-remembered dreams in the case of Nightmare Disorder, and repeated arousals during REM sleep with vocalizations or complex motor behavior in the case of REM Sleep Behavior Disorder. Restless Legs Syndrome is characterized by recurrent or persistent urges to move the legs in response to unpleasant sensations. Circadian Rhythm Sleep-Wake Disorder is characterized by a mismatch between the individual's schedule and natural sleep-wake patterns. Finally, Insomnia Disorder is characterized by a predominant complaint of dissatisfaction with sleep quality or quantity, associated with difficulty falling asleep, maintaining sleep, or early-morning awakening.

Hypersomnolence that occurs exclusively during, and is better explained by, any of these sleep disorders does not warrant a separate diagnosis of Hypersomnolence Disorder. If the severity of the hypersomnolence exceeds what would be expected from another sleep disorder or occurs at times other than when that sleep disorder is present, a comorbid diagnosis of Hypersomnolence Disorder may be appropriate.

The next step in the assessment is to consider whether the hypersomnolence is actually a symptom of another mental disorder. A number of mental disorders may include prominent symptoms of hypersomnolence, especially in Major Depressive Episodes With Atypical Features, as seen in Major Depressive Disorder, Bipolar I Disorder, and Bipolar II Disorder. If the daytime fatigue is adequately explained by the mental disorder, only the mental disorder is diagnosed and an additional diagnosis of Hypersomnolence Disorder is not made. If, however, the hypersomnolence predominates in the clinical picture and warrants clinical attention, then a comorbid diagnosis of Hypersomnolence Disorder may be appropriate. Similarly, a number of general medical conditions, such as mononucleosis, may be characterized by daytime fatigue. An additional diagnosis of Hypersomnolence Disorder may also be appropriate in such cases if the degree of hypersomnolence is not adequately explained by the general medical condition.

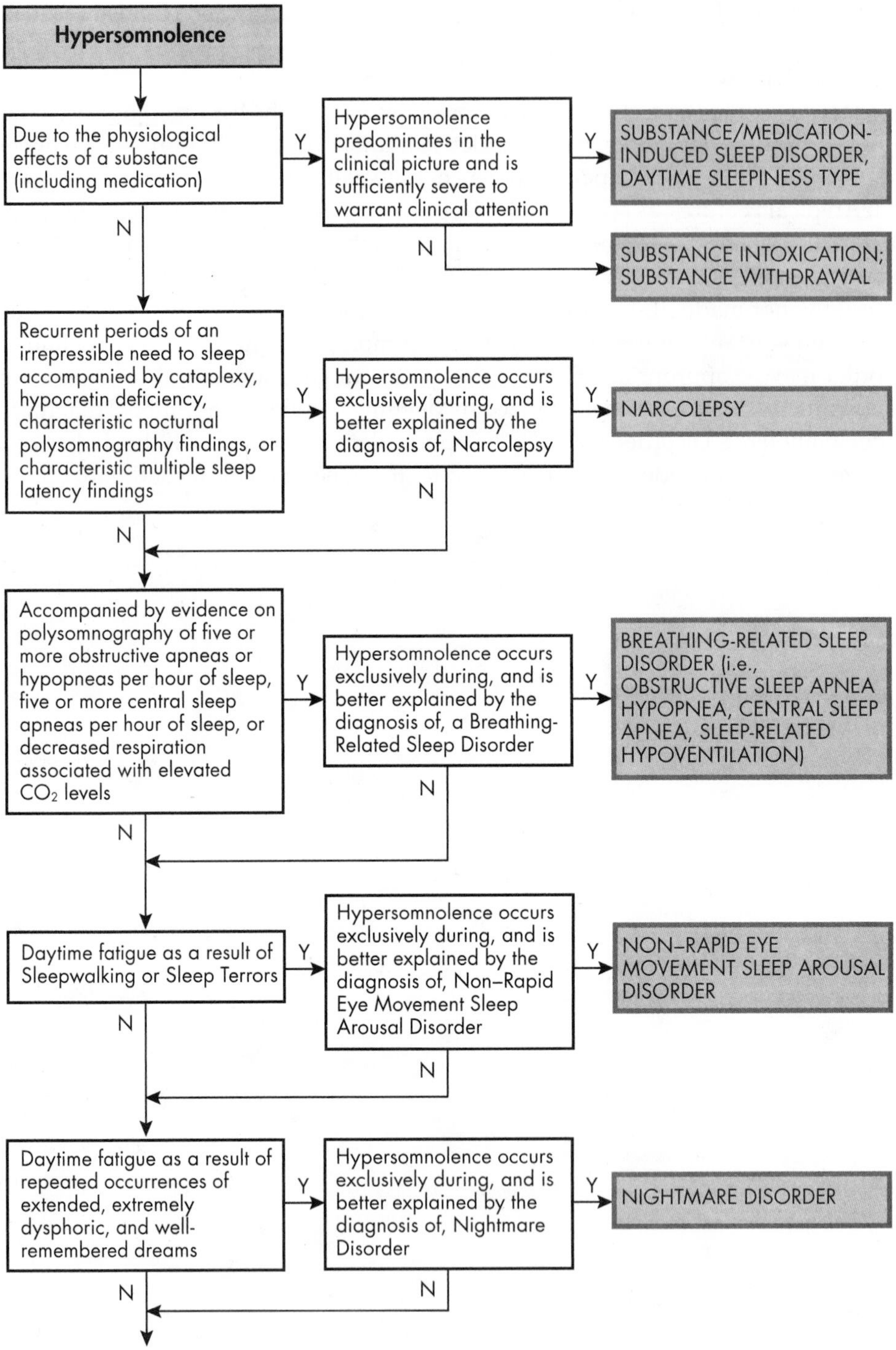
Hypersomnolence
Due to the physiological effects of a substance (including medication)
Y
Hypersomnolence predominates in the clinical picture and is sufficiently severe to warrant clinical attention
Y
SUBSTANCE/MEDICATION-INDUCED SLEEP DISORDER, DAYTIME SLEEPINESS TYPE
N
SUBSTANCE INTOXICATION; SUBSTANCE WITHDRAWAL
N
Recurrent periods of an irrepressible need to sleep accompanied by cataplexy, hypocretin deficiency, characteristic nocturnal polysomnography findings, or characteristic multiple sleep latency findings
Y
Hypersomnolence occurs exclusively during, and is better explained by the diagnosis of, Narcolepsy
Y
NARCOLEPSY
N
N
Accompanied by evidence on polysomnography of five or more obstructive apneas or hypopneas per hour of sleep, five or more central sleep apneas per hour of sleep, or decreased respiration associated with elevated CO2 levels
Y
Hypersomnolence occurs exclusively during, and is better explained by the diagnosis of, a Breathing-Related Sleep Disorder
Y
BREATHING-RELATED SLEEP DISORDER (i.e., OBSTRUCTIVE SLEEP APNEA HYPOPNEA, CENTRAL SLEEP APNEA, SLEEP-RELATED HYPOVENTILATION)
N
N
Daytime fatigue as a result of Sleepwalking or Sleep Terrors
Y
Hypersomnolence occurs exclusively during, and is better explained by the diagnosis of, Non–Rapid Eye Movement Sleep Arousal Disorder
Y
NON–RAPID EYE MOVEMENT SLEEP AROUSAL DISORDER
N
N
Daytime fatigue as a result of repeated occurrences of extended, extremely dysphoric, and well-remembered dreams
Y
Hypersomnolence occurs exclusively during, and is better explained by the diagnosis of, Nightmare Disorder
Y
NIGHTMARE DISORDER
N
N

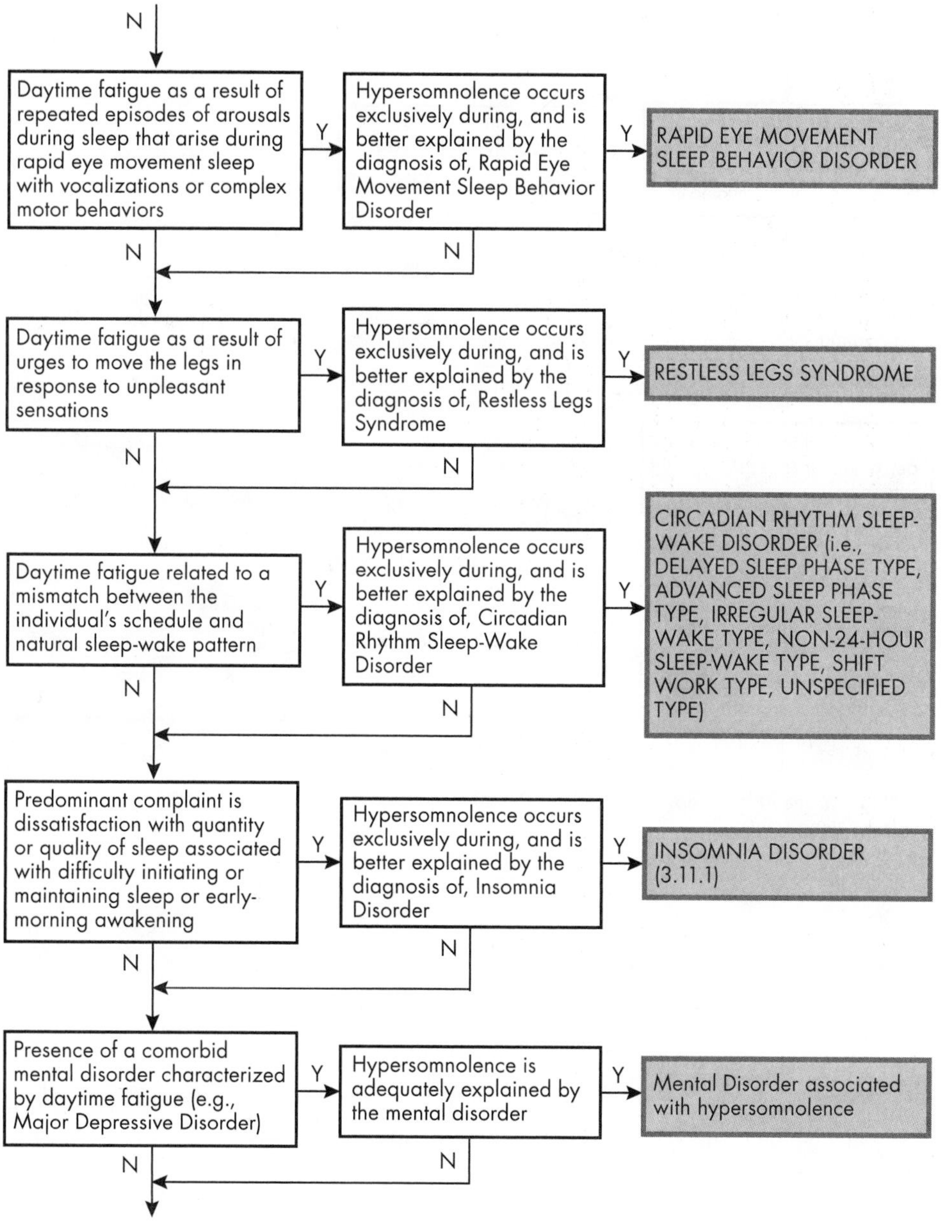
N
Daytime fatigue as a result of repeated episodes of arousals during sleep that arise during rapid eye movement sleep with vocalizations or complex motor behaviors
Y
Hypersomnolence occurs exclusively during, and is better explained by the diagnosis of, Rapid Eye Movement Sleep Behavior Disorder
Y
RAPID EYE MOVEMENT SLEEP BEHAVIOR DISORDER
N
N
Daytime fatigue as a result of urges to move the legs in response to unpleasant sensations
Y
Hypersomnolence occurs exclusively during, and is better explained by the diagnosis of, Restless Legs Syndrome
Y
RESTLESS LEGS SYNDROME
N
N
Daytime fatigue related to a mismatch between the individual's schedule and natural sleep-wake pattern
Y
Hypersomnolence occurs exclusively during, and is better explained by the diagnosis of, Circadian Rhythm Sleep-Wake Disorder
Y
CIRCADIAN RHYTHM SLEEP-WAKE DISORDER (i.e., DELAYED SLEEP PHASE TYPE, ADVANCED SLEEP PHASE TYPE, IRREGULAR SLEEP-WAKE TYPE, NON-24-HOUR SLEEP-WAKE TYPE, SHIFT WORK TYPE, UNSPECIFIED TYPE)
N
N
Predominant complaint is dissatisfaction with quantity or quality of sleep associated with difficulty initiating or maintaining sleep or early-morning awakening
Y
Hypersomnolence occurs exclusively during, and is better explained by the diagnosis of, Insomnia Disorder
Y
INSOMNIA DISORDER (3.11.1)
N
N
Presence of a comorbid mental disorder characterized by daytime fatigue (e.g., Major Depressive Disorder)
Y
Hypersomnolence is adequately explained by the mental disorder
Y
Mental Disorder associated with hypersomnolence
N
N

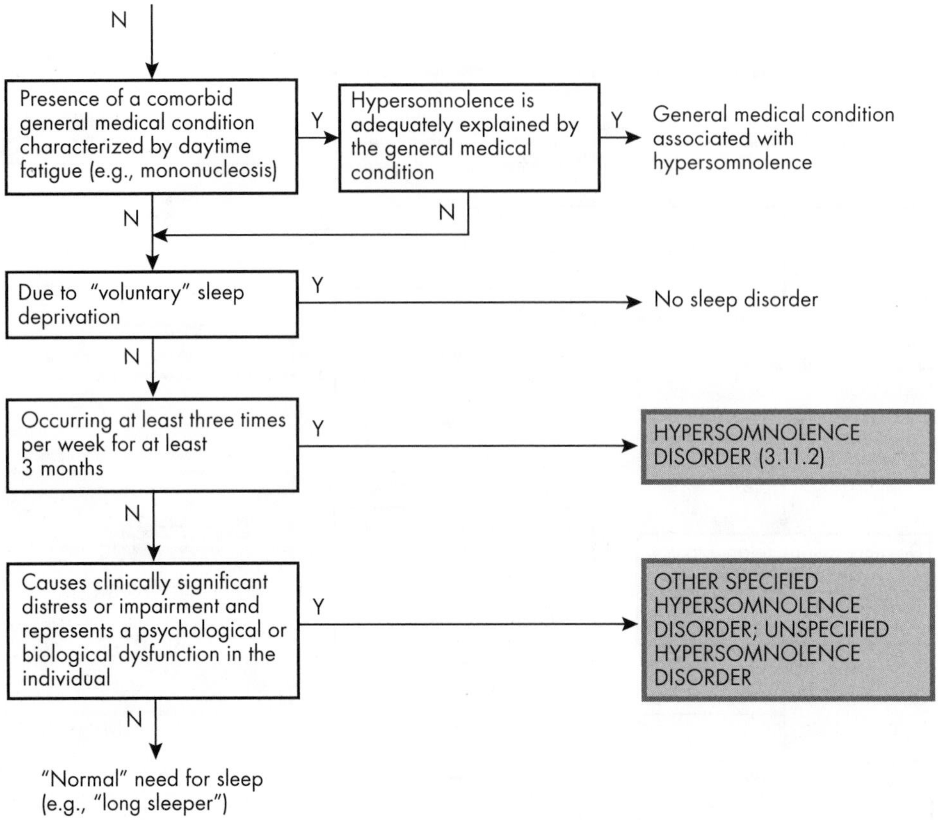
N
Presence of a comorbid general medical condition characterized by daytime fatigue (e.g., mononucleosis)
Y
Hypersomnolence is adequately explained by the general medical condition
Y
General medical condition associated with hypersomnolence
N
N
Due to "voluntary" sleep deprivation
Y
No sleep disorder
N
Occurring at least three times per week for at least 3 months
Y
HYPERSOMNOLENCE DISORDER (3.11.2)
N
Causes clinically significant distress or impairment and represents a psychological or biological dysfunction in the individual
Y
OTHER SPECIFIED HYPERSOMNOLENCE DISORDER; UNSPECIFIED HYPERSOMNOLENCE DISORDER
N
"Normal" need for sleep (e.g., "long sleeper")

2.21 Decision Tree for Sexual Dysfunction in a Female

The major difficulty in evaluating sexual dysfunctions in both women and men is that there are no accepted guidelines for determining what is "normal" sexual functioning. The threshold for normal sexual functioning varies with the woman's age and prior sexual experience, the availability and novelty of partners, and the expectations and standards characteristic of the woman's cultural, ethnic, or religious group. Successful arousal and orgasm require a level of sexual stimulation that is adequate in focus, intensity, and duration. A diagnosis of Female Sexual Interest/Arousal Disorder or Female Orgasmic Disorder therefore requires a clinical judgment that the woman has experienced adequate stimulation. Moreover, occasional sexual dysfunction is an inherent part of human sexuality and is not indicative of a disorder unless it is persistent (i.e., lasting for at least 6 months) or recurrent and results in marked distress or interpersonal difficulty.

Once the clinical judgment has been made that the sexual dysfunction is clinically significant, the next task is to determine its underlying etiology. The possible etiologies include psychological factors, general medical conditions, the side effects of many prescribed medications, and the consequence of drug abuse. This evaluation can be difficult because very often more than one etiology contributes to the sexual dysfunction. Before deciding that a sexual dysfunction is mediated entirely by psychological factors, you need to consider the possible contribution of a general medical condition or substance (including medication side effects), especially because these etiologies often have specific treatment implications (e.g., discontinuation of the offending medication). Also, you need to remember that the identification of a specific etiological general medical condition, medication, or drug of abuse does not negate the important contribution of psychological factors to the etiology of the sexual dysfunction.

Sexual problems are also commonly associated with a number of mental disorders (e.g., Depressive Disorders, Anxiety Disorders, Schizophrenia Spectrum and Other Psychotic Disorders). An additional diagnosis of a sexual dysfunction is not given if the sexual problems are better explained by the mental disorder. For example, low sexual desire occurring only during a Major Depressive Episode would not justify a separate diagnosis of Female Sexual Interest/Arousal Disorder. Both diagnoses can be given only if the low sexual desire is judged to be independent of the depressive disorder (i.e., it precedes the onset of the Major Depressive Episode or persists long after the depression has remitted). Similarly, sexual dysfunction that is better explained as a consequence of severe relationship distress would be diagnosed as a relational problem rather than a sexual dysfunction unless evidence demonstrated that the sexual dysfunction occurred independently of the relational problem.

After substances, general medical conditions, and relationship distress have been considered and ruled out, the focus then goes to the primary sexual dysfunctions themselves. In DSM-5, the female version of the DSM-IV-TR category Hypoactive Sexual Desire Disorder and the DSM-IV-TR category Female Sexual Arousal Disorder have been combined into a single diagnostic category called Female Sexual Interest/Arousal Disorder, reflecting evidence that sexual desire and sexual arousal are often not separable concepts in woman. Thus, Female Sexual Interest/Arousal Disorder covers a wide variety of problems, including reduced interest in sexual activity, reduced frequency of erotic thoughts or fantasies, reduced frequency of initiation of sexual activity, reduced sexual excitement or pleasure during sexual activity, reduced interest or arousal in response to erotic cues, and reduced genital and nongenital sensations during sexual activity. Female Orgasmic Disorder includes marked delay in achieving orgasm, marked infrequency or absence of orgasm, or markedly reduced intensity of orgasmic sensations. The DSM-5 category Genito-Pelvic Pain/Penetration Disorder combines two DSM-IV-TR categories (i.e., Vaginismus and Dyspareunia) and includes difficulties with having vaginal intercourse or penetration; marked vulvovaginal or pelvic pain during intercourse or penetration attempts; marked fear or anxiety about vulvovaginal or pelvic pain in anticipation of, during, or as a result of vaginal penetration; or marked tensing or tightening of the pelvic floor muscles during attempted vaginal penetration.

If a sexual dysfunction does not meet criteria for one of the sexual dysfunctions described above (perhaps because of inadequate frequency or duration) or occurs as part of a maladaptive response to a psychosocial stressor, a diagnosis of an Adjustment Disorder may be appropriate.

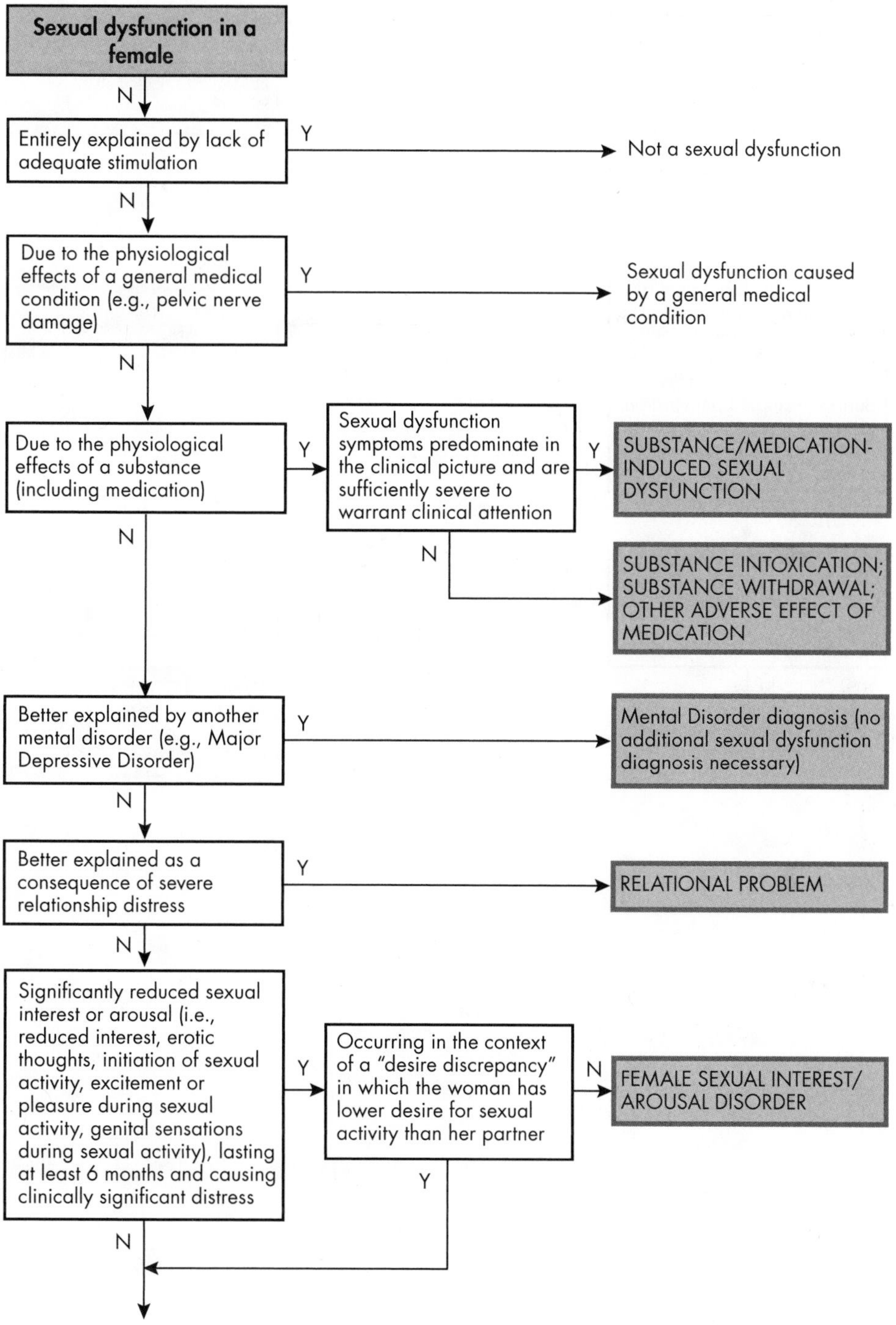
Sexual dysfunction in a female
N
Entirely explained by lack of adequate stimulation
Y
Not a sexual dysfunction
N
Due to the physiological effects of a general medical condition (e.g., pelvic nerve damage)
Y
Sexual dysfunction caused by a general medical condition
N
Due to the physiological effects of a substance (including medication)
Y
Sexual dysfunction symptoms predominate in the clinical picture and are sufficiently severe to warrant clinical attention
Y
SUBSTANCE/MEDICATION-INDUCED SEXUAL DYSFUNCTION
N
SUBSTANCE INTOXICATION; SUBSTANCE WITHDRAWAL; OTHER ADVERSE EFFECT OF MEDICATION
N
Better explained by another mental disorder (e.g., Major Depressive Disorder)
Y
Mental Disorder diagnosis (no additional sexual dysfunction diagnosis necessary)
N
Better explained as a consequence of severe relationship distress
Y
RELATIONAL PROBLEM
N
Significantly reduced sexual interest or arousal (i.e., reduced interest, erotic thoughts, initiation of sexual activity, excitement or pleasure during sexual activity, genital sensations during sexual activity), lasting at least 6 months and causing clinically significant distress
Y
Occurring in the context of a "desire discrepancy" in which the woman has lower desire for sexual activity than her partner
N
FEMALE SEXUAL INTEREST/ AROUSAL DISORDER
Y
N

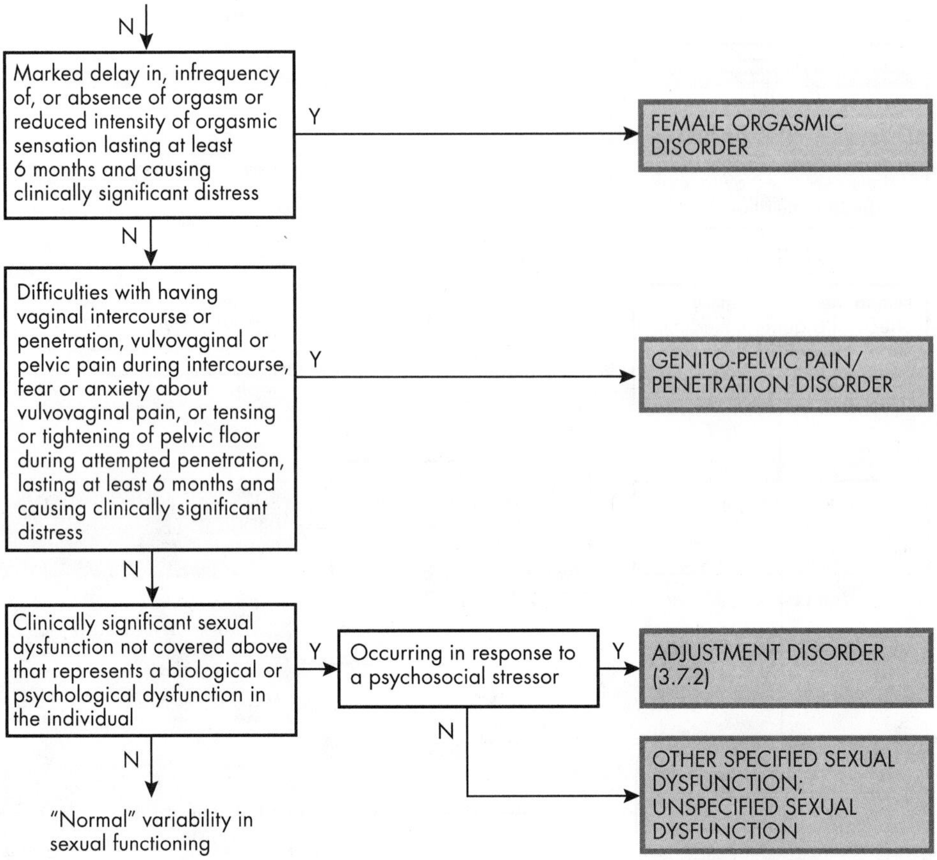
N
Marked delay in, infrequency of, or absence of orgasm or reduced intensity of orgasmic sensation lasting at least 6 months and causing clinically significant distress
Y
FEMALE ORGASMIC DISORDER
N
Difficulties with having vaginal intercourse or penetration, vulvovaginal or pelvic pain during intercourse, fear or anxiety about vulvovaginal pain, or tensing or tightening of pelvic floor during attempted penetration, lasting at least 6 months and causing clinically significant distress
Y
GENITO-PELVIC PAIN/ PENETRATION DISORDER
N
Clinically significant sexual dysfunction not covered above that represents a biological or psychological dysfunction in the individual
Y
Occurring in response to a psychosocial stressor
Y
ADJUSTMENT DISORDER (3.7.2)
N
OTHER SPECIFIED SEXUAL DYSFUNCTION; UNSPECIFIED SEXUAL DYSFUNCTION
N
"Normal" variability in sexual functioning

2.22 Decision Tree for Sexual Dysfunction in a Male

The major difficulty in evaluating sexual dysfunctions in both men and women is that there are no accepted guidelines for determining what is "normal" sexual functioning. The threshold for normal sexual functioning varies with the man's age and prior sexual experience, the availability and novelty of partners, and the expectations and standards characteristic of the man's cultural, ethnic, or religious group. Successful arousal and orgasm require a level of sexual stimulation that is adequate in focus, intensity, and duration. A diagnosis of Erectile Disorder or Delayed Ejaculation therefore requires a clinical judgment that the man has experienced adequate stimulation. Moreover, occasional sexual dysfunction is an inherent part of human sexuality and is not indicative of a disorder unless it is persistent (i.e., lasting for at least 6 months) or recurrent and results in marked distress or interpersonal difficulty.

Once the clinical judgment has been made that the sexual dysfunction is clinically significant, the next task is to determine its underlying etiology. The possible etiologies include psychological factors, general medical conditions, the side effects of many prescribed medications, and the consequence of drug abuse. This evaluation can be difficult because very often more than one etiology contributes to the sexual dysfunction. For example, it is not uncommon for someone who develops mild erectile dysfunction as a result of a general medical condition (e.g., vascular problems) to develop other sexual dysfunctions (e.g., low desire) as a psychological consequence. Before deciding that any sexual dysfunction is mediated strictly by psychological factors, you need to consider the possible contribution of a general medical condition or substance (including medication side effects), especially because these etiologies often have specific treatment implications (e.g., discontinuation of the offending medication). Also, you need to remember that the identification of a specific etiological general medical condition, medication, or drug of abuse does not negate the important contribution of psychological factors to the etiology of the dysfunction.

Sexual problems are also commonly associated with a number of mental disorders (e.g., Depressive Disorders, Anxiety Disorders, Schizophrenia Spectrum and Other Psychotic Disorders). An additional diagnosis of a sexual dysfunction is not given if the sexual problems are better explained by the mental disorder. For example, low sexual desire occurring only during a Major Depressive Episode would not warrant a separate diagnosis of Male Hypoactive Sexual Desire Disorder. Both diagnoses can be given only if the low sexual desire is judged to be independent of the depressive disorder (i.e., it precedes the onset of the Major Depressive Episode or persists long after the depression has remitted). Similarly, sexual dysfunction that is better explained as a consequence of severe relationship distress would be diagnosed as a relational problem rather than a sexual dysfunction unless evidence demonstrated that the sexual dysfunction occurred independently of the relational problem.

The primary sexual dysfunctions of males are organized based on when during the sexual response cycle the problem occurs. Male Hypoactive Sexual Desire Disorder is related to the initial phase, sexual desire. Erectile Disorder is related to the second phase, sexual arousal. Delayed Ejaculation and Premature (Early) Ejaculation are for problems that occur in the third phase, orgasm. Not infrequently, problems occur in more than one phase of the sexual response cycle. Because the phases of the sexual response cycle occur in sequence, successful functioning in one phase generally requires successful functioning in the previous phases (e.g., orgasm requires some level of arousal, which requires some level of desire). However, anticipation of the recurrence of problems in a later phase (e.g., difficulty ejaculating) often leads to problems in an earlier phase (e.g., consequent erectile dysfunction or low sexual desire).

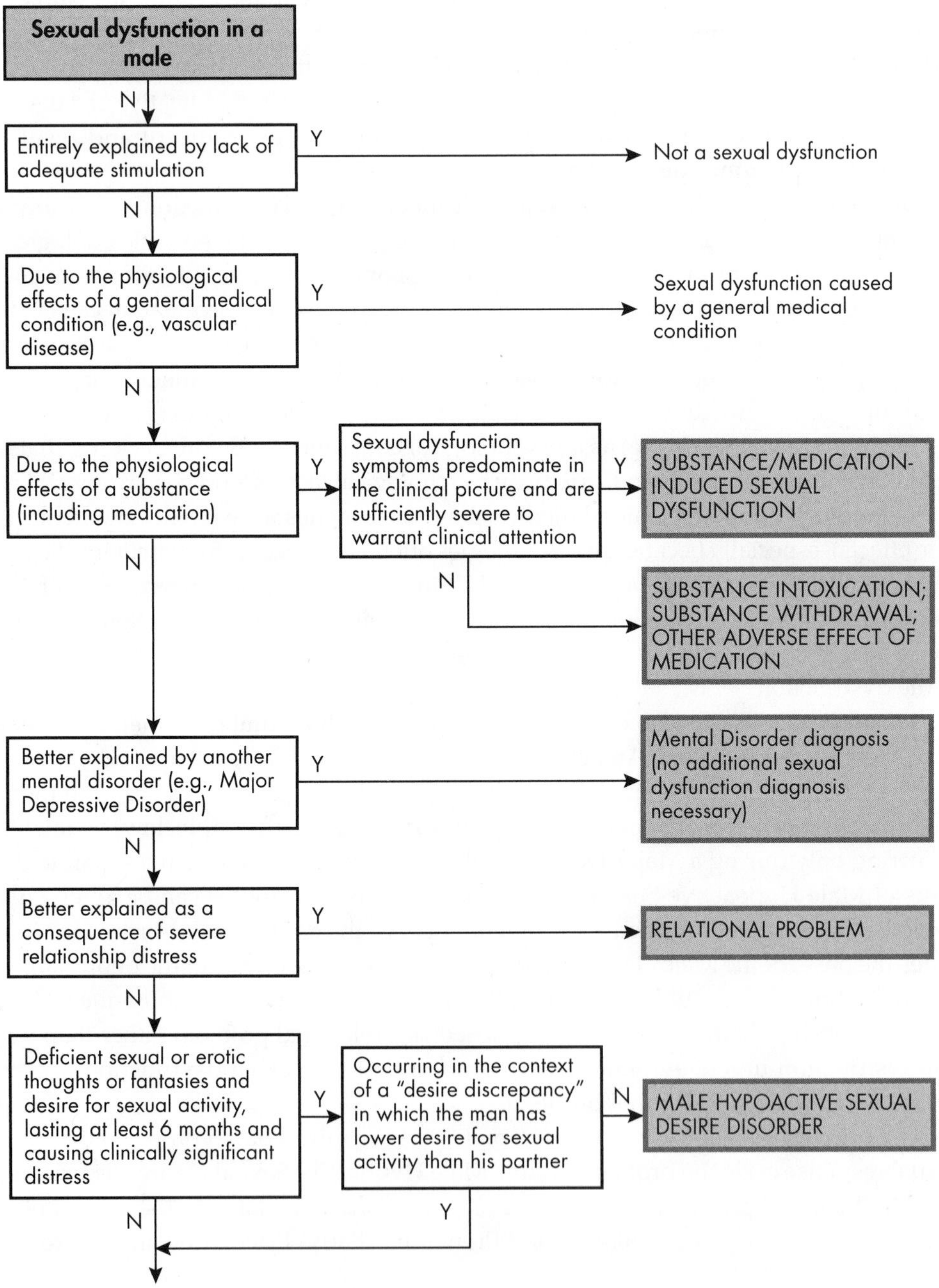

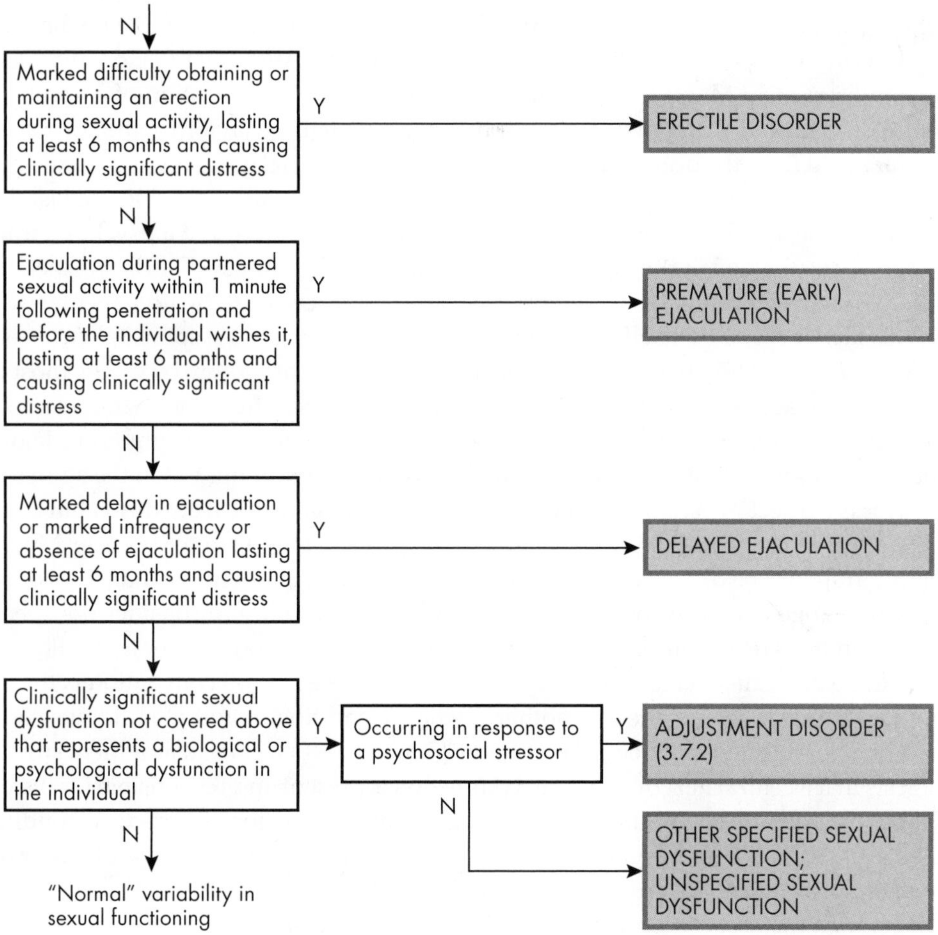
N
Marked difficulty obtaining or maintaining an erection during sexual activity, lasting at least 6 months and causing clinically significant distress
Y
ERECTILE DISORDER
N
Ejaculation during partnered sexual activity within 1 minute following penetration and before the individual wishes it, lasting at least 6 months and causing clinically significant distress
Y
PREMATURE (EARLY) EJACULATION
N
Marked delay in ejaculation or marked infrequency or absence of ejaculation lasting at least 6 months and causing clinically significant distress
Y
DELAYED EJACULATION
N
Clinically significant sexual dysfunction not covered above that represents a biological or psychological dysfunction in the individual
Y
Occurring in response to a psychosocial stressor
Y
ADJUSTMENT DISORDER (3.7.2)
N
OTHER SPECIFIED SEXUAL DYSFUNCTION; UNSPECIFIED SEXUAL DYSFUNCTION
N
"Normal" variability in sexual functioning

2.23 Decision Tree for Aggressive Behavior

Although aggressive behavior is a defining feature of only a handful of DSM-5 disorders (i.e., Intermittent Explosive Disorder, Conduct Disorder, Antisocial Personality Disorder, and Disruptive Mood Dysregulation Disorder), it is a complication of a number of mental disorders. It is important to note that most violent behavior occurs for reasons very far afield from the domain of mental illness (e.g., material gain, status, sadistic pleasure, revenge, furthering a political or religious cause). This is reflected in the last decision in the tree, in which aggressive behavior that does not represent a psychological or biological dysfunction in the individual is considered to be nonpsychiatric antisocial behavior. Moreover, even when the aggressive behavior is associated with a mental disorder, this fact does not by itself absolve the individual of criminal responsibility.

Among the DSM-5 disorders, the Substance-Related Disorders are by far the most frequent cause of aggressive behavior. Aggression can also result from the cognitive impairment and reduction in impulse control that is characteristic of Delirium and Major or Mild Neurocognitive Disorder Due to Another Medical Condition. When the aggressive behavior is a direct physiological consequence of a general medical condition but occurs in the absence of cognitive impairment, Personality Change Due to Another Medical Condition should be diagnosed. One issue that sometimes arises in the diagnosis of Personality Change Due to Another Medical Condition is whether to consider nonspecific medical findings (e.g., neurological soft signs, diffuse slowing on electroencephalogram) as evidence of a causative general medical condition. The DSM-5 convention is to diagnose Personality Change Due to Another Medical Condition only if the findings constitute a diagnosable general medical condition. However, when clinical judgment strongly suggests that a central nervous system dysfunction is present and responsible for the personality change but no specific diagnosis can be made, the general medical condition called Unspecified Condition of Brain can be indicated as the causative disorder and coded as an additional disorder (ICD-9-CM: 348.9, ICD-10-CM: G93.9).

Although the association is much less prominent, episodes of aggressive behavior may occur at somewhat elevated rates in individuals with Schizophrenia, other Psychotic Disorder, and Bipolar Disorder. A long-standing pattern of aggressive behavior suggests that the behavior is part of a Personality Disorder (e.g., Antisocial Personality Disorder, Borderline Personality Disorder). Aggressive behavior in children can occur in the context of a number of disorders. When it occurs as part of a pattern of antisocial behavior in a child, the diagnosis of Conduct Disorder applies. If the aggressive behavior occurs in the context of severe temper outbursts that are grossly out of proportion in intensity or duration to the situation or provocation, with persistent anger and irritability between the outbursts, the new DSM-5 diagnosis Disruptive Mood Dysregulation Disorder should be considered. Much less commonly, aggressive behavior can be associated with other childhood disorders, including Oppositional Defiant Disorder, Attention-Deficit/Hyperactivity Disorder, Separation Anxiety Disorder, Autism Spectrum Disorder, and Intellectual Disability (Intellectual Developmental Disorder).

Recurrent episodes of aggressive behavior (i.e., verbal aggression or physical aggression against people, animals, or property) that is not accounted for by any other mental disorder (including a Personality Disorder) may qualify the individual for a diagnosis of Intermittent Explosive Disorder if the minimum requirements are met for the frequency of outbursts (twice weekly for 3 months for verbal or physical aggression that does not result in injury or destruction of property, or alternatively three outbursts in a 12-month period resulting in injury or damage to property).

Aggressive behavior can also occur in response to a stressor. If the stressor is of a traumatic nature, the aggressive behavior might be part of the syndrome of Posttraumatic Stress Disorder (or Acute Stress Disorder if the duration is less than 1 month). Otherwise, aggressive behavior can be a manifestation of an Adjustment Disorder.

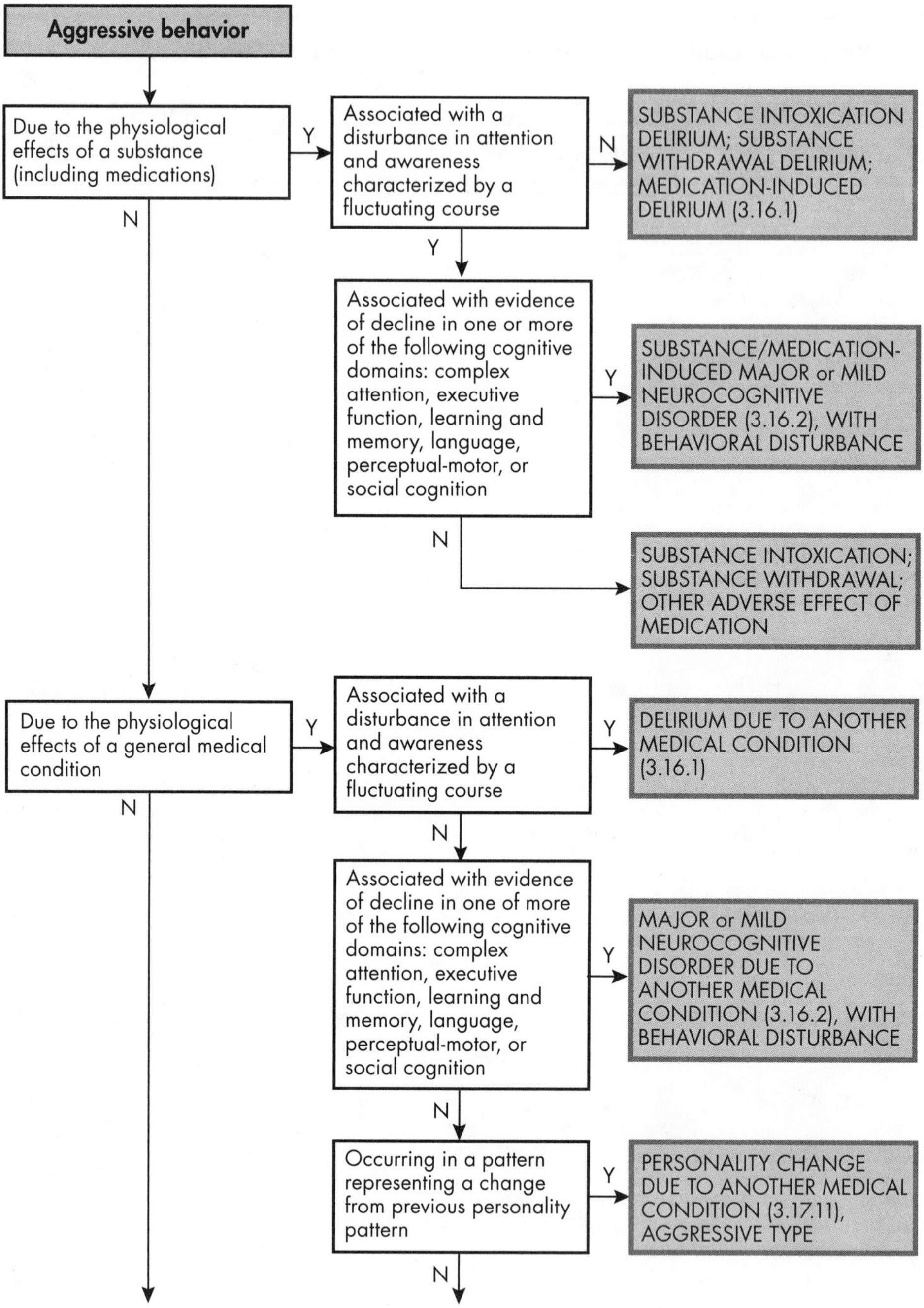
Aggressive behavior
Due to the physiological effects of a substance (including medications)
Y
Associated with a disturbance in attention and awareness characterized by a fluctuating course
N
SUBSTANCE INTOXICATION DELIRIUM; SUBSTANCE WITHDRAWAL DELIRIUM; MEDICATION-INDUCED DELIRIUM (3.16.1)
Y
Associated with evidence of decline in one or more of the following cognitive domains: complex attention, executive function, learning and memory, language, perceptual-motor, or social cognition
Y
SUBSTANCE/MEDICATION-INDUCED MAJOR or MILD NEUROCOGNITIVE DISORDER (3.16.2), WITH BEHAVIORAL DISTURBANCE
N
SUBSTANCE INTOXICATION; SUBSTANCE WITHDRAWAL; OTHER ADVERSE EFFECT OF MEDICATION
N
Due to the physiological effects of a general medical condition
Y
Associated with a disturbance in attention and awareness characterized by a fluctuating course
Y
DELIRIUM DUE TO ANOTHER MEDICAL CONDITION (3.16.1)
N
Associated with evidence of decline in one of more of the following cognitive domains: complex attention, executive function, learning and memory, language, perceptual-motor, or social cognition
Y
MAJOR or MILD NEUROCOGNITIVE DISORDER DUE TO ANOTHER MEDICAL CONDITION (3.16.2), WITH BEHAVIORAL DISTURBANCE
N
Occurring in a pattern representing a change from previous personality pattern
Y
PERSONALITY CHANGE DUE TO ANOTHER MEDICAL CONDITION (3.17.11), AGGRESSIVE TYPE
N
N

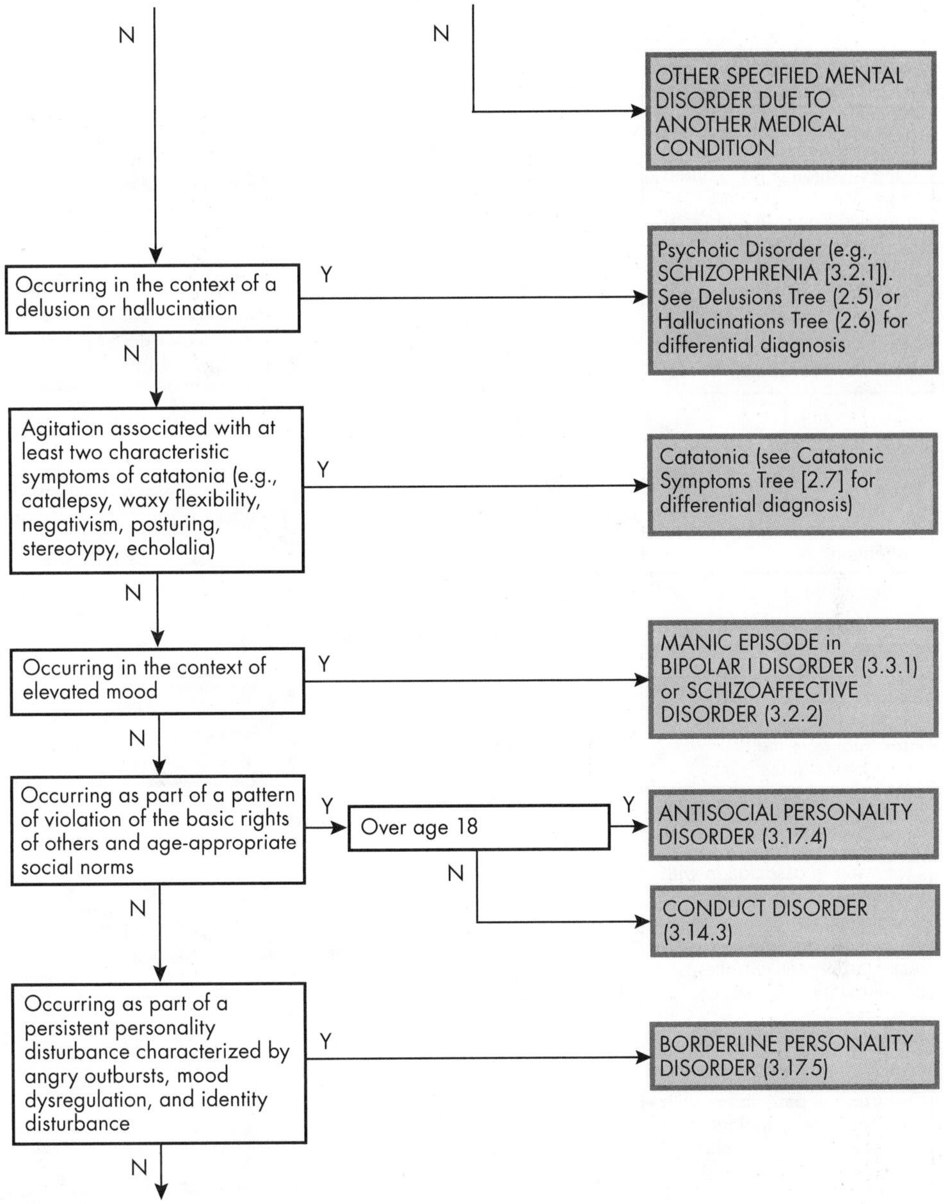
N
N
OTHER SPECIFIED MENTAL DISORDER DUE TO ANOTHER MEDICAL CONDITION
Occurring in the context of a delusion or hallucination
Y
Psychotic Disorder (e.g., SCHIZOPHRENIA [3.2.1]). See Delusions Tree (2.5) or Hallucinations Tree (2.6) for differential diagnosis
N
Agitation associated with at least two characteristic symptoms of catatonia (e.g., catalepsy, waxy flexibility, negativism, posturing, stereotypy, echolalia)
Y
Catatonia (see Catatonic Symptoms Tree [2.7] for differential diagnosis)
N
Occurring in the context of elevated mood
Y
MANIC EPISODE in BIPOLAR I DISORDER (3.3.1) or SCHIZOAFFECTIVE DISORDER (3.2.2)
N
Occurring as part of a pattern of violation of the basic rights of others and age-appropriate social norms
Y
Over age 18
Y
ANTISOCIAL PERSONALITY DISORDER (3.17.4)
N
CONDUCT DISORDER (3.14.3)
N
Occurring as part of a persistent personality disturbance characterized by angry outbursts, mood dysregulation, and identity disturbance
Y
BORDERLINE PERSONALITY DISORDER (3.17.5)
N

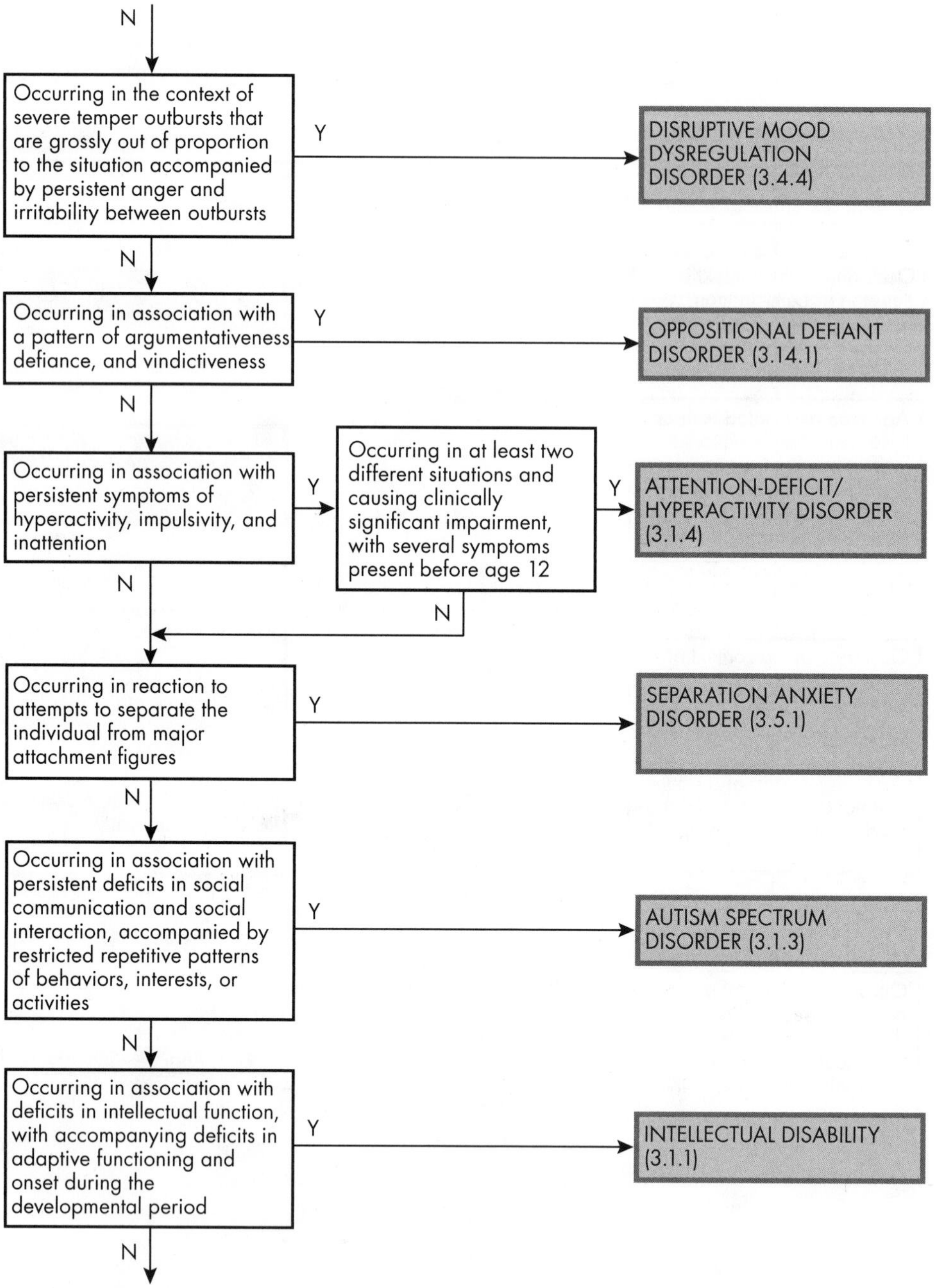
N
Occurring in the context of severe temper outbursts that are grossly out of proportion to the situation accompanied by persistent anger and irritability between outbursts
Y
DISRUPTIVE MOOD DYSREGULATION DISORDER (3.4.4)
N
Occurring in association with a pattern of argumentativeness defiance, and vindictiveness
Y
OPPOSITIONAL DEFIANT DISORDER (3.14.1)
N
Occurring in association with persistent symptoms of hyperactivity, impulsivity, and inattention
Y
Occurring in at least two different situations and causing clinically significant impairment, with several symptoms present before age 12
Y
ATTENTION-DEFICIT/ HYPERACTIVITY DISORDER (3.1.4)
N
N
Occurring in reaction to attempts to separate the individual from major attachment figures
Y
SEPARATION ANXIETY DISORDER (3.5.1)
N
Occurring in association with persistent deficits in social communication and social interaction, accompanied by restricted repetitive patterns of behaviors, interests, or activities
Y
AUTISM SPECTRUM DISORDER (3.1.3)
N
Occurring in association with deficits in intellectual function, with accompanying deficits in adaptive functioning and onset during the developmental period
Y
INTELLECTUAL DISABILITY (3.1.1)
N

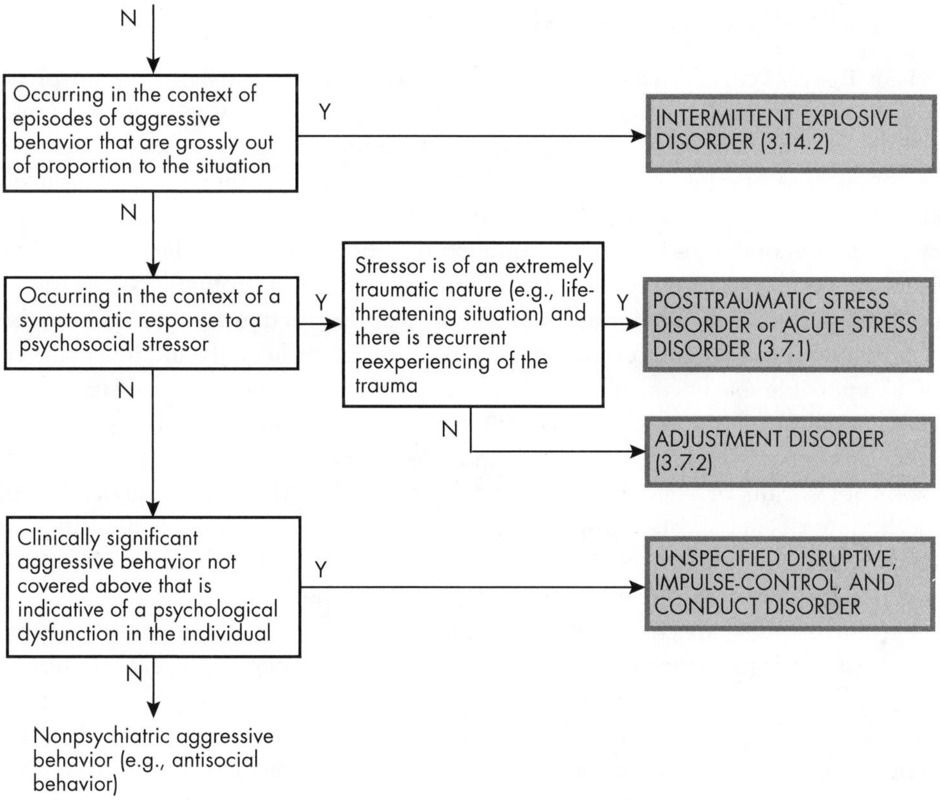
N
Occurring in the context of episodes of aggressive behavior that are grossly out of proportion to the situation
Y
INTERMITTENT EXPLOSIVE DISORDER (3.14.2)
N
Occurring in the context of a symptomatic response to a psychosocial stressor
Y
Stressor is of an extremely traumatic nature (e.g., life-threatening situation) and there is recurrent reexperiencing of the trauma
Y
POSTTRAUMATIC STRESS DISORDER or ACUTE STRESS DISORDER (3.7.1)
N
ADJUSTMENT DISORDER (3.7.2)
N
Clinically significant aggressive behavior not covered above that is indicative of a psychological dysfunction in the individual
Y
UNSPECIFIED DISRUPTIVE, IMPULSE-CONTROL, AND CONDUCT DISORDER
N
Nonpsychiatric aggressive behavior (e.g., antisocial behavior)

2.24 Decision Tree for Impulsivity or Impulse-Control Problems

Decision tree 2.24 covers two related symptoms: the trait of impulsivity and the problem of diminished impulse control. Impulsivity involves the tendency to act on a whim, displaying behavior characterized by little or no forethought, reflection, or consideration of consequences. A number of DSM-5 disorders are characterized by excessive impulsivity. Other disorders are characterized by problems in controlling certain impulses (e.g., the impulse to pull out one's hair in Trichotillomania, the impulse to binge in Binge-Eating Disorder). Both excessive impulsivity and impairment in controlling specific impulses can lead to impulsive behavior that can be both self-destructive and harmful to others.

Substance use is a common and devastating cause of impulsivity and must be considered as a possible sole or contributory factor in every presentation of impulsive behavior. General medical conditions can also result in the disinhibition of impulse control, which is often accompanied by poor judgment and other cognitive symptoms warranting a diagnosis of Delirium or Major or Mild Neurocognitive Disorder. When a general medical condition results in persistent impulsivity that occurs in the absence of clinically significant cognitive impairment, the diagnosis is Personality Change Due to Another Medical Condition (usually of the Disinhibited or Aggressive Type).

Certain disorders are characterized by impulsivity that is confined exclusively to the episode of the disturbance. Once substance use and a general medical condition are ruled out, the next step is to determine whether the presentation includes symptoms that would lead to a diagnosis of a Bipolar Disorder, Depressive Disorder, Schizophrenia or one of the other psychotic disorders, or Posttraumatic Stress Disorder or Acute Stress Disorder. Generalized impulsivity that has an early onset and persistent course is most likely to be associated with Attention-Deficit/Hyperactivity Disorder, Conduct Disorder, Antisocial Personality Disorder, or Borderline Personality Disorder.

A wide range of DSM-5 disorders are characterized by specific behaviors that can be conceptualized as manifestations of impaired impulse control. These include Gambling Disorder, in which the person's ability to control gambling behavior is impaired; Bulimia Nervosa and Binge-Eating Disorder, which are characterized by out-of-control binge eating; Pyromania and Kleptomania, which are characterized by an inability to resist impulses to, respectively, set fires and steal objects of little value; Trichotillomania and Excoriation Disorder, characterized by an inability to control impulses to, respectively, pull out one's hair or pick one's skin; and Intermittent Explosive Disorder, characterized by an intermittent inability to resist aggressive impulses.

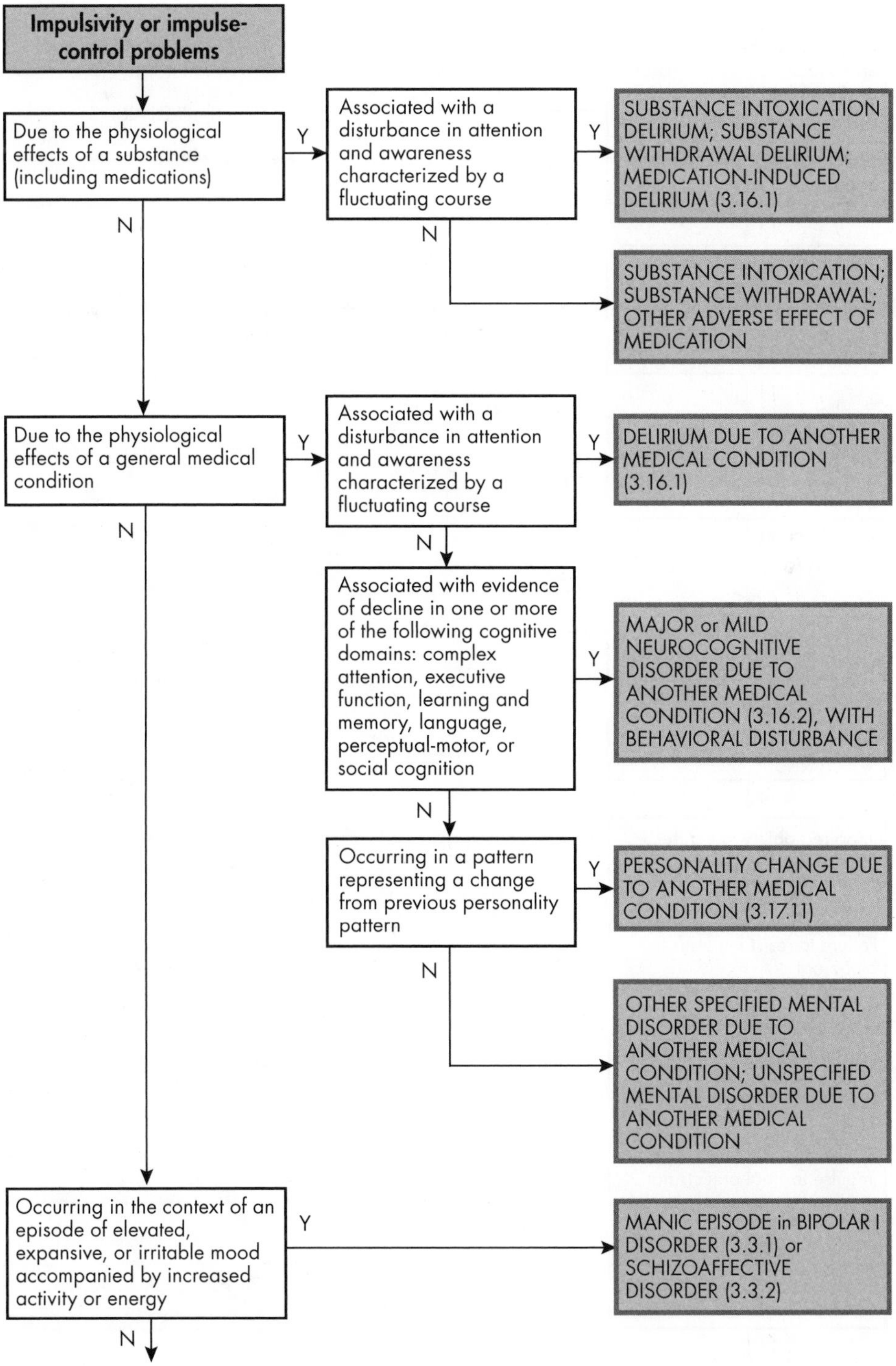
Impulsivity or impulse-control problems
Due to the physiological effects of a substance (including medications)
Y
N
Associated with a disturbance in attention and awareness characterized by a fluctuating course
Y
N
SUBSTANCE INTOXICATION DELIRIUM; SUBSTANCE WITHDRAWAL DELIRIUM; MEDICATION-INDUCED DELIRIUM (3.16.1)
SUBSTANCE INTOXICATION; SUBSTANCE WITHDRAWAL; OTHER ADVERSE EFFECT OF MEDICATION
Due to the physiological effects of a general medical condition
Y
N
Associated with a disturbance in attention and awareness characterized by a fluctuating course
Y
N
DELIRIUM DUE TO ANOTHER MEDICAL CONDITION (3.16.1)
Associated with evidence of decline in one or more of the following cognitive domains: complex attention, executive function, learning and memory, language, perceptual-motor, or social cognition
Y
N
MAJOR or MILD NEUROCOGNITIVE DISORDER DUE TO ANOTHER MEDICAL CONDITION (3.16.2), WITH BEHAVIORAL DISTURBANCE
Occurring in a pattern representing a change from previous personality pattern
Y
N
PERSONALITY CHANGE DUE TO ANOTHER MEDICAL CONDITION (3.17.11)
OTHER SPECIFIED MENTAL DISORDER DUE TO ANOTHER MEDICAL CONDITION; UNSPECIFIED MENTAL DISORDER DUE TO ANOTHER MEDICAL CONDITION
Occurring in the context of an episode of elevated, expansive, or irritable mood accompanied by increased activity or energy
Y
N
MANIC EPISODE in BIPOLAR I DISORDER (3.3.1) or SCHIZOAFFECTIVE DISORDER (3.3.2)

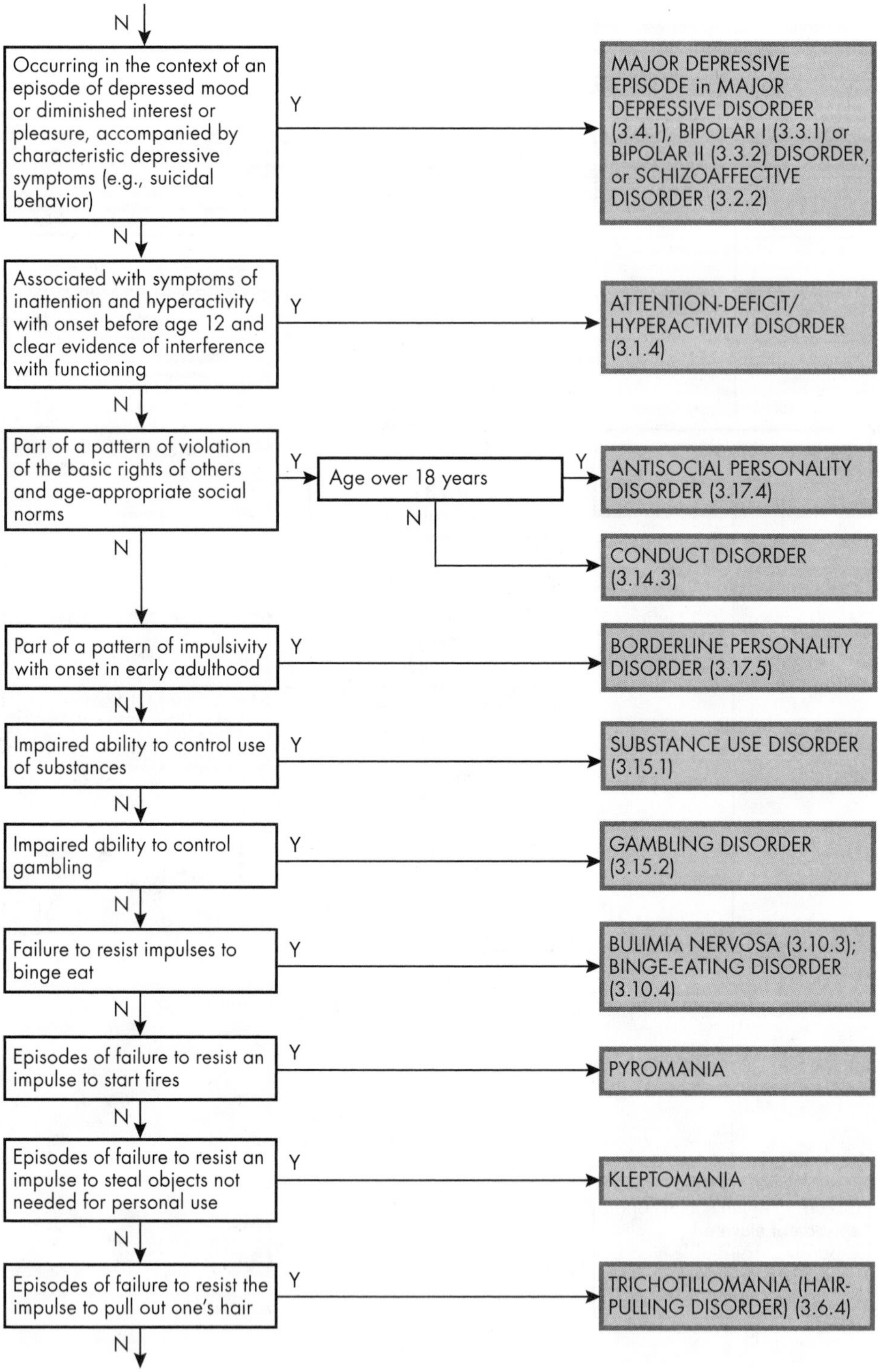
N
Occurring in the context of an episode of depressed mood or diminished interest or pleasure, accompanied by characteristic depressive symptoms (e.g., suicidal behavior)
Y
MAJOR DEPRESSIVE EPISODE in MAJOR DEPRESSIVE DISORDER (3.4.1), BIPOLAR I (3.3.1) or BIPOLAR II (3.3.2) DISORDER, or SCHIZOAFFECTIVE DISORDER (3.2.2)
N
Associated with symptoms of inattention and hyperactivity with onset before age 12 and clear evidence of interference with functioning
Y
ATTENTION-DEFICIT/ HYPERACTIVITY DISORDER (3.1.4)
N
Part of a pattern of violation of the basic rights of others and age-appropriate social norms
Y
Age over 18 years
Y
ANTISOCIAL PERSONALITY DISORDER (3.17.4)
N
CONDUCT DISORDER (3.14.3)
N
Part of a pattern of impulsivity with onset in early adulthood
Y
BORDERLINE PERSONALITY DISORDER (3.17.5)
N
Impaired ability to control use of substances
Y
SUBSTANCE USE DISORDER (3.15.1)
N
Impaired ability to control gambling
Y
GAMBLING DISORDER (3.15.2)
N
Failure to resist impulses to binge eat
Y
BULIMIA NERVOSA (3.10.3); BINGE-EATING DISORDER (3.10.4)
N
Episodes of failure to resist an impulse to start fires
Y
PYROMANIA
N
Episodes of failure to resist an impulse to steal objects not needed for personal use
Y
KLEPTOMANIA
N
Episodes of failure to resist the impulse to pull out one's hair
Y
TRICHOTILLOMANIA (HAIR-PULLING DISORDER) (3.6.4)
N

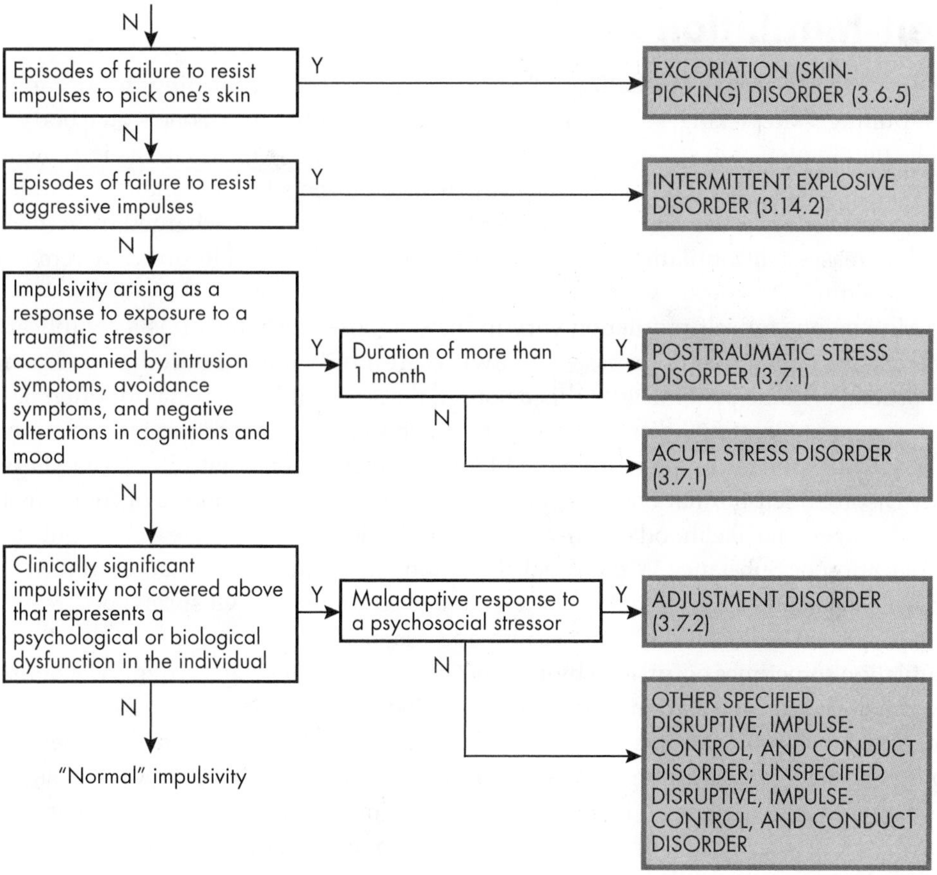
N
Episodes of failure to resist impulses to pick one's skin
Y
EXCORIATION (SKIN-PICKING) DISORDER (3.6.5)
N
Episodes of failure to resist aggressive impulses
Y
INTERMITTENT EXPLOSIVE DISORDER (3.14.2)
N
Impulsivity arising as a response to exposure to a traumatic stressor accompanied by intrusion symptoms, avoidance symptoms, and negative alterations in cognitions and mood
Y
Duration of more than 1 month
Y
POSTTRAUMATIC STRESS DISORDER (3.7.1)
N
ACUTE STRESS DISORDER (3.7.1)
N
Clinically significant impulsivity not covered above that represents a psychological or biological dysfunction in the individual
Y
Maladaptive response to a psychosocial stressor
Y
ADJUSTMENT DISORDER (3.7.2)
N
OTHER SPECIFIED DISRUPTIVE, IMPULSE-CONTROL, AND CONDUCT DISORDER; UNSPECIFIED DISRUPTIVE, IMPULSE-CONTROL, AND CONDUCT DISORDER
N
"Normal" impulsivity

2.25 Decision Tree for Self-Injury or Self-Mutilation

Self-injurious and self-mutilating behaviors include cutting, burning, head banging, hair pulling, skin picking, self-biting, and hitting of various parts of one's own body. Notably, the frequency of self-mutilation appears to be greatest in situations in which the individual is confined (e.g., in a hospital, prison, children's home). Therefore, an interesting dilemma is presented when a patient who is about to be discharged from the hospital increases self-mutilating behaviors, which may in fact be reinforced by remaining in that setting.

Motivations for self-mutilation vary in the diagnoses for which it is a complication. The most frequent diagnosis associated with self-mutilation is Borderline Personality Disorder. For some patients with this disorder, the self-mutilating behavior often occurs as a means of "treating" dissociative states wherein the patient returns to feeling alive only when experiencing pain or seeing blood. In other patients with Borderline Personality Disorder, self-mutilation is a means of "treating" intense dysphoria or counteracting intense anger. The likelihood of self-mutilative episodes is greatly increased by Substance Intoxication or Substance Withdrawal. The motivation for self-mutilation in psychotic patients is usually a delusional belief (e.g., the need to punish evil spirits) or a response to a command hallucination. In Delirium and Major Neurocognitive Disorder, the self-mutilation sometimes occurs as a by-product of the confusion (e.g., struggling against restraints). The self-mutilation that infrequently occurs as a complication of Obsessive-Compulsive Disorder results from the inability to resist the constant need to perform a compulsive act (e.g., cleaning hands raw as a result of a hand-washing compulsion). In Trichotillomania, there is an inability to resist the impulse to pull out one's hair, which may result in patches of hair loss. Similar failure to resist impulses to pick one's skin in Excoriation Disorder leads to noticeable skin lesions. In Sexual Masochism Disorder, the motivation for the self-mutilation is sexual pleasure.

Stereotypies, which can result in self-injury, are the central component of Stereotypic Movement Disorder. When Stereotypic Movement Disorder results in clinically significant self-injury, this can be indicated by specifying "with self-injurious behavior." Stereotypies are not infrequent in Intellectual Disability (Intellectual Developmental Disorder) and should be diagnosed separately as Stereotypic Movement Disorder only if they are not better explained by the underlying cause of the Intellectual Disability.

Self-mutilating behavior is sometimes a manifestation of Factitious Disorder or Malingering. The patient learns that cutting or burning will result in a desired hospitalization or prevent an undesired discharge. Factitious Disorder and Malingering are differentiated based on whether the feigned behavior occurs in the absence of obvious external rewards; if so, the diagnosis is Factitious Disorder. If the feigned self-injurious behavior only occurs in the presence of obvious external rewards, Malingering is diagnosed instead.

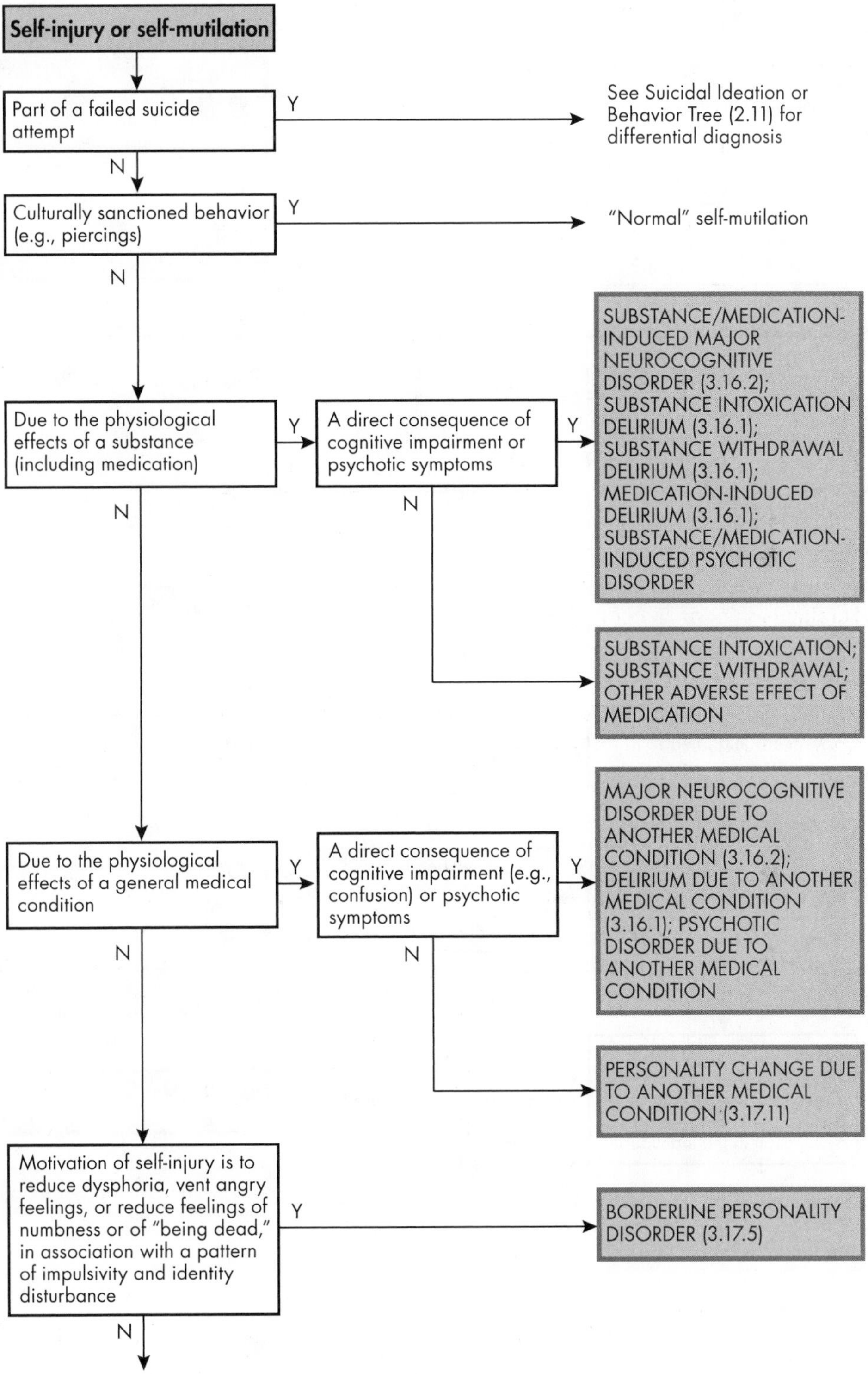
Self-injury or self-mutilation
Part of a failed suicide attempt
Y
See Suicidal Ideation or Behavior Tree (2.11) for differential diagnosis
N
Culturally sanctioned behavior (e.g., piercings)
Y
"Normal" self-mutilation
N
Due to the physiological effects of a substance (including medication)
Y
A direct consequence of cognitive impairment or psychotic symptoms
Y
SUBSTANCE/MEDICATION-INDUCED MAJOR NEUROCOGNITIVE DISORDER (3.16.2); SUBSTANCE INTOXICATION DELIRIUM (3.16.1); SUBSTANCE WITHDRAWAL DELIRIUM (3.16.1); MEDICATION-INDUCED DELIRIUM (3.16.1); SUBSTANCE/MEDICATION-INDUCED PSYCHOTIC DISORDER
N
SUBSTANCE INTOXICATION; SUBSTANCE WITHDRAWAL; OTHER ADVERSE EFFECT OF MEDICATION
N
Due to the physiological effects of a general medical condition
Y
A direct consequence of cognitive impairment (e.g., confusion) or psychotic symptoms
Y
MAJOR NEUROCOGNITIVE DISORDER DUE TO ANOTHER MEDICAL CONDITION (3.16.2); DELIRIUM DUE TO ANOTHER MEDICAL CONDITION (3.16.1); PSYCHOTIC DISORDER DUE TO ANOTHER MEDICAL CONDITION
N
PERSONALITY CHANGE DUE TO ANOTHER MEDICAL CONDITION (3.17.11)
N
Motivation of self-injury is to reduce dysphoria, vent angry feelings, or reduce feelings of numbness or of "being dead," in association with a pattern of impulsivity and identity disturbance
Y
BORDERLINE PERSONALITY DISORDER (3.17.5)
N

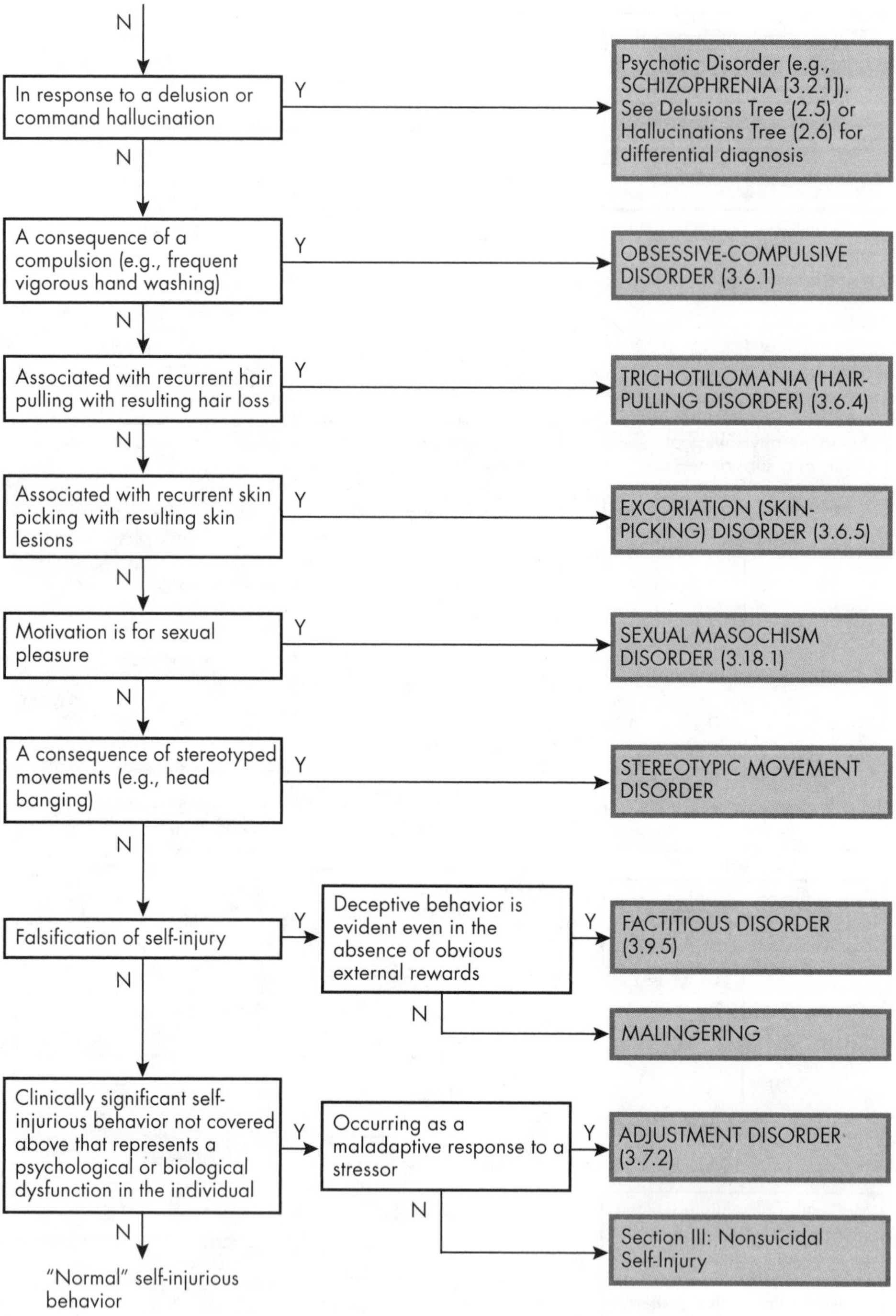
N
In response to a delusion or command hallucination
Y
Psychotic Disorder (e.g., SCHIZOPHRENIA [3.2.1]). See Delusions Tree (2.5) or Hallucinations Tree (2.6) for differential diagnosis
N
A consequence of a compulsion (e.g., frequent vigorous hand washing)
Y
OBSESSIVE-COMPULSIVE DISORDER (3.6.1)
N
Associated with recurrent hair pulling with resulting hair loss
Y
TRICHOTILLOMANIA (HAIR-PULLING DISORDER) (3.6.4)
N
Associated with recurrent skin picking with resulting skin lesions
Y
EXCORIATION (SKIN-PICKING) DISORDER (3.6.5)
N
Motivation is for sexual pleasure
Y
SEXUAL MASOCHISM DISORDER (3.18.1)
N
A consequence of stereotyped movements (e.g., head banging)
Y
STEREOTYPIC MOVEMENT DISORDER
N
Falsification of self-injury
Y
Deceptive behavior is evident even in the absence of obvious external rewards
Y
FACTITIOUS DISORDER (3.9.5)
N
MALINGERING
N
Clinically significant self-injurious behavior not covered above that represents a psychological or biological dysfunction in the individual
Y
Occurring as a maladaptive response to a stressor
Y
ADJUSTMENT DISORDER (3.7.2)
N
Section III: Nonsuicidal Self-Injury
N
"Normal" self-injurious behavior

2.26 Decision Tree for Excessive Substance Use

Many individuals can take substances without having any clinically significant problems that would warrant a DSM-5 diagnosis. However, substance-related disorders are among the most common and impairing of the mental disorders. Because substance-related presentations are so frequently encountered in mental health, substance treatment, and primary care settings, a substance-related disorder must be considered in every differential diagnosis.

In DSM-5, the term *substance-related* refers to disorders associated with drugs of abuse, the side effects of medication, and toxin-induced states. There are two types of substance-related diagnoses in DSM-5: the Substance Use Disorders, which describe a pattern of problematic substance use, and the Substance-Induced Disorders (comprising Substance Intoxication, Substance Withdrawal, and Substance/Medication-Induced Mental Disorders), which describe behavioral syndromes that are caused by the direct effect of a substance on the central nervous system (CNS). More often than not, Substance-Induced Disorders occur in the context of an accompanying Substance Use Disorder, and when this occurs, both should be diagnosed. The method for recording these diagnoses depends on the requirements of the ICD-9-CM or ICD-10-CM coding system. If a diagnosis is made while ICD-9-CM is in effect (i.e., up to October 1, 2014), two diagnoses are given (e.g., Severe Alcohol Use Disorder and Alcohol Withdrawal). If a diagnosis is made while ICD-10-CM is in effect (i.e., beginning October 1, 2014, or after), then a single combined diagnosis is given (e.g., Severe Alcohol Use Disorder With Alcohol Withdrawal). See the recording procedures for Substance-Induced Disorders in DSM-5 for more information. For this reason, the decision tree starts off with a decision point that highlights the fact that Substance Use Disorders and Substance-Induced Disorders are often comorbid, and clearly indicates that if a Substance Use Disorder is present and there is evidence that the substance has caused psychiatric symptoms because of its direct effect on the CNS, the remainder of the tree must be reviewed to determine the differential diagnosis of the relevant Substance-Induced Disorder.

Substance Intoxication and Substance Withdrawal can be characterized by psychopathology that mimics other disorders contained in DSM-5 and must always be considered in the differential diagnosis of every condition (see Step 2 in Chapter 1). The Substance/Medication-Induced Mental Disorders (e.g., Substance/Medication-Induced Psychotic Disorder, Substance/Medication-Induced Bipolar and Related Disorder, and so forth) have been included in DSM-5 for presentations in which a particular symptom, such as delusions, hallucinations, or mania, predominate in the clinical picture and warrant clinical attention. For example, virtually every individual withdrawing from cocaine will experience some dysphoric mood, and in most situations a diagnosis of Cocaine Withdrawal will suffice. However, were the individual to become suicidally depressed, the diagnosis of Cocaine-Induced Depressive Disorder may be more appropriate. Often, more than one symptom (e.g., depressed mood and anxiety) may be prominent enough to be a focus of clinical attention. In such situations, it is generally preferable to give just one substance/medication-induced diagnosis indicating the predominating symptom.

The psychiatric sequelae to substance/medication use can occur in any of four contexts: 1) as an acute effect of Substance Intoxication, 2) as an acute effect of Substance Withdrawal, 3) as a medication side effect not necessarily related to Substance Intoxication or Substance Withdrawal, and 4) as an effect that endures even after Substance Intoxication or Substance Withdrawal has abated (in the case of Substance/Medication-Induced Major or Mild Neurocognitive Disorder and Hallucinogen Persisting Perception Disorder).

Delirium Due to Multiple Etiologies and Major or Mild Neurocognitive Disorder Due to Multiple Etiologies have been included in DSM-5 (and in this decision tree) to emphasize that very often these conditions have multiple interacting etiologies, including substances. A common (and sometimes devastating) error is to assume your job is finished once you have identified a substance as a contributing etiology to the Delirium or the Major or Mild Neurocognitive Disorder and therefore to miss the associated contribution of head trauma or another medical condition.

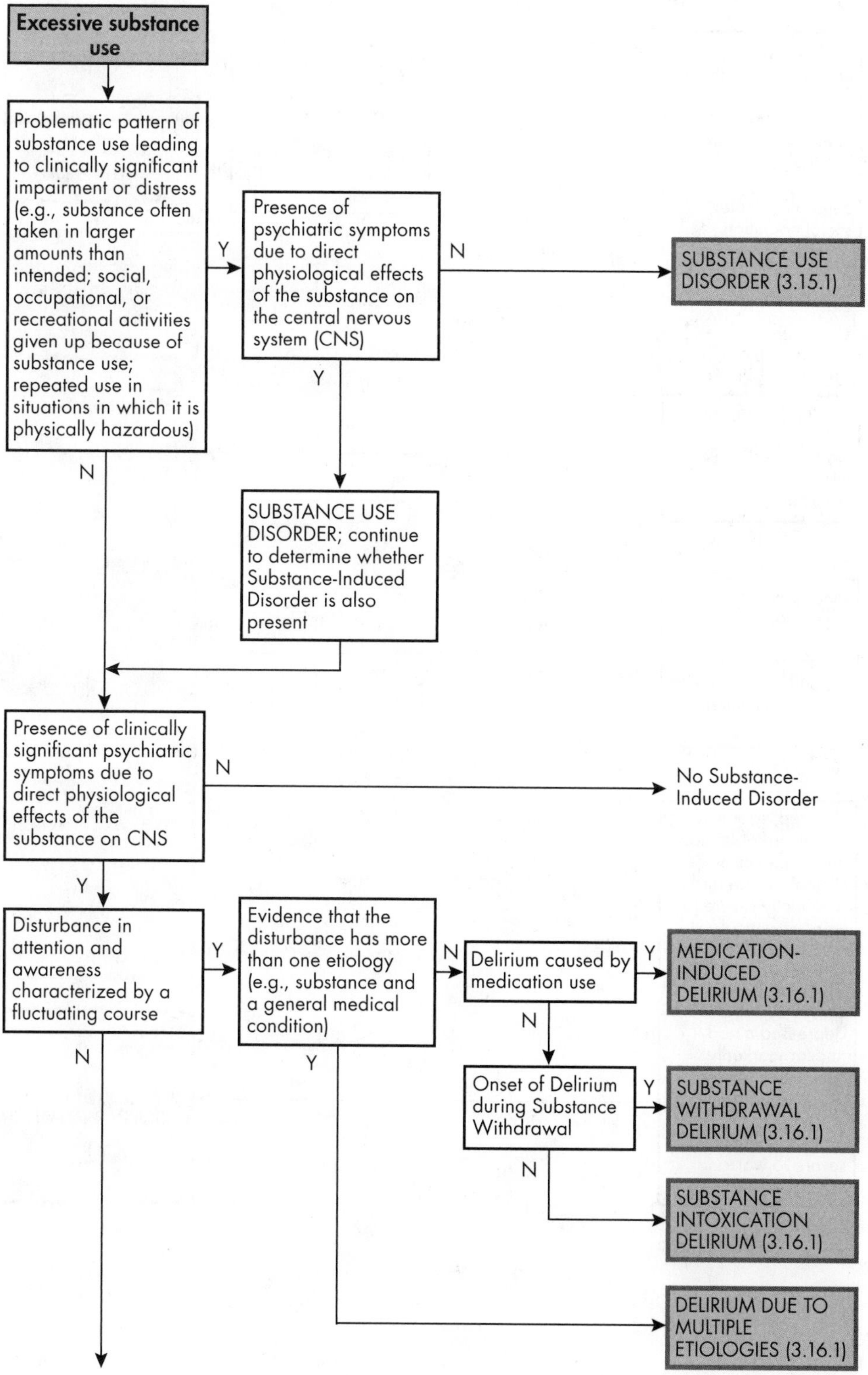
Excessive substance use
Problematic pattern of substance use leading to clinically significant impairment or distress (e.g., substance often taken in larger amounts than intended; social, occupational, or recreational activities given up because of substance use; repeated use in situations in which it is physically hazardous)
Y
Presence of psychiatric symptoms due to direct physiological effects of the substance on the central nervous system (CNS)
N
SUBSTANCE USE DISORDER (3.15.1)
Y
SUBSTANCE USE DISORDER; continue to determine whether Substance-Induced Disorder is also present
N
Presence of clinically significant psychiatric symptoms due to direct physiological effects of the substance on CNS
N
No Substance-Induced Disorder
Y
Disturbance in attention and awareness characterized by a fluctuating course
Y
Evidence that the disturbance has more than one etiology (e.g., substance and a general medical condition)
N
Delirium caused by medication use
Y
MEDICATION-INDUCED DELIRIUM (3.16.1)
N
Onset of Delirium during Substance Withdrawal
Y
SUBSTANCE WITHDRAWAL DELIRIUM (3.16.1)
N
SUBSTANCE INTOXICATION DELIRIUM (3.16.1)
Y
DELIRIUM DUE TO MULTIPLE ETIOLOGIES (3.16.1)
N

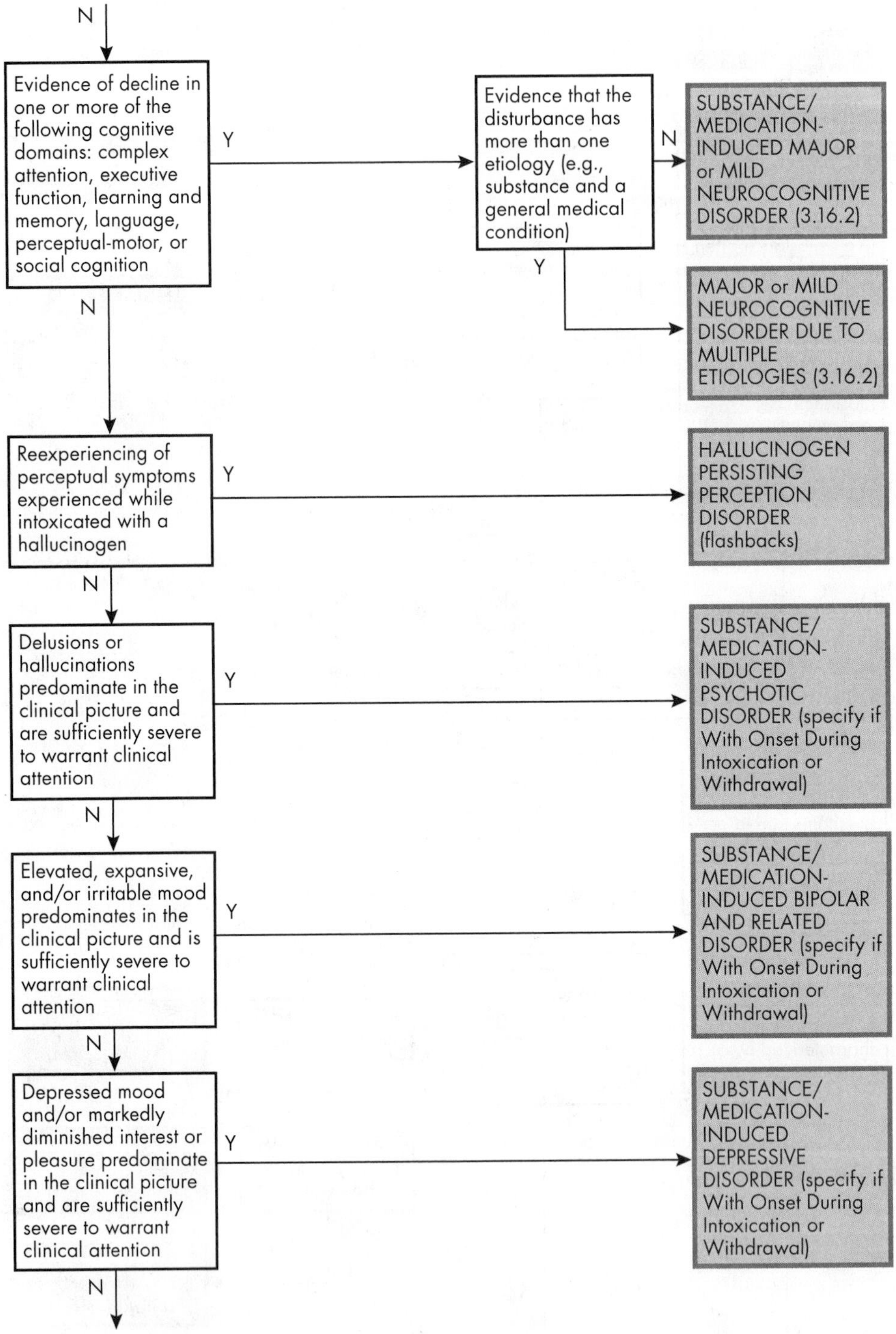
N
Evidence of decline in one or more of the following cognitive domains: complex attention, executive function, learning and memory, language, perceptual-motor, or social cognition
Y
Evidence that the disturbance has more than one etiology (e.g., substance and a general medical condition)
N
SUBSTANCE/ MEDICATION-INDUCED MAJOR or MILD NEUROCOGNITIVE DISORDER (3.16.2)
Y
MAJOR or MILD NEUROCOGNITIVE DISORDER DUE TO MULTIPLE ETIOLOGIES (3.16.2)
N
Reexperiencing of perceptual symptoms experienced while intoxicated with a hallucinogen
Y
HALLUCINOGEN PERSISTING PERCEPTION DISORDER (flashbacks)
N
Delusions or hallucinations predominate in the clinical picture and are sufficiently severe to warrant clinical attention
Y
SUBSTANCE/ MEDICATION-INDUCED PSYCHOTIC DISORDER (specify if With Onset During Intoxication or Withdrawal)
N
Elevated, expansive, and/or irritable mood predominates in the clinical picture and is sufficiently severe to warrant clinical attention
Y
SUBSTANCE/ MEDICATION-INDUCED BIPOLAR AND RELATED DISORDER (specify if With Onset During Intoxication or Withdrawal)
N
Depressed mood and/or markedly diminished interest or pleasure predominate in the clinical picture and are sufficiently severe to warrant clinical attention
Y
SUBSTANCE/ MEDICATION-INDUCED DEPRESSIVE DISORDER (specify if With Onset During Intoxication or Withdrawal)
N

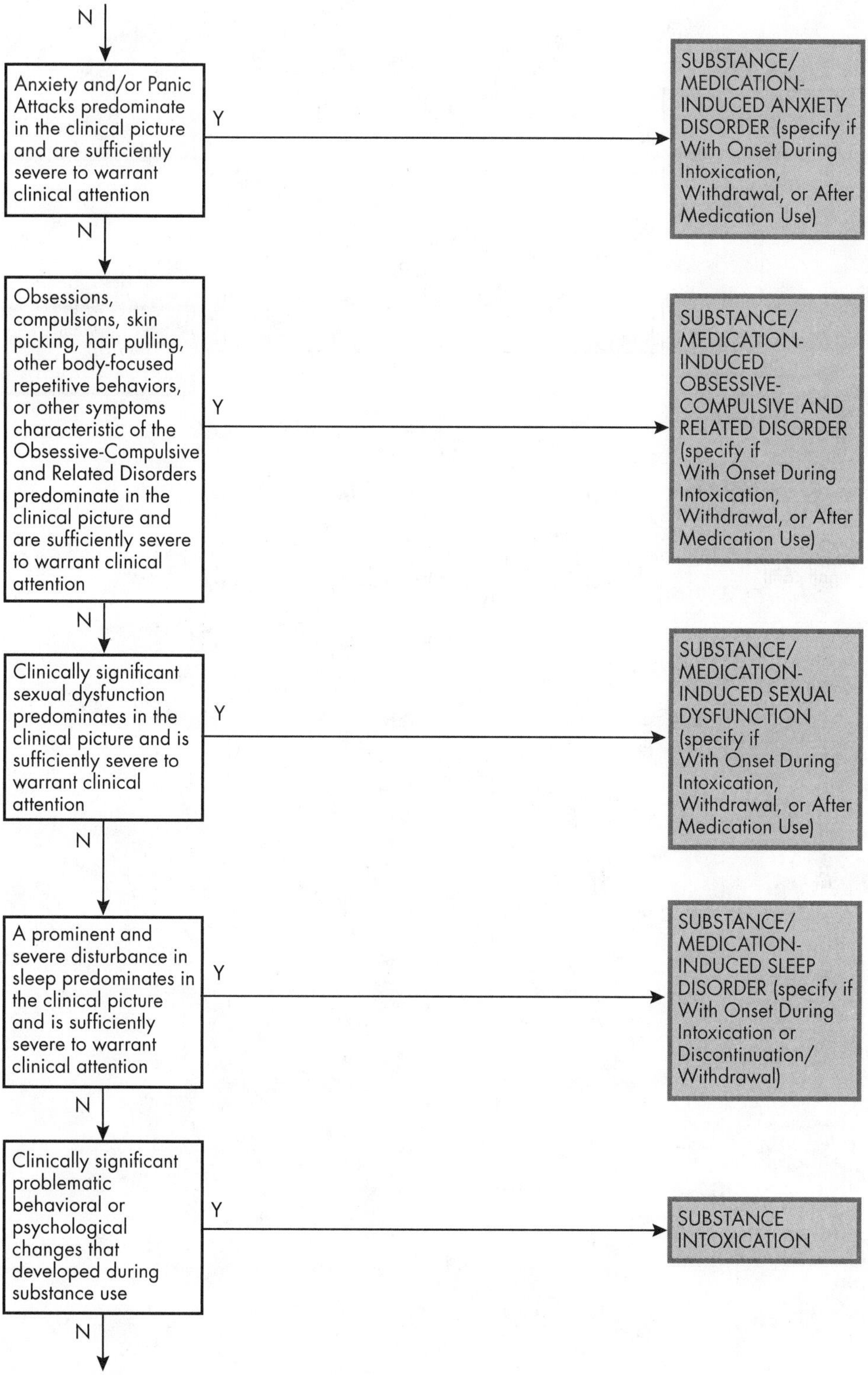
N
Anxiety and/or Panic Attacks predominate in the clinical picture and are sufficiently severe to warrant clinical attention
Y
SUBSTANCE/ MEDICATION-INDUCED ANXIETY DISORDER (specify if With Onset During Intoxication, Withdrawal, or After Medication Use)
N
Obsessions, compulsions, skin picking, hair pulling, other body-focused repetitive behaviors, or other symptoms characteristic of the Obsessive-Compulsive and Related Disorders predominate in the clinical picture and are sufficiently severe to warrant clinical attention
Y
SUBSTANCE/ MEDICATION-INDUCED OBSESSIVE-COMPULSIVE AND RELATED DISORDER (specify if With Onset During Intoxication, Withdrawal, or After Medication Use)
N
Clinically significant sexual dysfunction predominates in the clinical picture and is sufficiently severe to warrant clinical attention
Y
SUBSTANCE/ MEDICATION-INDUCED SEXUAL DYSFUNCTION (specify if With Onset During Intoxication, Withdrawal, or After Medication Use)
N
A prominent and severe disturbance in sleep predominates in the clinical picture and is sufficiently severe to warrant clinical attention
Y
SUBSTANCE/ MEDICATION-INDUCED SLEEP DISORDER (specify if With Onset During Intoxication or Discontinuation/ Withdrawal)
N
Clinically significant problematic behavioral or psychological changes that developed during substance use
Y
SUBSTANCE INTOXICATION
N

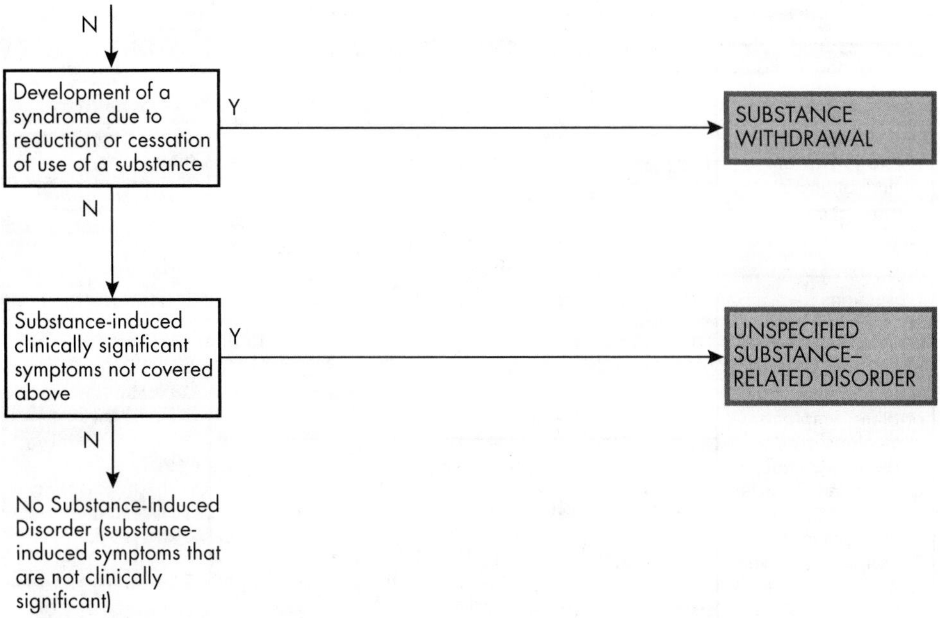
N
Development of a syndrome due to reduction or cessation of use of a substance
Y
SUBSTANCE WITHDRAWAL
N
Substance-induced clinically significant symptoms not covered above
Y
UNSPECIFIED SUBSTANCE–RELATED DISORDER
N
No Substance-Induced Disorder (substance-induced symptoms that are not clinically significant)

2.27 Decision Tree for Memory Loss

Memory loss can be characterized by difficulty in laying down new memories and/or in the recall of previous memories. The various aspects of memory functioning may be tested separately. These include 1) registration (the ability of the patient to repeat numbers or words immediately after hearing them), 2) short-term recall (the ability of the patient to repeat the names of three unrelated objects after a period of several minutes), 3) recognition (the ability of the patient to retrieve previously forgotten names if provided with clues), and 4) remote memory (the ability of the patient to recall important personal or historical events). The differential decisions in this tree concern whether the etiology of the memory loss is the direct physiological effect on the central nervous system of substance/medication use or a general medical condition, whether it is an associated feature of another mental disorder, or whether the memory loss is a dissociative phenomenon (e.g., as in Posttraumatic Stress Disorder or a Dissociative Disorder).

Memory impairment is one of the types of cognitive impairment that characterize Delirium and Major or Mild Neurocognitive Disorder. The hallmark of Delirium is a fluctuating course of clouding of consciousness characterized by a disturbance in attention (i.e., reduced ability to direct, focus, sustain, and shift attention) and awareness (i.e., reduced orientation to the environment). The definition of Delirium also requires an accompanying disturbance in cognition (which can take the form of memory impairment, language, visuospatial ability, or perception). Neurocognitive Disorder is defined as a decline in one or more neurocognitive domains, which DSM-5 specifies as including complex attention, executive functioning, learning and memory, language, perceptual-motor, and social cognition. Although such cognitive impairment occurs on a continuum, DSM-5 has split the dimension into two categorical disorders: Major Neurocognitive Disorder and Mild Neurocognitive Disorder. Major Neurocognitive Disorder is characterized by a significant decline in cognition that is so severe as to interfere with independence. In Mild Neurocognitive Disorder, the cognitive decline is limited to being only at a "modest" level of severity. The diagnosis is made when the individual, a knowledgeable informant, or the clinician notices a mild decline in the patient's cognitive function; this decline must be accompanied by evidence of a modest impairment in cognitive performance preferably documented by standardized neuropsychological testing or another quantified clinical assessment.

Memory impairment associated with substance use can be either temporary (as in Substance Intoxication, Substance Withdrawal, Substance Intoxication Delirium or Substance Withdrawal Delirium, and Other Adverse Effect of Medication) or persistent (as in Substance/Medication-Induced Major or Mild Neurocognitive Disorder, which requires the cognitive impairments to persist beyond the usual duration of acute intoxication or withdrawal).

Memory impairment is also a common associated feature of a number of mental disorders. For example, memory impairment occurring in the context of a Major Depressive Episode can be so severe as to resemble an irreversible dementing process. Frequently, it is only when the memory impairment resolves after antidepressant treatment that it becomes clear that there was no comorbid Major Neurocognitive Disorder. This differential is further complicated by the fact that the medication (e.g., lithium) being taken by the patient may also contribute to memory problems.

Dissociation is a disruption in the usually integrated functions of consciousness, memory, identity, or perception of the environment. Memory loss, especially for traumatic events, is a feature of Dissociative Amnesia and Dissociative Identity Disorder, as well as of Posttraumatic Stress Disorder and Acute Stress Disorder. Particularly when someone has been exposed to an event that is both physically and psychologically traumatic (e.g., car accident), it can be difficult to tease apart whether the memory loss is a psychological reaction to the events or is due to direct damage to the brain. Moreover, especially in forensic situations, feigned claims of memory loss may be used in an attempt to deny responsibility. In such cases, the diagnosis is either Factitious Disorder or Malingering, with Factitious Disorder diagnosed when the feigned memory loss is evident even in the absence of obvious external rewards. Otherwise, Malingering (which is not considered to be a mental disorder) is diagnosed.

It should also be noted that virtually everyone wishes that his or her memory were better than it is and that this longing usually becomes more poignant as people get older and begin having more difficulty commanding their memories. Before considering the disorders on this decision tree, it must be determined that the memory loss is sufficiently severe to be clinically significant and that it is more severe than might be expected given the person's previous memory functioning and the norms for his or her age.

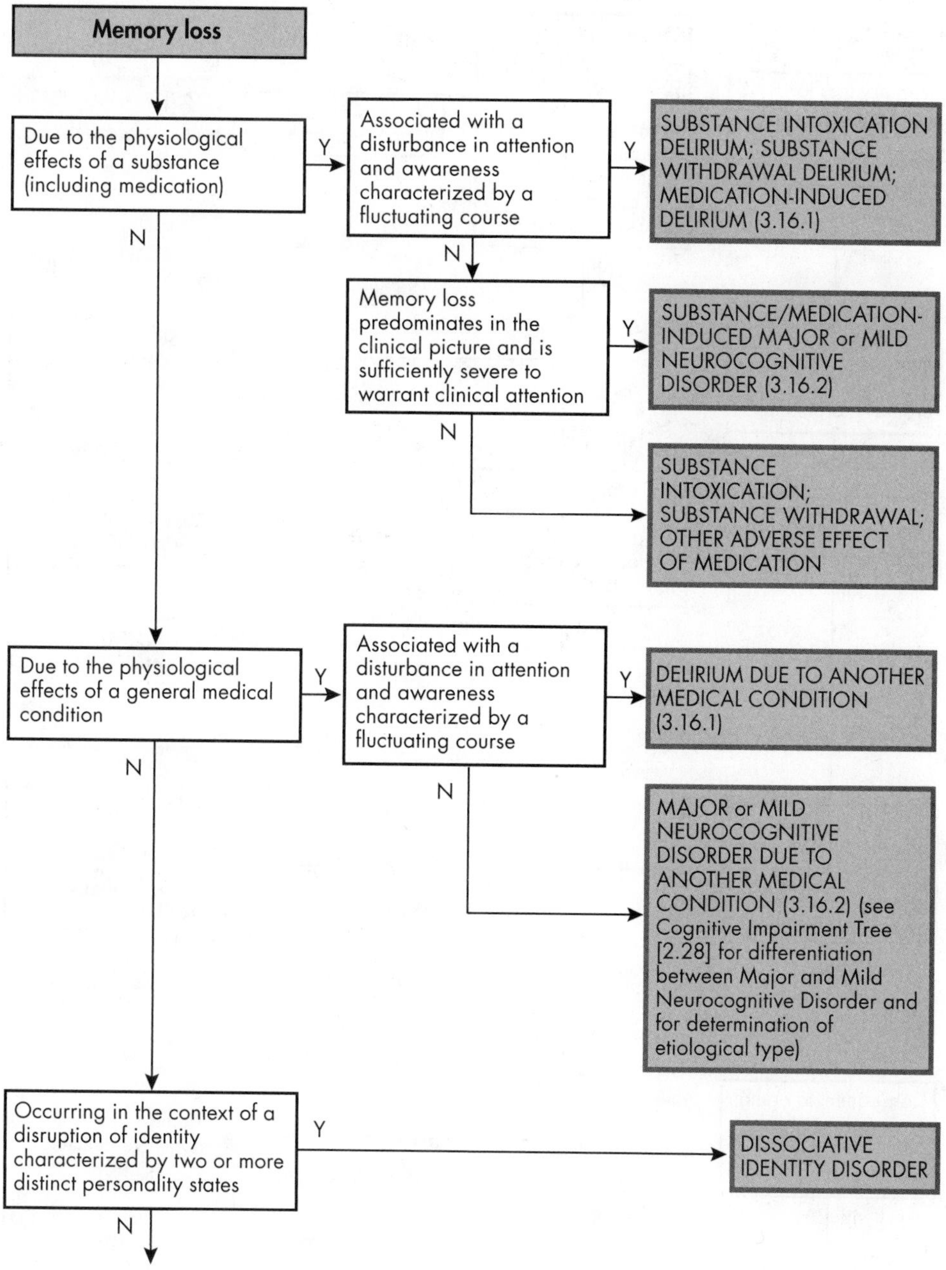
Memory loss
Due to the physiological effects of a substance (including medication)
Y
Associated with a disturbance in attention and awareness characterized by a fluctuating course
Y
SUBSTANCE INTOXICATION DELIRIUM; SUBSTANCE WITHDRAWAL DELIRIUM; MEDICATION-INDUCED DELIRIUM (3.16.1)
N
Memory loss predominates in the clinical picture and is sufficiently severe to warrant clinical attention
Y
SUBSTANCE/MEDICATION-INDUCED MAJOR or MILD NEUROCOGNITIVE DISORDER (3.16.2)
N
SUBSTANCE INTOXICATION; SUBSTANCE WITHDRAWAL; OTHER ADVERSE EFFECT OF MEDICATION
N
Due to the physiological effects of a general medical condition
Y
Associated with a disturbance in attention and awareness characterized by a fluctuating course
Y
DELIRIUM DUE TO ANOTHER MEDICAL CONDITION (3.16.1)
N
MAJOR or MILD NEUROCOGNITIVE DISORDER DUE TO ANOTHER MEDICAL CONDITION (3.16.2) (see Cognitive Impairment Tree [2.28] for differentiation between Major and Mild Neurocognitive Disorder and for determination of etiological type)
N
Occurring in the context of a disruption of identity characterized by two or more distinct personality states
Y
DISSOCIATIVE IDENTITY DISORDER
N

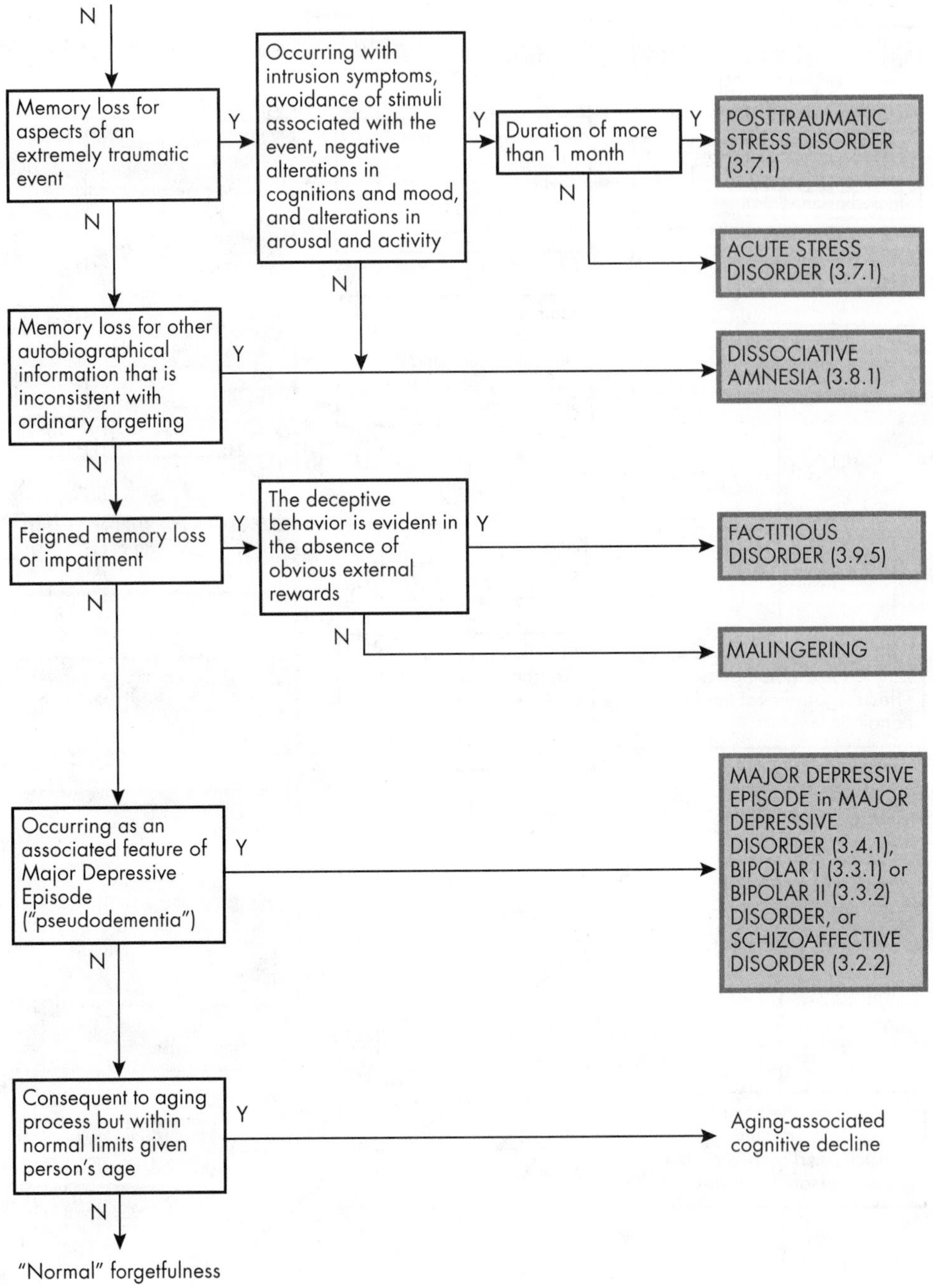
N
Memory loss for aspects of an extremely traumatic event
Y
Occurring with intrusion symptoms, avoidance of stimuli associated with the event, negative alterations in cognitions and mood, and alterations in arousal and activity
Y
Duration of more than 1 month
Y
POSTTRAUMATIC STRESS DISORDER (3.7.1)
N
ACUTE STRESS DISORDER (3.7.1)
N
N
Memory loss for other autobiographical information that is inconsistent with ordinary forgetting
Y
DISSOCIATIVE AMNESIA (3.8.1)
N
Feigned memory loss or impairment
Y
The deceptive behavior is evident in the absence of obvious external rewards
Y
FACTITIOUS DISORDER (3.9.5)
N
MALINGERING
N
Occurring as an associated feature of Major Depressive Episode ("pseudodementia")
Y
MAJOR DEPRESSIVE EPISODE in MAJOR DEPRESSIVE DISORDER (3.4.1), BIPOLAR I (3.3.1) or BIPOLAR II (3.3.2) DISORDER, or SCHIZOAFFECTIVE DISORDER (3.2.2)
N
Consequent to aging process but within normal limits given person's age
Y
Aging-associated cognitive decline
N
"Normal" forgetfulness

2.28 Decision Tree for Cognitive Impairment

Although *cognitive impairment* is a broad term that can include impairment in virtually any cognitive function, in the context of this decision tree, the term is referring to impairment in one of the cognitive domains listed in the criteria for Major or Mild Neurocognitive Disorder: complex attention, executive function, learning and memory, language, perceptual-motor, or social cognition. If cognitive impairment is restricted to memory loss, you should refer to the decision tree for memory loss (2.27) for the differential diagnosis.

The pattern of cognitive impairments that defines the Delirium syndrome is rather specific. The hallmark of Delirium is a clouding of consciousness characterized by a disturbance in attention (i.e., a reduced ability to direct, focus, sustain, and shift attention) and awareness (i.e., by reduced orientation to the environment) that develops over a short period of time and fluctuates in severity during the course of a day. The definition of Delirium also requires an accompanying disturbance in cognition (which can take the form of memory impairment, language, visuospatial ability, or perception). Once the syndrome of Delirium is established, the actual DSM-5 diagnosis depends on the etiology; Delirium can be due to multiple etiologies (Delirium Due to Multiple Etiologies), to the physiological effects of a substance or medication (Substance Intoxication Delirium, Substance Withdrawal Delirium, Medication-Induced Delirium), or to the physiological effects of a general medical condition (Delirium Due to Another Medical Condition).

Significant cognitive impairment also occurs in the context of various mental disorders. Although cognitive impairment is not one of the defining symptoms of Schizophrenia, cognitive symptoms, especially decrements in declarative and working memory, language function, and other executive functions, are extremely common and are a major contributor to the poor long-term functioning that often characterizes Schizophrenia. Similarly, although many individuals in the midst of a Manic Episode feel more confident in their cognitive abilities, in between mood episodes there may be significant cognitive impairment that has a negative impact on long-term functioning. Depressive Disorders, such as Major Depressive Disorder and Persistent Depressive Disorder (Dysthymia), are characterized by diminished ability to think or concentrate that in some cases can be so severe as to resemble a dementing illness ("pseudodementia"). Difficulty with concentration is common during the dysphoric periods in Premenstrual Dysphoric Disorder, and is also part of the symptomatic pictures of Posttraumatic Stress Disorder, Acute Stress Disorder, and Generalized Anxiety Disorder. Inattention and distractibility are defining features of Attention-Deficit/Hyperactivity Disorder. Because Major or Mild Neurocognitive Disorder may still occur comorbidly with these conditions, the decision tree instructs you to keep moving down toward Neurocognitive Disorder if not all of the cognitive symptoms that are part of the presenting picture are accounted for by the mental disorder.

Neurocognitive Disorders are divided into Major and Mild Neurocognitive Disorder and typed by etiology. They differ based on whether the individual has a substantial impairment in cognitive functions that interferes with independence (Major Neurocognitive Disorder) or has modest declines in functions that are insufficiently severe to interfere with the capacity for independence in everyday activities (Mild Neurocognitive Disorder). Because of the relatively greater clinical importance of Major Neurocognitive Disorder, this decision tree provides the decision points for determining the etiological type only for this condition. The same decision points would apply to the determination of the etiological type for Mild Neurocognitive Disorder as well.

As was the case for Delirium, if the Major Neurocognitive Disorder has more than one contributing etiological factor, Major Neurocognitive Disorder Due to Multiple Etiologies is diagnosed. Otherwise, decision points are given for the various specific medical etiologies, starting with Parkinson's disease, then followed by traumatic brain injury, HIV infection, Huntington's disease, prion disease (e.g., Creutzfeldt-Jakob disease), frontotemporal lobar degeneration (e.g., Pick's disease), Lewy body disease, vascular disease, and Alzheimer's disease. Several etiologies (i.e., Parkinson's disease, frontotemporal lobar degeneration, Lewy body disease, vascular disease, and Alzheimer's disease) must be further specified as being "probable" or "possible" based on specific diagnostic criteria. If another medical etiology is responsible for the Major Neurocognitive Disorder (e.g., multiple sclerosis), Major Neurocognitive Disorder Due to Another Medical Condition is diagnosed. Finally, if the Major Neurocognitive Disorder is caused by the physiological effects of a substance that persist beyond acute intoxication or withdrawal, Substance/Medication-Induced Major Neurocognitive Disorder is diagnosed. If the etiology for Major or Mild Neurocognitive Disorder cannot be determined, then Unspecified Neurocognitive Disorder is diagnosed.

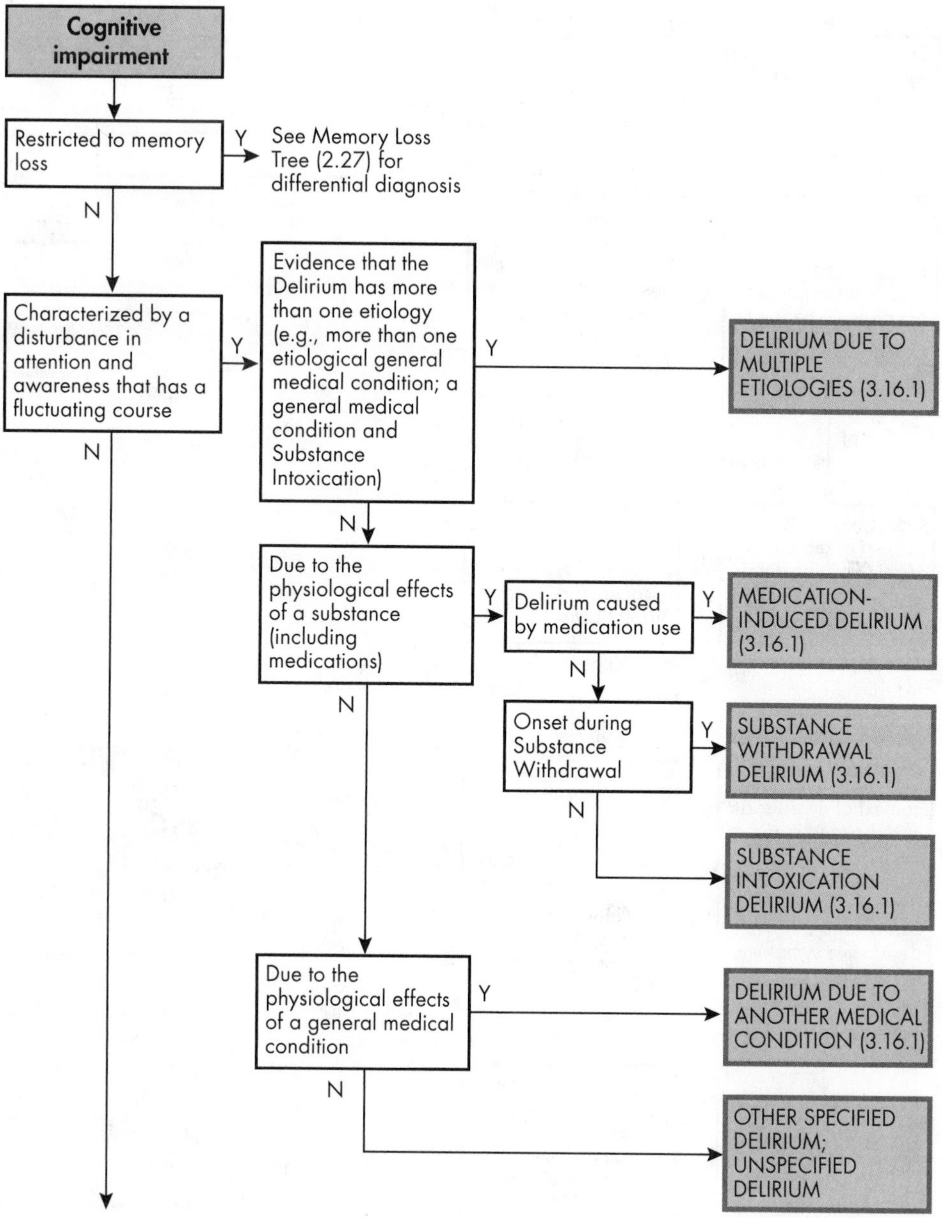
Cognitive impairment
Restricted to memory loss
Y
See Memory Loss Tree (2.27) for differential diagnosis
N
Characterized by a disturbance in attention and awareness that has a fluctuating course
Y
Evidence that the Delirium has more than one etiology (e.g., more than one etiological general medical condition; a general medical condition and Substance Intoxication)
Y
DELIRIUM DUE TO MULTIPLE ETIOLOGIES (3.16.1)
N
Due to the physiological effects of a substance (including medications)
Y
Delirium caused by medication use
Y
MEDICATION-INDUCED DELIRIUM (3.16.1)
N
Onset during Substance Withdrawal
Y
SUBSTANCE WITHDRAWAL DELIRIUM (3.16.1)
N
SUBSTANCE INTOXICATION DELIRIUM (3.16.1)
N
Due to the physiological effects of a general medical condition
Y
DELIRIUM DUE TO ANOTHER MEDICAL CONDITION (3.16.1)
N
OTHER SPECIFIED DELIRIUM; UNSPECIFIED DELIRIUM
N

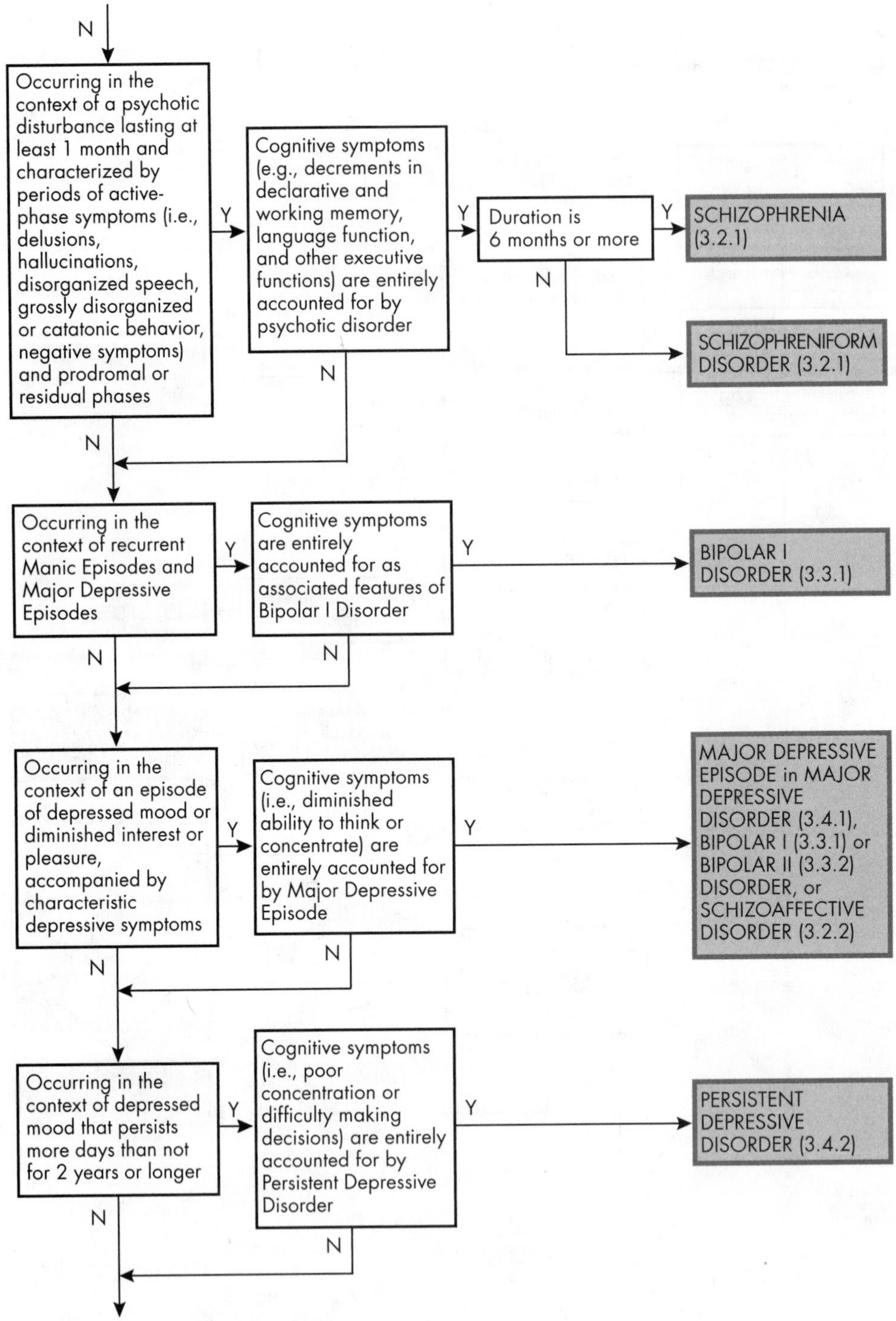
N
Occurring in the context of a psychotic disturbance lasting at least 1 month and characterized by periods of active-phase symptoms (i.e., delusions, hallucinations, disorganized speech, grossly disorganized or catatonic behavior, negative symptoms) and prodromal or residual phases
Y
Cognitive symptoms (e.g., decrements in declarative and working memory, language function, and other executive functions) are entirely accounted for by psychotic disorder
Y
Duration is 6 months or more
Y
SCHIZOPHRENIA (3.2.1)
N
SCHIZOPHRENIFORM DISORDER (3.2.1)
N
N
Occurring in the context of recurrent Manic Episodes and Major Depressive Episodes
Y
Cognitive symptoms are entirely accounted for as associated features of Bipolar I Disorder
Y
BIPOLAR I DISORDER (3.3.1)
N
N
Occurring in the context of an episode of depressed mood or diminished interest or pleasure, accompanied by characteristic depressive symptoms
Y
Cognitive symptoms (i.e., diminished ability to think or concentrate) are entirely accounted for by Major Depressive Episode
Y
MAJOR DEPRESSIVE EPISODE in MAJOR DEPRESSIVE DISORDER (3.4.1), BIPOLAR I (3.3.1) or BIPOLAR II (3.3.2) DISORDER, or SCHIZOAFFECTIVE DISORDER (3.2.2)
N
N
Occurring in the context of depressed mood that persists more days than not for 2 years or longer
Y
Cognitive symptoms (i.e., poor concentration or difficulty making decisions) are entirely accounted for by Persistent Depressive Disorder
Y
PERSISTENT DEPRESSIVE DISORDER (3.4.2)
N
N

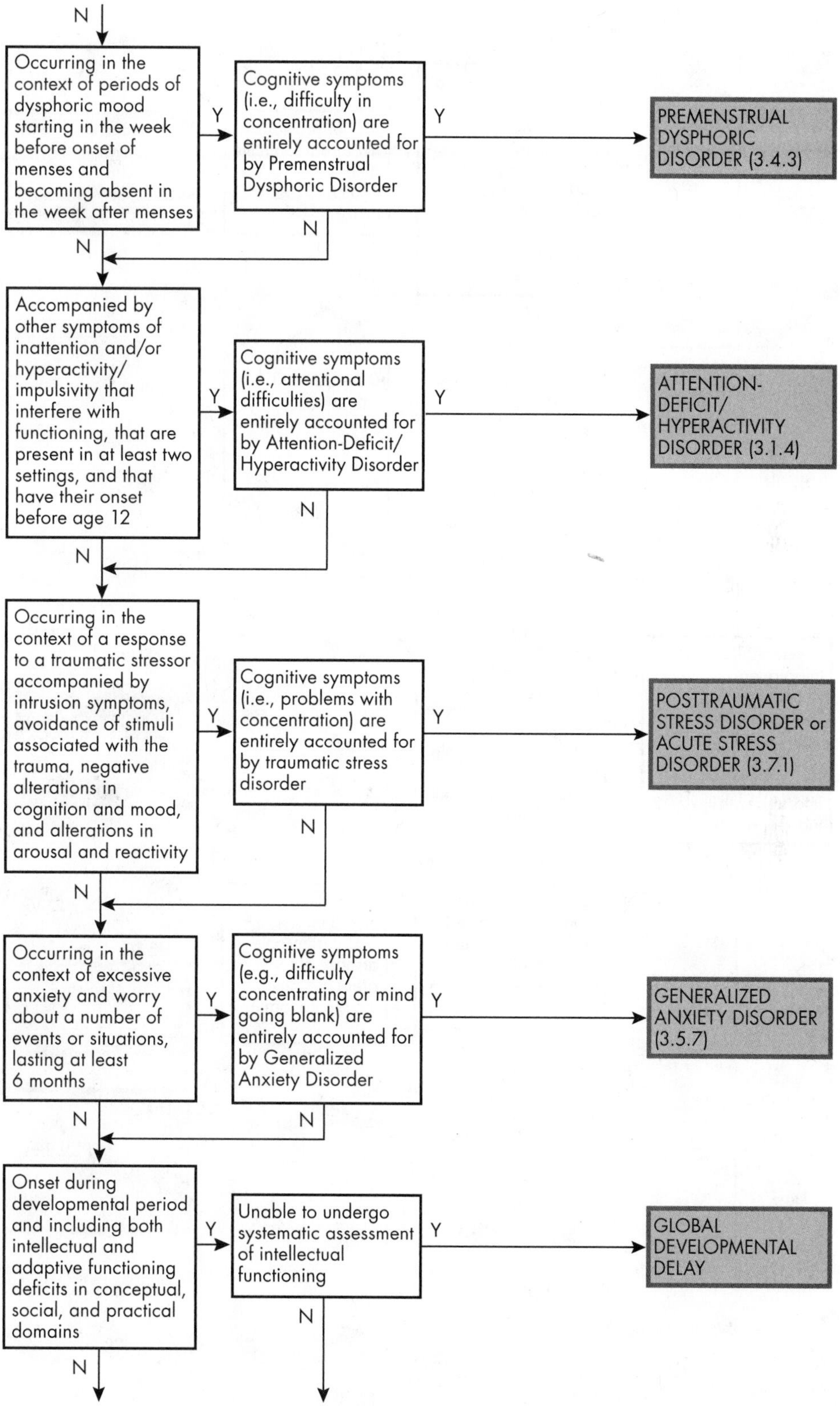
N
Occurring in the context of periods of dysphoric mood starting in the week before onset of menses and becoming absent in the week after menses
Y
Cognitive symptoms (i.e., difficulty in concentration) are entirely accounted for by Premenstrual Dysphoric Disorder
Y
PREMENSTRUAL DYSPHORIC DISORDER (3.4.3)
N
N
Accompanied by other symptoms of inattention and/or hyperactivity/impulsivity that interfere with functioning, that are present in at least two settings, and that have their onset before age 12
Y
Cognitive symptoms (i.e., attentional difficulties) are entirely accounted for by Attention-Deficit/Hyperactivity Disorder
Y
ATTENTION-DEFICIT/HYPERACTIVITY DISORDER (3.1.4)
N
N
Occurring in the context of a response to a traumatic stressor accompanied by intrusion symptoms, avoidance of stimuli associated with the trauma, negative alterations in cognition and mood, and alterations in arousal and reactivity
Y
Cognitive symptoms (i.e., problems with concentration) are entirely accounted for by traumatic stress disorder
Y
POSTTRAUMATIC STRESS DISORDER or ACUTE STRESS DISORDER (3.7.1)
N
N
Occurring in the context of excessive anxiety and worry about a number of events or situations, lasting at least 6 months
Y
Cognitive symptoms (e.g., difficulty concentrating or mind going blank) are entirely accounted for by Generalized Anxiety Disorder
Y
GENERALIZED ANXIETY DISORDER (3.5.7)
N
N
Onset during developmental period and including both intellectual and adaptive functioning deficits in conceptual, social, and practical domains
Y
Unable to undergo systematic assessment of intellectual functioning
Y
GLOBAL DEVELOPMENTAL DELAY
N
N

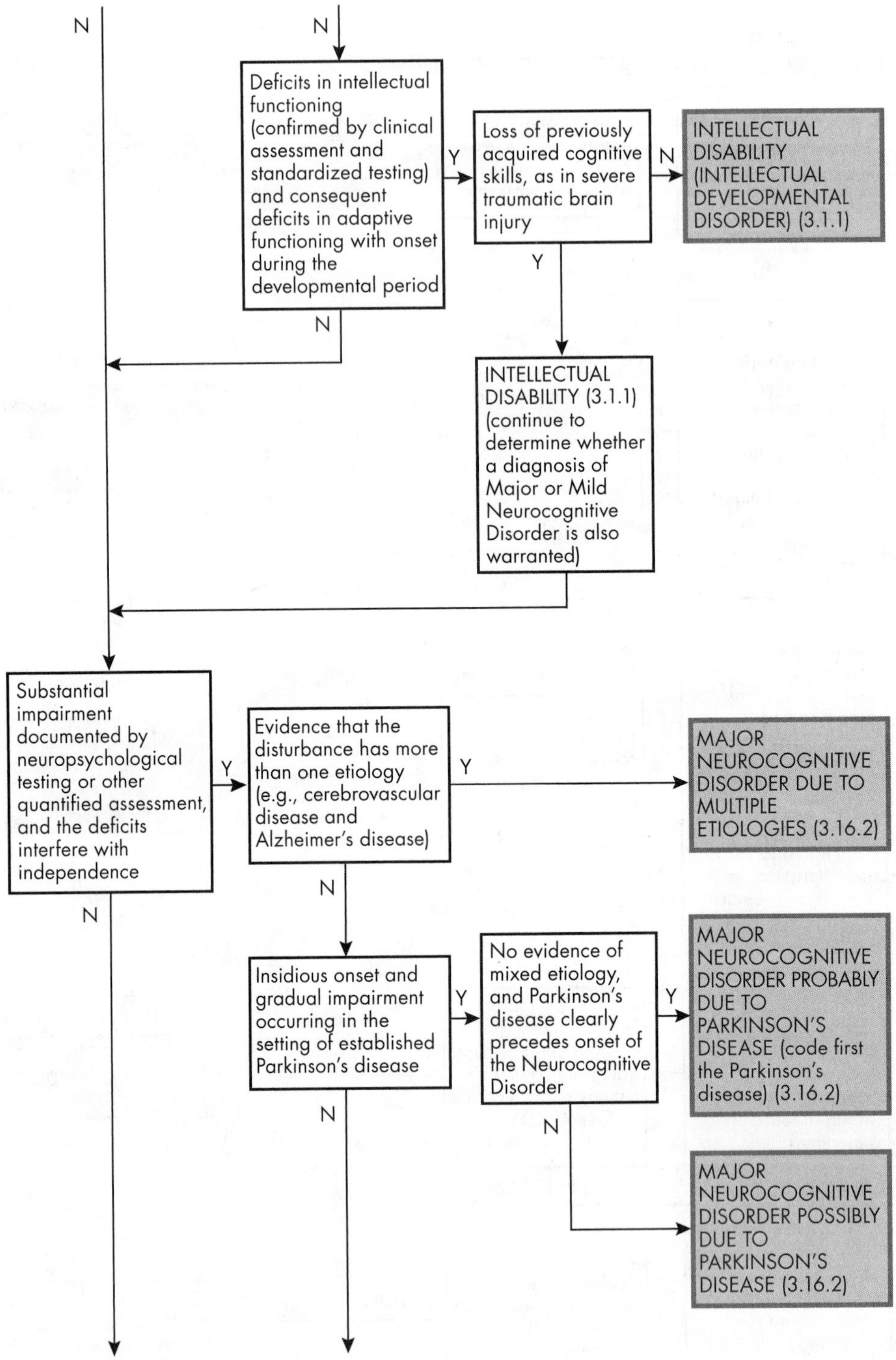
N
N
Deficits in intellectual functioning (confirmed by clinical assessment and standardized testing) and consequent deficits in adaptive functioning with onset during the developmental period
Y
Loss of previously acquired cognitive skills, as in severe traumatic brain injury
N
INTELLECTUAL DISABILITY (INTELLECTUAL DEVELOPMENTAL DISORDER) (3.1.1)
Y
N
INTELLECTUAL DISABILITY (3.1.1) (continue to determine whether a diagnosis of Major or Mild Neurocognitive Disorder is also warranted)
Substantial impairment documented by neuropsychological testing or other quantified assessment, and the deficits interfere with independence
Y
Evidence that the disturbance has more than one etiology (e.g., cerebrovascular disease and Alzheimer's disease)
Y
MAJOR NEUROCOGNITIVE DISORDER DUE TO MULTIPLE ETIOLOGIES (3.16.2)
N
N
Insidious onset and gradual impairment occurring in the setting of established Parkinson's disease
Y
No evidence of mixed etiology, and Parkinson's disease clearly precedes onset of the Neurocognitive Disorder
Y
MAJOR NEUROCOGNITIVE DISORDER PROBABLY DUE TO PARKINSON'S DISEASE (code first the Parkinson's disease) (3.16.2)
N
N
MAJOR NEUROCOGNITIVE DISORDER POSSIBLY DUE TO PARKINSON'S DISEASE (3.16.2)

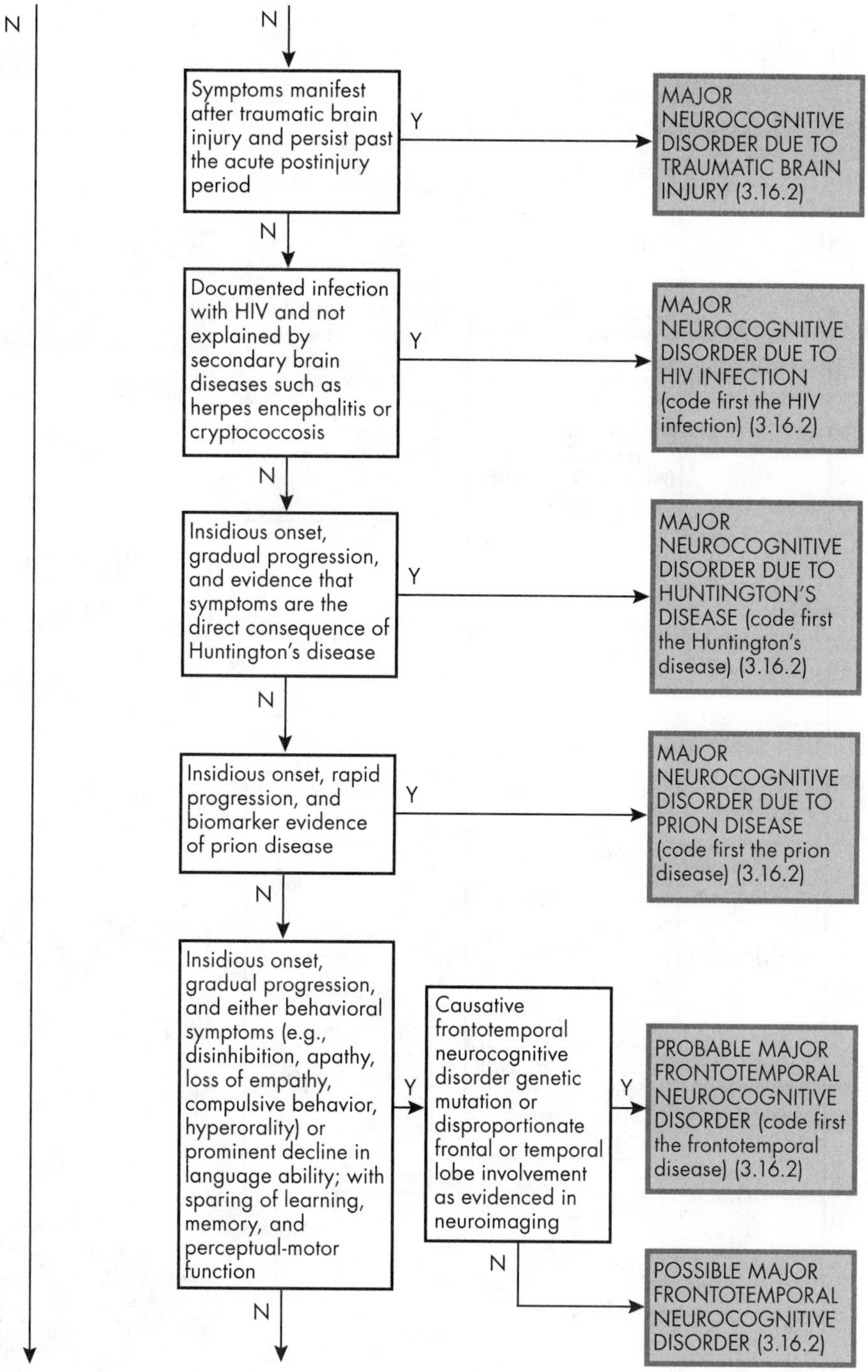
N
N
Symptoms manifest after traumatic brain injury and persist past the acute postinjury period
Y
MAJOR NEUROCOGNITIVE DISORDER DUE TO TRAUMATIC BRAIN INJURY (3.16.2)
N
Documented infection with HIV and not explained by secondary brain diseases such as herpes encephalitis or cryptococcosis
Y
MAJOR NEUROCOGNITIVE DISORDER DUE TO HIV INFECTION (code first the HIV infection) (3.16.2)
N
Insidious onset, gradual progression, and evidence that symptoms are the direct consequence of Huntington's disease
Y
MAJOR NEUROCOGNITIVE DISORDER DUE TO HUNTINGTON'S DISEASE (code first the Huntington's disease) (3.16.2)
N
Insidious onset, rapid progression, and biomarker evidence of prion disease
Y
MAJOR NEUROCOGNITIVE DISORDER DUE TO PRION DISEASE (code first the prion disease) (3.16.2)
N
Insidious onset, gradual progression, and either behavioral symptoms (e.g., disinhibition, apathy, loss of empathy, compulsive behavior, hyperorality) or prominent decline in language ability; with sparing of learning, memory, and perceptual-motor function
Y
Causative frontotemporal neurocognitive disorder genetic mutation or disproportionate frontal or temporal lobe involvement as evidenced in neuroimaging
Y
PROBABLE MAJOR FRONTOTEMPORAL NEUROCOGNITIVE DISORDER (code first the frontotemporal disease) (3.16.2)
N
POSSIBLE MAJOR FRONTOTEMPORAL NEUROCOGNITIVE DISORDER (3.16.2)
N

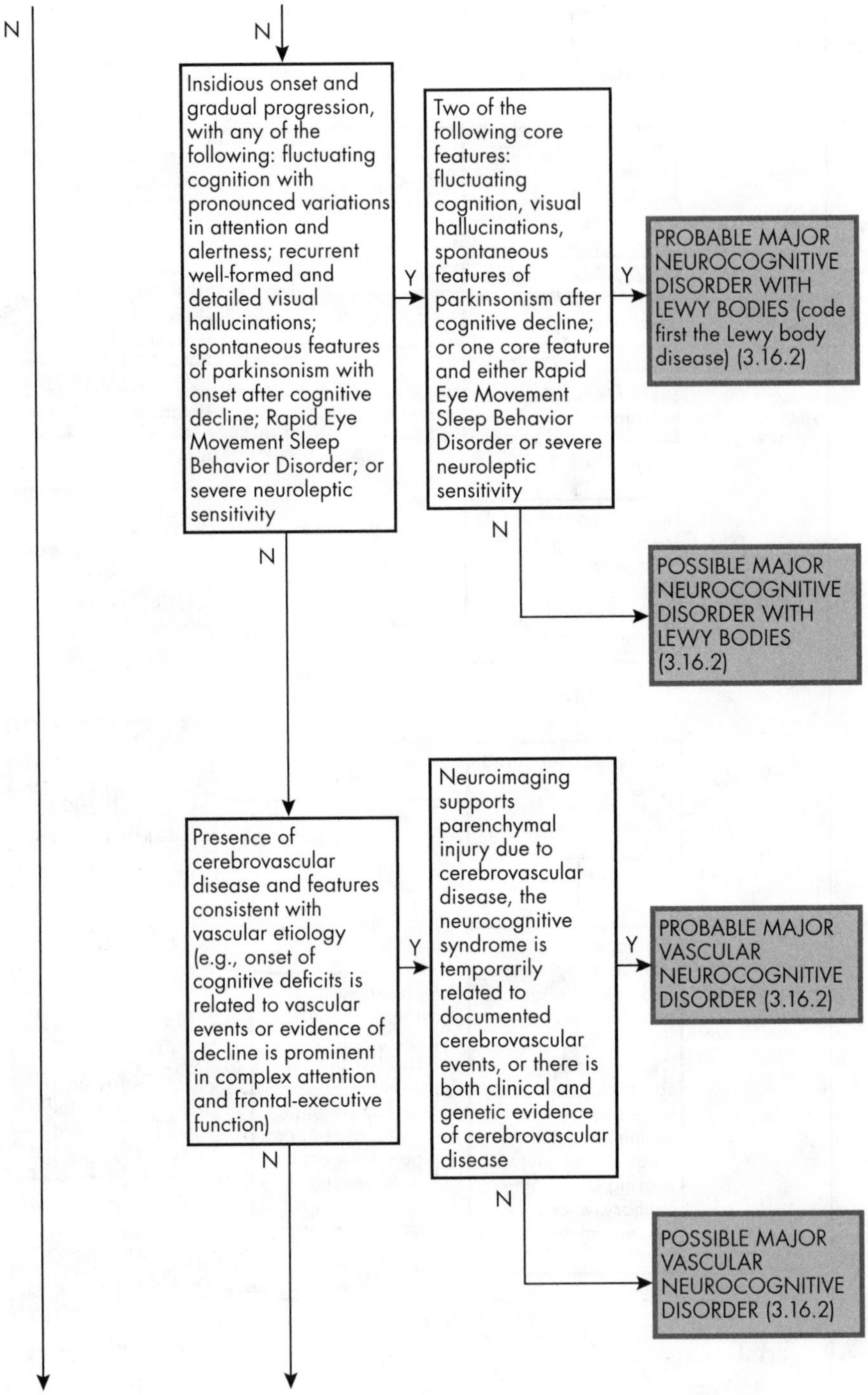
N
N
Insidious onset and gradual progression, with any of the following: fluctuating cognition with pronounced variations in attention and alertness; recurrent well-formed and detailed visual hallucinations; spontaneous features of parkinsonism with onset after cognitive decline; Rapid Eye Movement Sleep Behavior Disorder; or severe neuroleptic sensitivity
Y
Two of the following core features: fluctuating cognition, visual hallucinations, spontaneous features of parkinsonism after cognitive decline; or one core feature and either Rapid Eye Movement Sleep Behavior Disorder or severe neuroleptic sensitivity
Y
PROBABLE MAJOR NEUROCOGNITIVE DISORDER WITH LEWY BODIES (code first the Lewy body disease) (3.16.2)
N
POSSIBLE MAJOR NEUROCOGNITIVE DISORDER WITH LEWY BODIES (3.16.2)
N
Presence of cerebrovascular disease and features consistent with vascular etiology (e.g., onset of cognitive deficits is related to vascular events or evidence of decline is prominent in complex attention and frontal-executive function)
Y
Neuroimaging supports parenchymal injury due to cerebrovascular disease, the neurocognitive syndrome is temporarily related to documented cerebrovascular events, or there is both clinical and genetic evidence of cerebrovascular disease
Y
PROBABLE MAJOR VASCULAR NEUROCOGNITIVE DISORDER (3.16.2)
N
POSSIBLE MAJOR VASCULAR NEUROCOGNITIVE DISORDER (3.16.2)
N

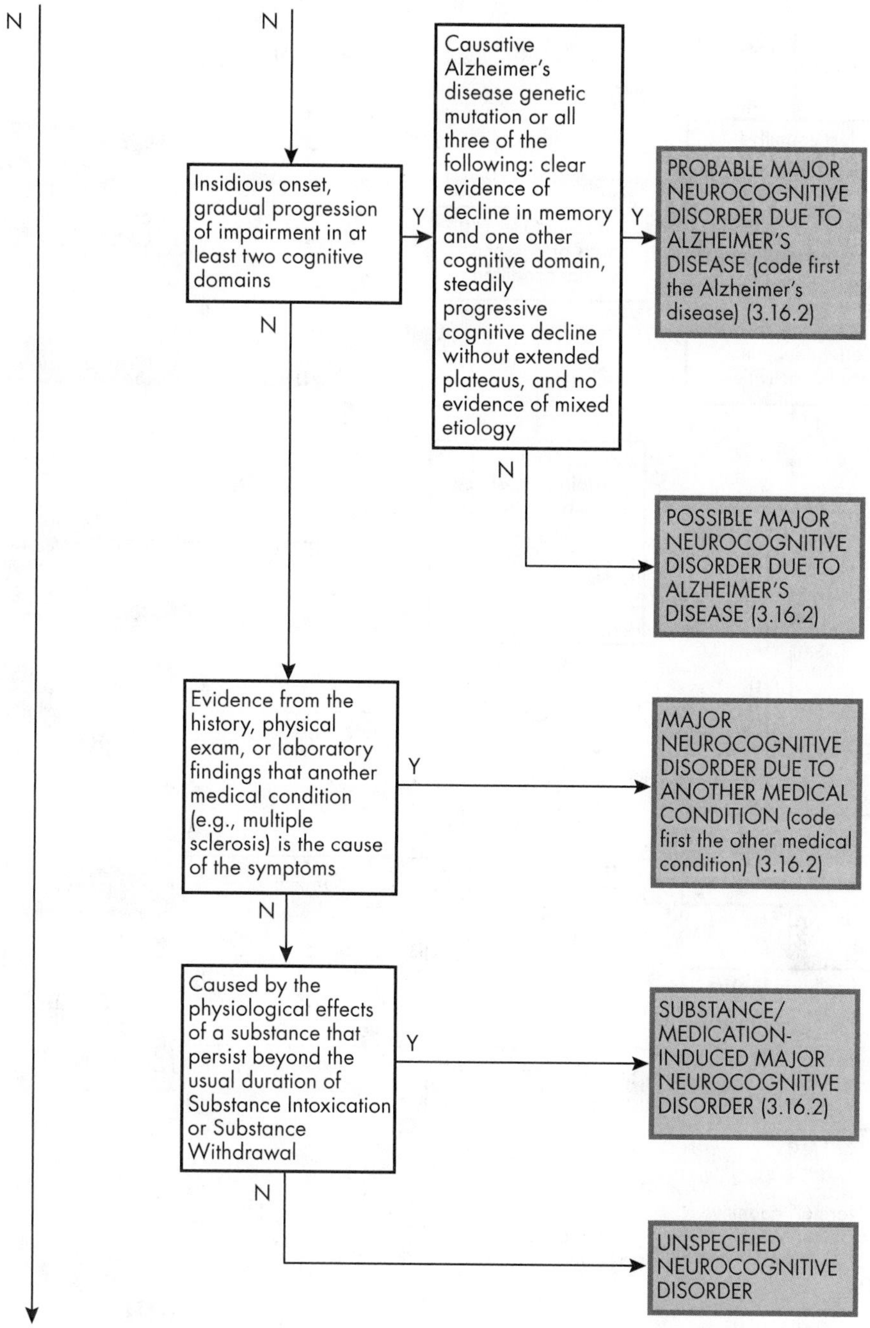
N
N
Insidious onset, gradual progression of impairment in at least two cognitive domains
Y
Causative Alzheimer's disease genetic mutation or all three of the following: clear evidence of decline in memory and one other cognitive domain, steadily progressive cognitive decline without extended plateaus, and no evidence of mixed etiology
Y
PROBABLE MAJOR NEUROCOGNITIVE DISORDER DUE TO ALZHEIMER'S DISEASE (code first the Alzheimer's disease) (3.16.2)
N
POSSIBLE MAJOR NEUROCOGNITIVE DISORDER DUE TO ALZHEIMER'S DISEASE (3.16.2)
N
Evidence from the history, physical exam, or laboratory findings that another medical condition (e.g., multiple sclerosis) is the cause of the symptoms
Y
MAJOR NEUROCOGNITIVE DISORDER DUE TO ANOTHER MEDICAL CONDITION (code first the other medical condition) (3.16.2)
N
Caused by the physiological effects of a substance that persist beyond the usual duration of Substance Intoxication or Substance Withdrawal
Y
SUBSTANCE/ MEDICATION-INDUCED MAJOR NEUROCOGNITIVE DISORDER (3.16.2)
N
UNSPECIFIED NEUROCOGNITIVE DISORDER

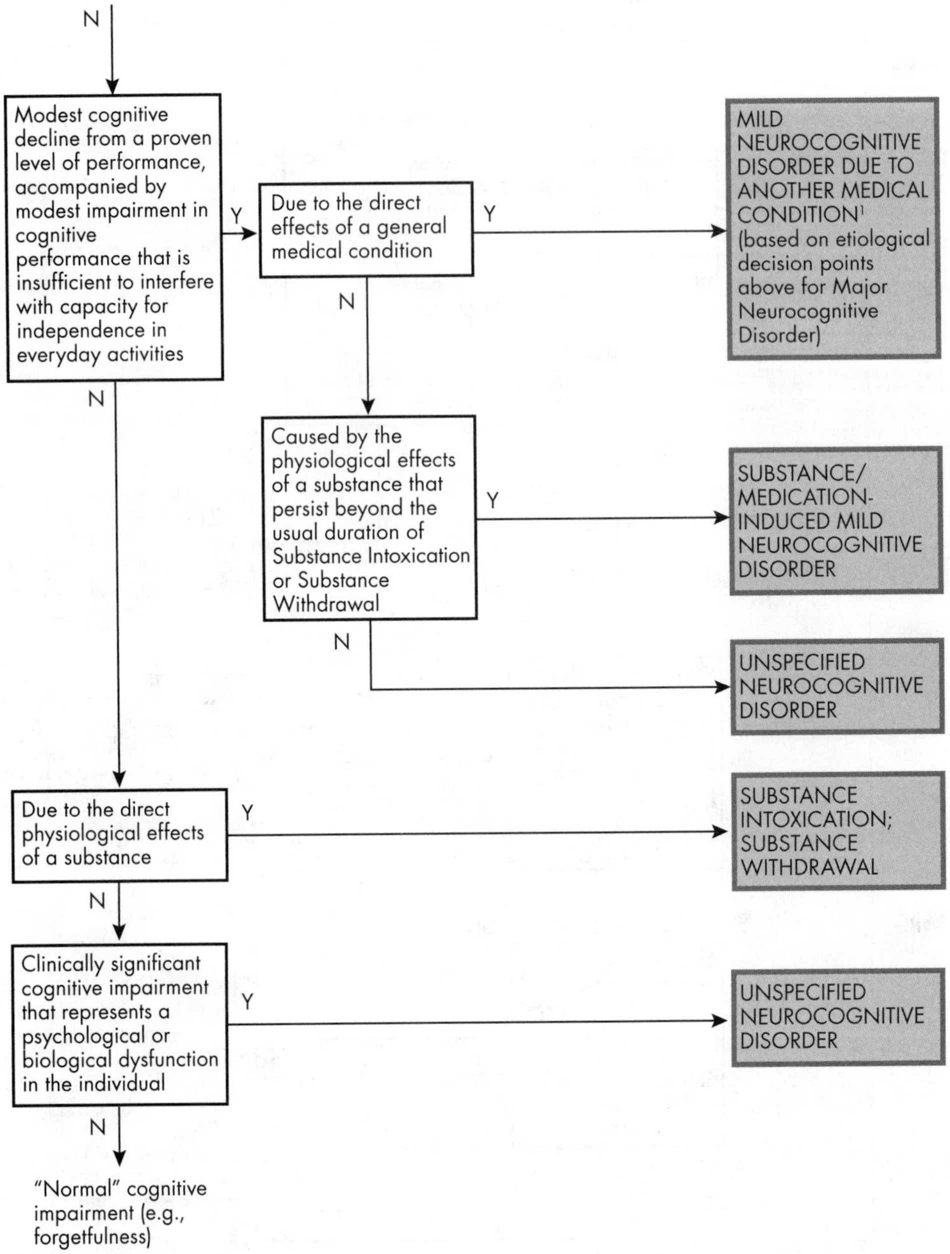

[1] The specific decision points for determining the various etiological types of Mild Neurocognitive Disorder have been omitted from this decision tree for brevity. Review the decision points for the various etiological types of Major Neurocognitive Disorder and consult the DSM-5 criteria.

2.29 Decision Tree for Etiological Medical Conditions

A crucial step in the evaluation of every patient is to consider the possibility that the symptoms are due to the direct physiological effect of a general medical condition (see Step 3 in Chapter 1). In fact, psychiatric symptoms are sometimes the first harbinger of a not-yet-diagnosed general medical condition. Determining that a general medical condition is responsible for the psychopathology has obvious treatment implications, because treatment of the general medical condition is itself important and often results in the remission of the psychiatric symptoms.

Not every behavioral symptom arising from a general medical condition warrants a diagnosis of a Mental Disorder Due to Another Medical Condition. Certainly, most patients who are experiencing anxiety, sadness, fatigue, or sleepless nights because of a general medical condition do not have a mental disorder that would be covered in this decision tree. The disorders in this tree should be considered only when the symptoms are sufficiently severe and prolonged to warrant clinical attention. Not uncommonly, the psychiatric presentation due to a general medical condition is characterized by a mixture of symptoms from more than one section of the classification (e.g., depression, anxiety, and sleep). In most cases, you should choose the diagnosis that reflects the most prominent aspect of the symptom presentation.

Delirium Due to Multiple Etiologies is included in DSM-5 (and in this tree) to emphasize that very often these conditions have multiple interacting etiologies. Moreover, the medications used to treat general medical conditions often have behavioral side effects that may be confused both with primary psychiatric symptoms and with the psychiatric manifestations of the general medical condition itself. This is particularly common in elderly individuals who may be taking a number of different medications and have a reduced ability to metabolize (or eliminate) them.

Major and Mild Neurocognitive Disorders, especially when persistent, are most often caused by a general medical condition and are subtyped based on the specific medical etiology. They differ based on whether the individual has a substantial impairment in cognitive functions that interferes with independence (i.e., Major Neurocognitive Disorder) or has modest declines in functions that are insufficiently severe to interfere with the capacity for independence in everyday activities (i.e., Mild Neurocognitive Disorder). Because of the relatively greater clinical importance of Major Neurocognitive Disorder, this decision tree provides the decision points for determining the etiological type only for this condition. The same decision points would apply to the determination of the etiological type for Mild Neurocognitive Disorder.

Finally, when communicating or recording the diagnoses in this tree, the actual name of the etiological general medical condition should be recorded rather than the generic term "due to another medical condition" (e.g., 293.83 [F06.32] Depressive Disorder Due to Hypothyroidism, With Major Depressive-Like Episode). In addition, it is mandatory to list (and code) the etiological general medical condition on diagnostic reporting forms immediately *before* the mental disorder due to another medical condition (e.g. 244.9 [E03.9] Hypothyroidism; 293.83 [F06.32] Depressive Disorder Due to Hypothyroidism, With Major Depressive-Like Episode).

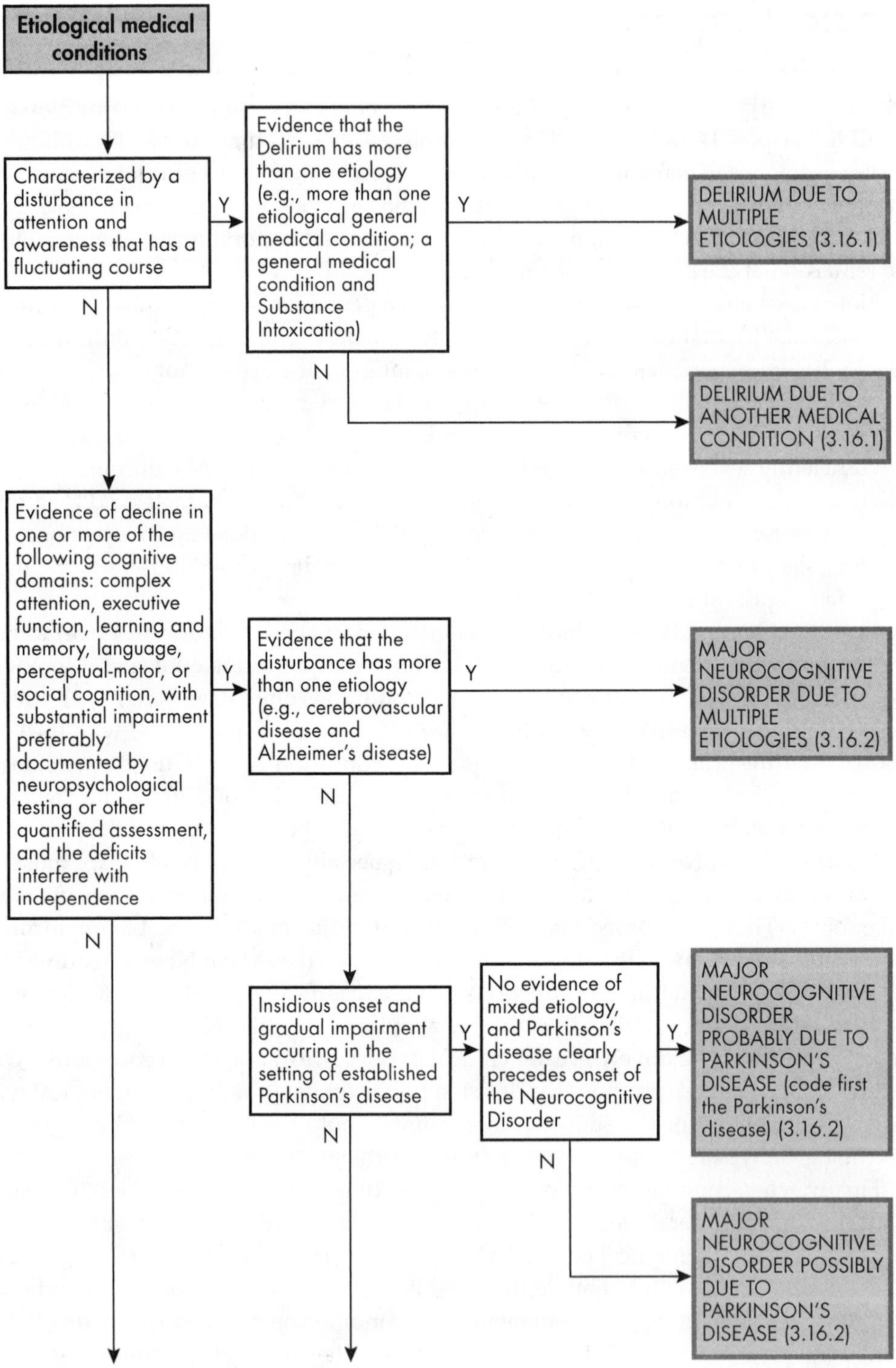
Etiological medical conditions
Characterized by a disturbance in attention and awareness that has a fluctuating course
Y
N
Evidence that the Delirium has more than one etiology (e.g., more than one etiological general medical condition; a general medical condition and Substance Intoxication)
Y
N
DELIRIUM DUE TO MULTIPLE ETIOLOGIES (3.16.1)
DELIRIUM DUE TO ANOTHER MEDICAL CONDITION (3.16.1)
Evidence of decline in one or more of the following cognitive domains: complex attention, executive function, learning and memory, language, perceptual-motor, or social cognition, with substantial impairment preferably documented by neuropsychological testing or other quantified assessment, and the deficits interfere with independence
Y
N
Evidence that the disturbance has more than one etiology (e.g., cerebrovascular disease and Alzheimer's disease)
Y
N
MAJOR NEUROCOGNITIVE DISORDER DUE TO MULTIPLE ETIOLOGIES (3.16.2)
Insidious onset and gradual impairment occurring in the setting of established Parkinson's disease
Y
N
No evidence of mixed etiology, and Parkinson's disease clearly precedes onset of the Neurocognitive Disorder
Y
N
MAJOR NEUROCOGNITIVE DISORDER PROBABLY DUE TO PARKINSON'S DISEASE (code first the Parkinson's disease) (3.16.2)
MAJOR NEUROCOGNITIVE DISORDER POSSIBLY DUE TO PARKINSON'S DISEASE (3.16.2)

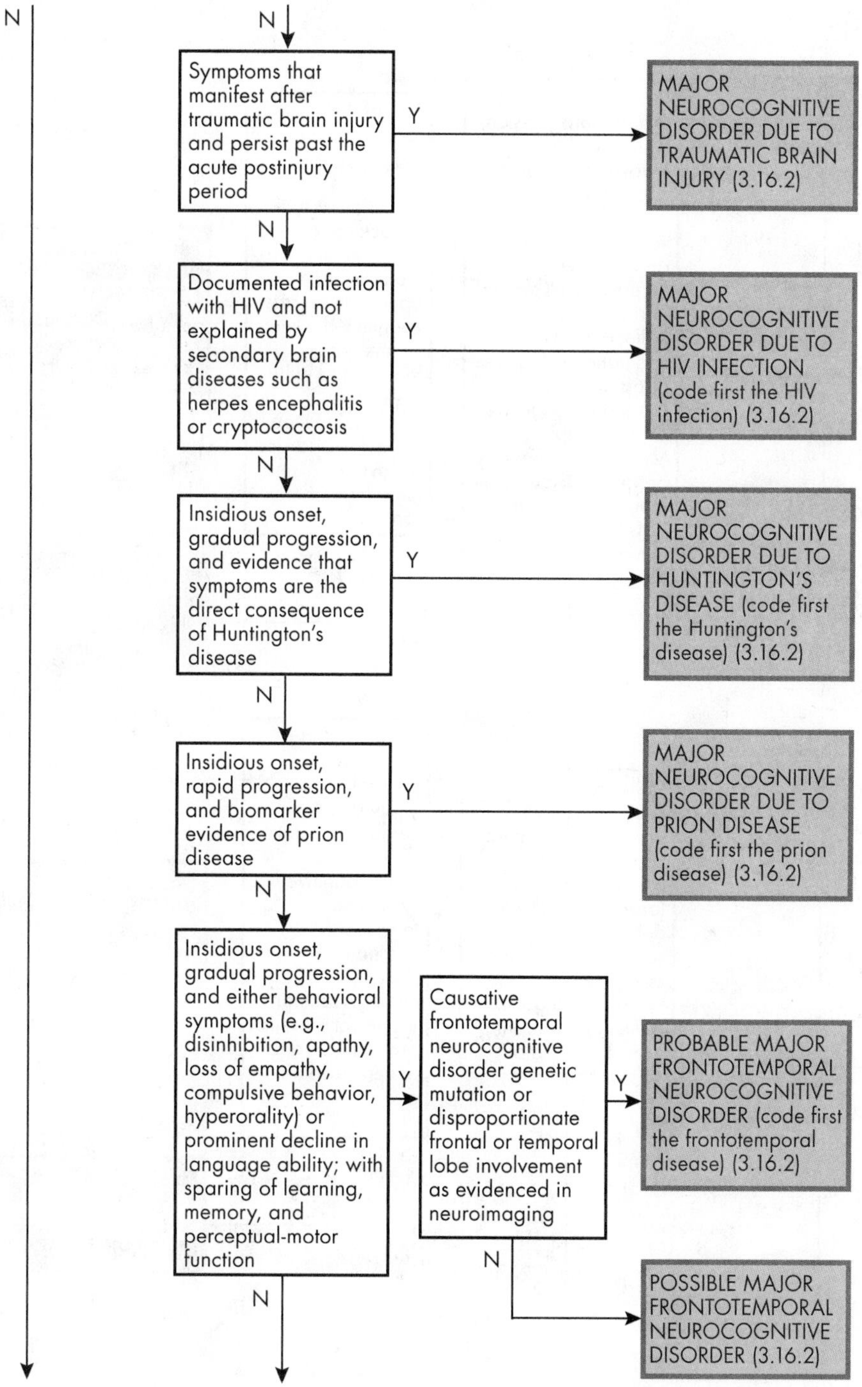
N
N
Symptoms that manifest after traumatic brain injury and persist past the acute postinjury period
Y
MAJOR NEUROCOGNITIVE DISORDER DUE TO TRAUMATIC BRAIN INJURY (3.16.2)
N
Documented infection with HIV and not explained by secondary brain diseases such as herpes encephalitis or cryptococcosis
Y
MAJOR NEUROCOGNITIVE DISORDER DUE TO HIV INFECTION (code first the HIV infection) (3.16.2)
N
Insidious onset, gradual progression, and evidence that symptoms are the direct consequence of Huntington's disease
Y
MAJOR NEUROCOGNITIVE DISORDER DUE TO HUNTINGTON'S DISEASE (code first the Huntington's disease) (3.16.2)
N
Insidious onset, rapid progression, and biomarker evidence of prion disease
Y
MAJOR NEUROCOGNITIVE DISORDER DUE TO PRION DISEASE (code first the prion disease) (3.16.2)
N
Insidious onset, gradual progression, and either behavioral symptoms (e.g., disinhibition, apathy, loss of empathy, compulsive behavior, hyperorality) or prominent decline in language ability; with sparing of learning, memory, and perceptual-motor function
Y
Causative frontotemporal neurocognitive disorder genetic mutation or disproportionate frontal or temporal lobe involvement as evidenced in neuroimaging
Y
PROBABLE MAJOR FRONTOTEMPORAL NEUROCOGNITIVE DISORDER (code first the frontotemporal disease) (3.16.2)
N
POSSIBLE MAJOR FRONTOTEMPORAL NEUROCOGNITIVE DISORDER (3.16.2)
N

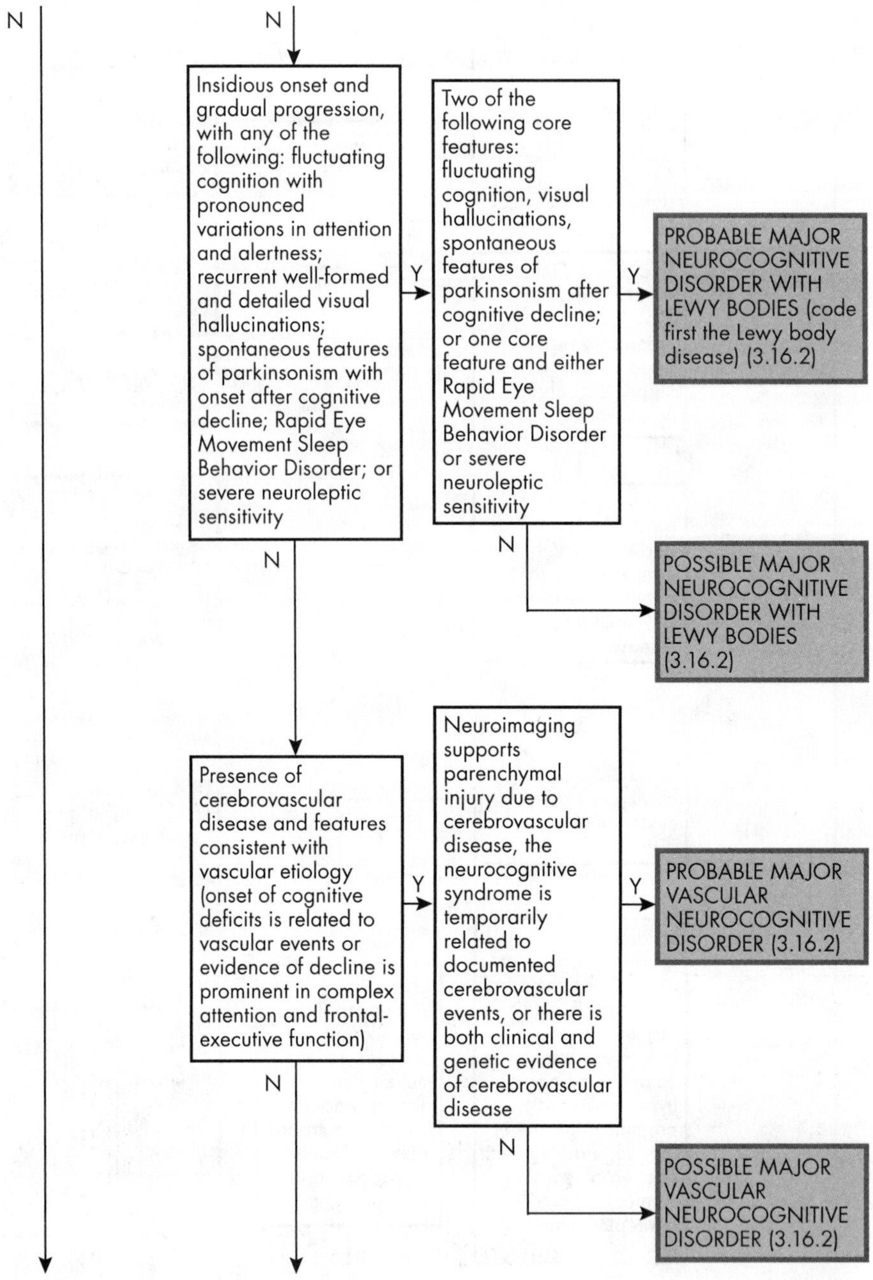
N
N
Insidious onset and gradual progression, with any of the following: fluctuating cognition with pronounced variations in attention and alertness; recurrent well-formed and detailed visual hallucinations; spontaneous features of parkinsonism with onset after cognitive decline; Rapid Eye Movement Sleep Behavior Disorder; or severe neuroleptic sensitivity
Y
Two of the following core features: fluctuating cognition, visual hallucinations, spontaneous features of parkinsonism after cognitive decline; or one core feature and either Rapid Eye Movement Sleep Behavior Disorder or severe neuroleptic sensitivity
Y
PROBABLE MAJOR NEUROCOGNITIVE DISORDER WITH LEWY BODIES (code first the Lewy body disease) (3.16.2)
N
POSSIBLE MAJOR NEUROCOGNITIVE DISORDER WITH LEWY BODIES (3.16.2)
N
Presence of cerebrovascular disease and features consistent with vascular etiology (onset of cognitive deficits is related to vascular events or evidence of decline is prominent in complex attention and frontal-executive function)
Y
Neuroimaging supports parenchymal injury due to cerebrovascular disease, the neurocognitive syndrome is temporarily related to documented cerebrovascular events, or there is both clinical and genetic evidence of cerebrovascular disease
Y
PROBABLE MAJOR VASCULAR NEUROCOGNITIVE DISORDER (3.16.2)
N
POSSIBLE MAJOR VASCULAR NEUROCOGNITIVE DISORDER (3.16.2)
N

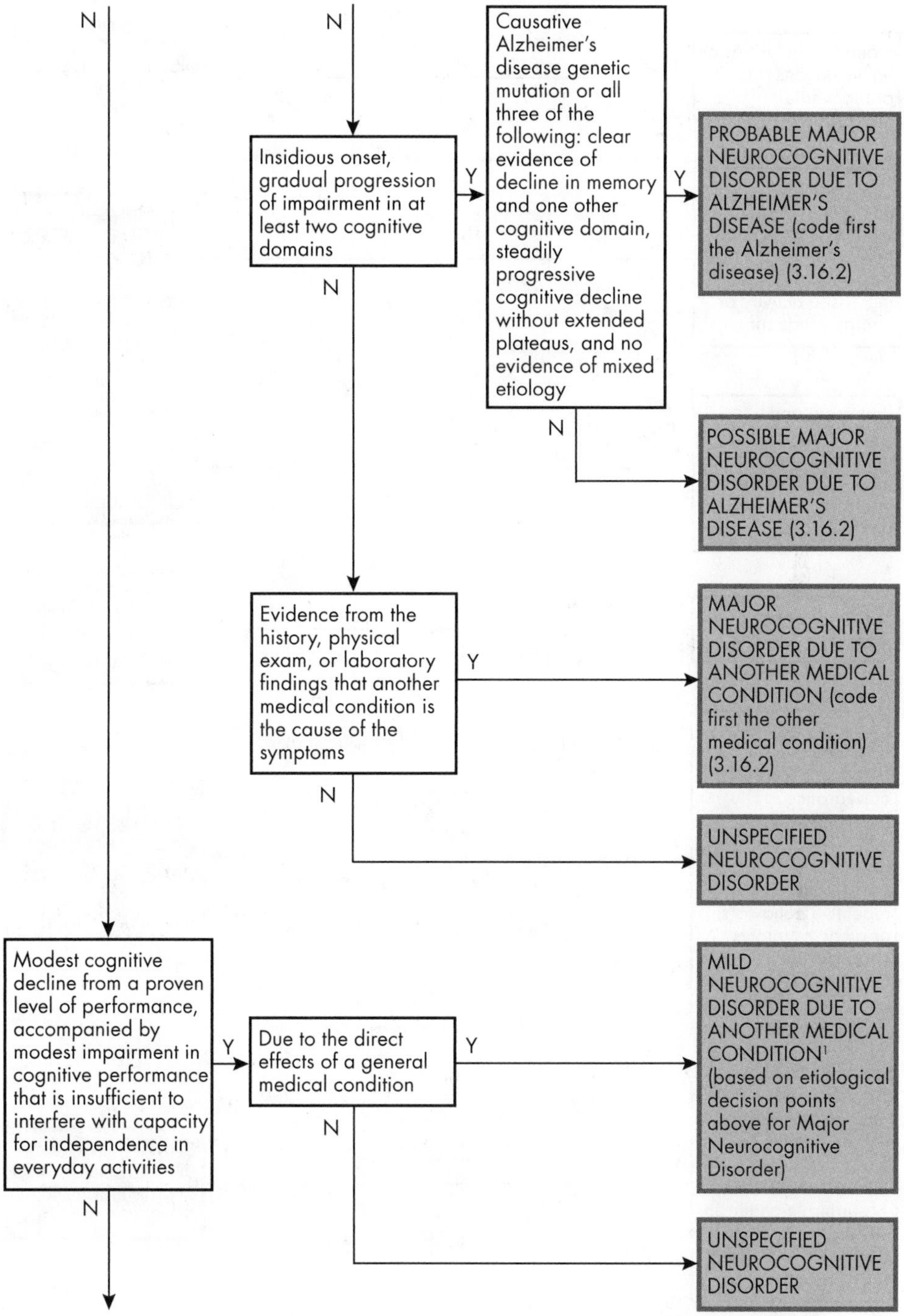

[1] The specific decision points for determining the various etiological types of Mild Neurocognitive Disorder have been omitted from this decision tree for brevity. Review the decision points for the various etiological types of Major Neurocognitive Disorder and consult the DSM-5 criteria.

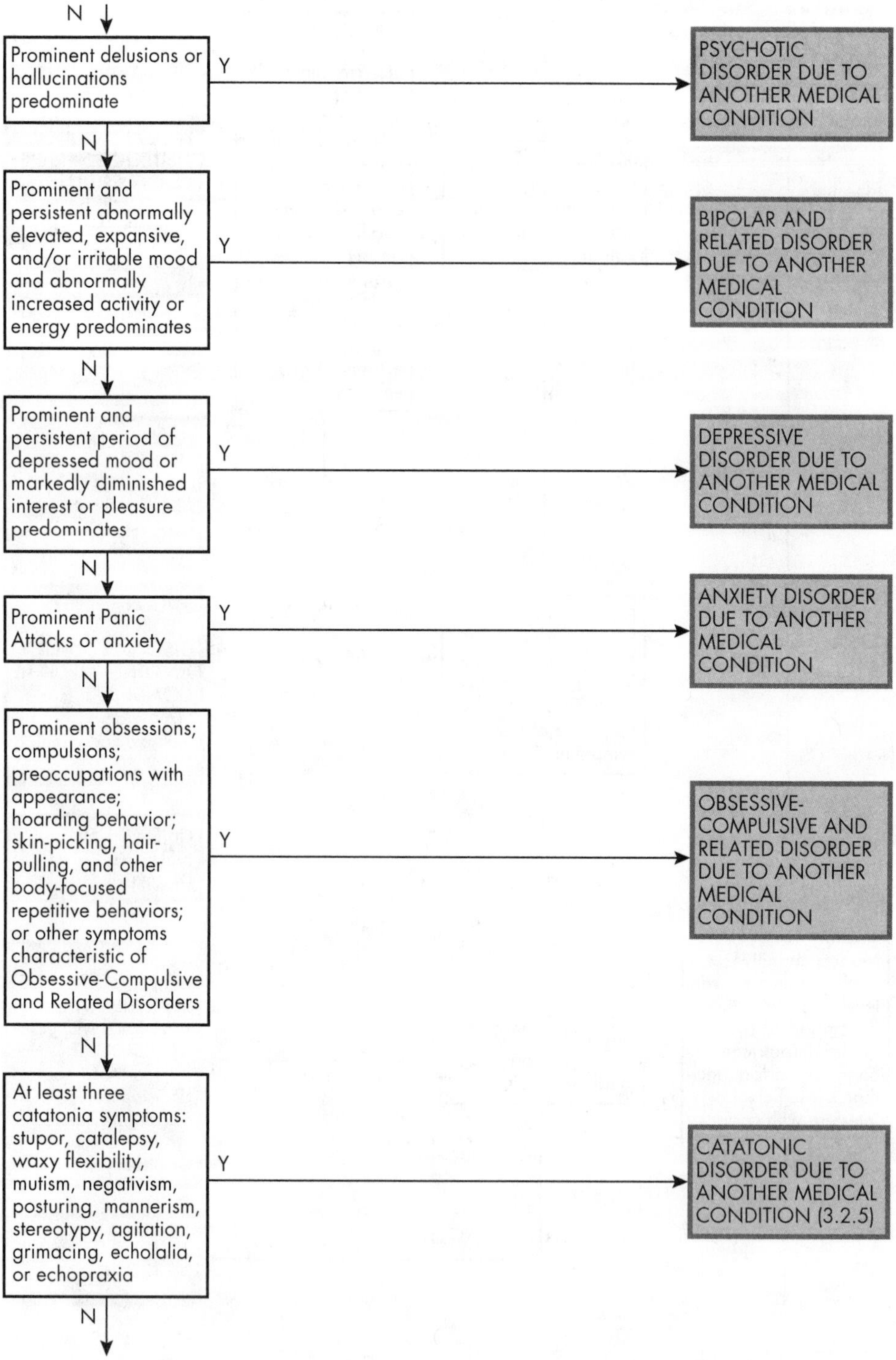
N
Prominent delusions or hallucinations predominate
Y
PSYCHOTIC DISORDER DUE TO ANOTHER MEDICAL CONDITION
N
Prominent and persistent abnormally elevated, expansive, and/or irritable mood and abnormally increased activity or energy predominates
Y
BIPOLAR AND RELATED DISORDER DUE TO ANOTHER MEDICAL CONDITION
N
Prominent and persistent period of depressed mood or markedly diminished interest or pleasure predominates
Y
DEPRESSIVE DISORDER DUE TO ANOTHER MEDICAL CONDITION
N
Prominent Panic Attacks or anxiety
Y
ANXIETY DISORDER DUE TO ANOTHER MEDICAL CONDITION
N
Prominent obsessions; compulsions; preoccupations with appearance; hoarding behavior; skin-picking, hair-pulling, and other body-focused repetitive behaviors; or other symptoms characteristic of Obsessive-Compulsive and Related Disorders
Y
OBSESSIVE-COMPULSIVE AND RELATED DISORDER DUE TO ANOTHER MEDICAL CONDITION
N
At least three catatonia symptoms: stupor, catalepsy, waxy flexibility, mutism, negativism, posturing, mannerism, stereotypy, agitation, grimacing, echolalia, or echopraxia
Y
CATATONIC DISORDER DUE TO ANOTHER MEDICAL CONDITION (3.2.5)
N

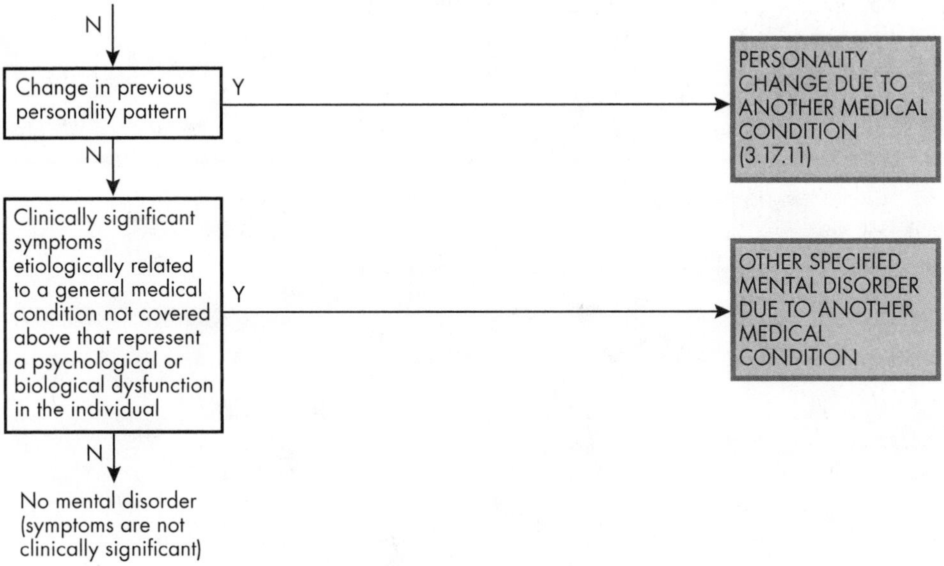
N
Change in previous personality pattern
Y
PERSONALITY CHANGE DUE TO ANOTHER MEDICAL CONDITION (3.17.11)
N
Clinically significant symptoms etiologically related to a general medical condition not covered above that represent a psychological or biological dysfunction in the individual
Y
OTHER SPECIFIED MENTAL DISORDER DUE TO ANOTHER MEDICAL CONDITION
N
No mental disorder (symptoms are not clinically significant)

3

Differential Diagnosis by the Tables

In contrast to the 29 decision trees included in Chapter 2, which use presenting symptoms as their starting points, the entry points to the 66 differential diagnosis tables included in this chapter are the DSM-5 disorders themselves. Although the practice of quickly arriving at a working diagnosis based on the gestalt of the patient has its pitfalls in terms of prematurely closing the clinician's mind to other equally valid possible diagnostic contenders, this is likely the method most often used by experienced clinicians. To help ensure that your working diagnosis is in fact the best diagnostic fit for your patient's clinical presentation, the disorder-oriented differential diagnosis tables can be invaluable in providing a comprehensive listing of those DSM-5 disorders that share important features with your initial working diagnosis so that these disorders can be considered and ruled out.

The first step is to locate the differential diagnosis table(s) corresponding to your working diagnosis (or diagnoses, if multiple diagnoses initially seem likely). In the list included at the end of this introduction, the differential diagnosis tables are grouped according to DSM-5 diagnostic class so that the relevant differential diagnosis table is easier to find. (An alphabetical index of differential diagnosis tables is also available at the end of this handbook.) Each disorder-oriented differential diagnosis table in this chapter includes two columns. The first left-hand entry in each table summarizes the definition of the index disorder to facilitate its differentiation from the other disorders in the table. The left-hand column lists those disorders (or nonpathological conditions) that share diagnostic features with the index disorder and thus need to be considered and ruled out as part of the differential diagnosis of the index disorder. For each such disorder or nonpathological condition in the differential diagnosis, the entry in the right-hand column indicates the diagnostic feature that differentiates it from the index disorder. For example, the differential diagnosis table for Separation Anxiety Disorder (Table 3.5.1) includes Agoraphobia in the differential diagnosis because both Separation Anxiety Disorder and Agoraphobia have anxiety and avoidance as shared diagnostic features, indicating that if a clinician is considering a diagnosis of Separation Anxiety Disorder based on the clinical presentation, Agoraphobia should also be considered as a possible explanatory disorder. The corresponding entry in the right-hand column explains how Separation Anxiety Disorder and Agoraphobia can be differentiated "[Agoraphobia] is characterized by anxiety about being trapped or incapacitated in places or situations from which escape is perceived as difficult in the event of panic-like symptoms or other incapacitating symptoms. In Separation Anxiety Disorder, the focus of the fear is on separation from major attachment figures."

Sometimes it may not be immediately obvious which diagnostic features the other disorders have in common with the index disorder that would justify their being included in the differential diagnosis table. In such cases, the entry in the right-hand column begins by stating what the putatively shared diagnostic feature is. For example, the differential diagnosis table for Avoidant/Restrictive Food Intake Disorder (ARFID; Table 3.10.1) includes Autism Spectrum Disorder, which may seem mysterious given that restrictive eating behavior is not part of the definition of Autism Spectrum Disorder. The entry in the right-hand column therefore begins by noting that Autism Spectrum Disorder "may be characterized by rigid eating behaviors and heightened sensory sensitivities," which is also a feature of ARFID, and then goes on to differentiate the two disorders by noting that "this often does not result in the level of impairment that would be required for a diagnosis of ARFID."

Multiple disorders are grouped in some tables to reduce the number of differential diagnosis tables. In some tables, such as Table 3.2.1, Schizophrenia or Schizophreniform Disorder, and Table 3.7.1, Posttraumatic Stress Disorder or Acute Stress Disorder, the disorders have been grouped together because they share virtually all the same diagnostic features except duration (which is noted in an accompanying footnote) and therefore share the same differential diagnosis list. In other tables, such as Table 3.1.2, Communication Disorders, a single differential diagnosis table is provided that covers all the disorders in that diagnostic grouping as if that were a single disorder. In these types of tables, if a disorder is included in the differential diagnosis list that pertains to only one of the disorders within that diagnostic grouping, it will be indicated in a parenthetical phrase. For example, in Table 3.1.2, although most of the differential diagnostic entries listed apply to all of the communication disorders, the entry for Autism Spectrum Disorder applies only to Social (Pragmatic) Communication Disorder. Therefore, the phrase "(as distinguished from Social [Pragmatic] Communication Disorder)" is included in that row of the table to indicate that this differentiation applies only to that disorder.

Some caveats should be kept in mind regarding the use of the tables. First, although the entries in the tables focus on the features that differentiate between disorders, given that only a minority of DSM-5 disorders (e.g., Bipolar I Disorder and Major Depressive Disorder) are by definition mutually exclusive, diagnostic comorbidity is the default position. Thus, unless otherwise stated, if the criteria are fully met for both the index disorder and a disorder in the table, both should be diagnosed.

Second, although the pertinent other specified and unspecified categories are not included in the differential diagnosis tables, they are an important consideration in the differential diagnosis for every disorder. Every experienced clinician knows that the complexity of practice offers many presentations that fall between the neatly defined DSM-5 disorders. Many patients do not present a clear picture that comfortably approximates the prototype for any of the disorders described in the DSM-5 criteria sets. Instead, patients often have clinical features that appear to be at the boundary between criteria sets or that satisfy the criteria for a number of possibly related disorders. It is important to recognize that a boundary patient is indeed a boundary patient and should not be shoehorned into a diagnosis that does not fit well. Such patients may require serial trials of treatment to help clarify the most appropriate diagnosis and plan of management.

Third, the differential diagnosis tables tend to focus on cross-sectional symptom presentations because these are the easiest to define and evaluate. Other factors that may be useful in guiding differential diagnosis include the patient's previous history, family history of psychopathology, course, biological test results, and responses to previous treatment trials. Especially in doubtful cases, these factors may tip the differential diagnostic balance one way or the other.

Differential diagnostic tables grouped by DSM-5 diagnostic class

Neurodevelopmental Disorders

3.1.1 Intellectual Disability (Intellectual Developmental Disorder)
3.1.2 Communication Disorders
3.1.3 Autism Spectrum Disorder
3.1.4 Attention-Deficit/Hyperactivity Disorder
3.1.5 Specific Learning Disorder
3.1.6 Tic Disorders

Schizophrenia Spectrum and Other Psychotic Disorders

3.2.1 Schizophrenia or Schizophreniform Disorder
3.2.2 Schizoaffective Disorder
3.2.3 Delusional Disorder
3.2.4 Brief Psychotic Disorder
3.2.5 Unspecified Catatonia

Bipolar and Related Disorders

3.3.1 Bipolar I Disorder
3.3.2 Bipolar II Disorder
3.3.3 Cyclothymic Disorder

Depressive Disorders

3.4.1 Major Depressive Disorder
3.4.2 Persistent Depressive Disorder (Dysthymia)
3.4.3 Premenstrual Dysphoric Disorder
3.4.4 Disruptive Mood Dysregulation Disorder

Differential diagnostic tables grouped by DSM-5 diagnostic class *(continued)*

Anxiety Disorders
3.5.1 Separation Anxiety Disorder
3.5.2 Selective Mutism
3.5.3 Specific Phobia
3.5.4 Social Anxiety Disorder (Social Phobia)
3.5.5 Panic Disorder
3.5.6 Agoraphobia
3.5.7 Generalized Anxiety Disorder

Obsessive-Compulsive and Related Disorders
3.6.1 Obsessive-Compulsive Disorder
3.6.2 Body Dysmorphic Disorder
3.6.3 Hoarding Disorder
3.6.4 Trichotillomania (Hair-Pulling Disorder)
3.6.5 Excoriation (Skin-Picking) Disorder

Trauma- and Stressor-Related Disorders
3.7.1 Posttraumatic Stress Disorder or Acute Stress Disorder
3.7.2 Adjustment Disorder

Dissociative Disorders
3.8.1 Dissociative Amnesia
3.8.2 Depersonalization/Derealization Disorder

Somatic Symptom and Related Disorders
3.9.1 Somatic Symptom Disorder
3.9.2 Illness Anxiety Disorder
3.9.3 Conversion Disorder (Functional Neurological Symptom Disorder)
3.9.4 Psychological Factors Affecting Other Medical Conditions
3.9.5 Factitious Disorder

Feeding and Eating Disorders
3.10.1 Avoidant/Restrictive Food Intake Disorder
3.10.2 Anorexia Nervosa
3.10.3 Bulimia Nervosa
3.10.4 Binge-Eating Disorder

Sleep-Wake Disorders
3.11.1 Insomnia Disorder
3.11.2 Hypersomnolence Disorder

Sexual Dysfunctions
3.12.1 Sexual Dysfunctions

Gender Dysphoria
3.13.1 Gender Dysphoria

Differential diagnostic tables grouped by DSM-5 diagnostic class *(continued)*

Disruptive, Impulse-Control, and Conduct Disorders
3.14.1 Oppositional Defiant Disorder
3.14.2 Intermittent Explosive Disorder
3.14.3 Conduct Disorder

Substance-Related and Addictive Disorders
3.15.1 Substance Use Disorders
3.15.2 Gambling Disorder

Neurocognitive Disorders
3.16.1 Delirium
3.16.2 Major or Mild Neurocognitive Disorder

Personality Disorders
3.17.1 Paranoid Personality Disorder
3.17.2 Schizoid Personality Disorder
3.17.3 Schizotypal Personality Disorder
3.17.4 Antisocial Personality Disorder
3.17.5 Borderline Personality Disorder
3.17.6 Histrionic Personality Disorder
3.17.7 Narcissistic Personality Disorder
3.17.8 Avoidant Personality Disorder
3.17.9 Dependent Personality Disorder
3.17.10 Obsessive-Compulsive Personality Disorder
3.17.11 Personality Change Due to Another Medical Condition

Paraphilic Disorders
3.18.1 Paraphilic Disorders

Neurodevelopmental Disorders

3.1.1 Differential Diagnosis for Intellectual Disability (Intellectual Developmental Disorder)

Intellectual Disability, which is characterized by global deficits in intellectual functions (such as reasoning, problem solving, planning, abstract thinking, judgment, academic learning, and learning from experience) and deficits in adaptive functioning that result in failure to meet developmental and sociocultural standards for personal independence and social responsibility, must be differentiated from...	In contrast to Intellectual Disability...
Specific Learning Disorder	Is characterized by an impairment confined to a specific area of academic achievement (e.g., reading, spelling, written expression, performing arithmetic calculations, mathematical reasoning). There are no deficits in intellectual and adaptive behavior.
Communication Disorders (i.e., Language Disorder, Speech Sound Disorder, Childhood-Onset Fluency Disorder [Stuttering], Social [Pragmatic] Communication Disorder)	Are characterized by impairments that are confined to speech or language problems. There are no deficits in intellectual and adaptive behavior.
Autism Spectrum Disorder	Is defined by the presence of persistent deficits in social communication and social interaction, along with restricted, repetitive patterns of behaviors, interests, or activities. Although there may be some impairment in social-communicative skills in Intellectual Disability, it is on par with deficits in other intellectual skills. Intellectual Disability is frequently comorbid with Autism Spectrum Disorder, and if criteria are met for both, both diagnoses should be given.

3.1.1 Differential Diagnosis for Intellectual Disability (Intellectual Developmental Disorder) *(continued)*

Major Neurocognitive Disorder	Is characterized by a significant cognitive decline from a previous level of performance in one or more cognitive domains such as executive function, learning, memory, and language. Both Major Neurocognitive Disorder and Intellectual Disability can be diagnosed if the onset of intellectual and adaptive deficits is during the developmental period.
Borderline intellectual functioning	Is characterized by a lesser degree of intellectual impairment (typically IQ around 70) or no problems in adaptive functioning if there are significant intellectual impairments (e.g., IQ is below 70).

3.1.2 Differential Diagnosis for Communication Disorders

Communication Disorders (i.e., Language Disorder, Speech Sound Disorder, Childhood-Onset Fluency Disorder [Stuttering], Social [Pragmatic] Communication Disorder) must be differentiated from…	In contrast to Communication Disorders…
Intellectual Disability (Intellectual Developmental Disorder)	Involves an overall impairment in intellectual functioning as opposed to only language impairment. A Communication Disorder can also be diagnosed if the language problems are in excess of those usually associated with Intellectual Disability.
Communication difficulties related to hearing impairment, a neurological deficit (e.g., Landau-Kleffner syndrome), a motor disorder (e.g., dysarthria), or a structural defect (e.g., cleft palate)	Are attributable to hearing impairment, a neurological deficit, a motor disorder, or a structural defect and are not in excess of that expected given the sensory or speech-motor deficit. A Communication Disorder can be diagnosed if the problems in communication are in excess of those usually associated with the deficits or disorders.
Selective Mutism	Is characterized by a lack of speech in some settings (e.g., in school, with strangers), whereas the child speaks normally in "safe" settings (e.g., at home). In a Communication Disorder, the communication problems are consistent across all settings. Some children with a Communication Disorder may develop Selective Mutism because of embarrassment about their speech deficits.
Tourette's Disorder (as distinguished from Childhood-Onset Fluency Disorder)	Is characterized by vocal tics and repetitive vocalizations that differ in nature and timing from the repetitive sounds of Childhood-Onset Fluency Disorder, which are characterized by broken words (i.e., pauses within a word), audible or silent blocking (i.e., filled or unfilled pauses in speech), circumlocutions (i.e., word substitutions to avoid problematic words), words produced with an excess of physical tension, and monosyllabic whole-word repetitions (e.g., "I-I-I-I see him").

3.1.2 Differential Diagnosis for Communication Disorders *(continued)*

Autism Spectrum Disorder (as distinguished from Social [Pragmatic] Communication Disorder)	Is characterized by restricted, repetitive patterns of behavior, interests, or activities in addition to social communication deficits, whereas in Social (Pragmatic) Communication Disorder, restricted, repetitive patterns of behavior, interests, or activities are absent.
Social Anxiety Disorder (Social Phobia) (as distinguished from Social [Pragmatic] Communication Disorder)	Is characterized by the lack of use of appropriately developed social communication skills because of anxiety, fear, or distress about social interactions. In Social (Pragmatic) Communication Disorder, these skills have never been present.
Normal dysfluencies or articulation difficulties in young children	Are developmentally appropriate.

3.1.3 Differential Diagnosis for Autism Spectrum Disorder

Autism Spectrum Disorder, which is characterized by persistent deficits in social communication and social interaction across multiple contexts, accompanied by restricted, repetitive patterns of behavior, interests, or activities, must be differentiated from…	In contrast to Autism Spectrum Disorder…
Rett's Disorder	Includes disruptions in social interactions during the regressive phase of this neurological condition (i.e., between ages 1 and 4), which is also characterized by deceleration in head growth, loss of hand movements, and poor coordination.
Schizophrenia	Childhood-onset Schizophrenia usually develops after a period of normal, or near-normal, development. The Schizophrenia prodromal state may include social impairment and atypical interests and beliefs, which could be confused with the social deficits seen in Autism Spectrum Disorder. Hallucinations and delusions, which are defining features of Schizophrenia, are not seen in Autism Spectrum Disorder.
Selective Mutism	Is characterized by normal early development and by appropriate social communication functioning in certain "safe" contexts and settings (e.g., at home with parents).
Language Disorder	Is characterized by a lack of qualitative impairment in social interaction, and the individual's range of interests and behaviors are not restricted.
Social (Pragmatic) Communication Disorder	Is characterized by impairment in social communication and social interactions without the restricted and repetitive behaviors or interests characteristic of Autism Spectrum Disorder.

3.1.3 Differential Diagnosis for Autism Spectrum Disorder *(continued)*

Intellectual Disability (Intellectual Developmental Disorder)	Involves general impairment in intellectual functioning; there is no discrepancy between the level of the social communicative skills and other intellectual skills. A diagnosis of Autism Spectrum Disorder in an individual with Intellectual Disability is appropriate when social communication and interaction are significantly impaired relative to the developmental level of the individual's nonverbal skills.
Stereotypic Movement Disorder	Occurs in the absence of impairment of social interaction and language development. Stereotypic Movement Disorder is generally not diagnosed if the stereotypy is part of Autism Spectrum Disorder; however, when stereotypies cause self-injury and become a focus of treatment, both diagnoses may be appropriate.

3.1.4 Differential Diagnosis for Attention-Deficit/Hyperactivity Disorder

Attention-Deficit/Hyperactivity Disorder (ADHD), which is characterized by symptoms of inattention, hyperactivity, and impulsivity that are inconsistent with developmental level and that negatively impact social and academic/occupational activities, must be differentiated from…	In contrast to Attention-Deficit/Hyperactivity Disorder…
Normative behaviors in active children	Are consistent with developmental level.
Understimulating environments	Lead to inattention that is related to boredom.
Oppositional Defiant Disorder	May be characterized by resistance to work or school tasks because of a refusal to submit to others' demands, which is accompanied by negativity, hostility, and defiance. In ADHD, however, the aversion to school or mentally demanding tasks is due to difficulty in sustaining mental effort, forgetting instructions, and impulsivity.
Intermittent Explosive Disorder	Is also characterized by high levels of impulsive behavior, but unlike ADHD, there are episodes of serious aggression toward others. An additional diagnosis of Intermittent Explosive Disorder can be made if the recurrent impulsive aggressive outbursts are in excess of those usually seen in ADHD and warrant independent clinical attention.
Conduct Disorder	May be characterized by high levels of impulsivity, but there is also a pattern of antisocial behavior.
Stereotypic Movement Disorder	Is characterized by repetitive motor behavior that may resemble the increased motor behavior in ADHD. In contrast to ADHD, however, the motor behavior is generally fixed and repetitive (e.g., body rocking, self-biting), whereas the fidgetiness and restlessness in ADHD are typically generalized.

3.1.4 Differential Diagnosis for Attention-Deficit/Hyperactivity Disorder *(continued)*

Specific Learning Disorder	May be characterized by inattentive behavior because of frustration, lack of interest, or limited ability. However, inattention in individuals with Specific Learning Disorder who do not have ADHD is not impairing outside of schoolwork.
Intellectual Disability (Intellectual Developmental Disorder)	May be characterized by symptoms of inattention, hyperactivity, and impulsivity among children placed in academic settings that are inappropriate to their intellectual ability. Individuals with Intellectual Disability without ADHD do not have symptoms during nonacademic tasks. A diagnosis of ADHD in individuals with Intellectual Disability requires that the inattention or hyperactivity be excessive for the individual's mental age.
Autism Spectrum Disorder	May be characterized by social disengagement and social isolation due to deficits in social communication, as well as temper tantrums due to an inability to tolerate a change from the expected course of events, whereas social dysfunction and peer rejection in ADHD are related to symptoms of inattention and hyperactivity, and misbehavior and temper tantrums are related to impulsivity or poor self-control.
Disinhibited Social Engagement Disorder	Is characterized by social disinhibition, but not the full ADHD symptom cluster. Children with Disinhibited Social Engagement Disorder also have a history of extremes of insufficient care.
Disruptive Mood Dysregulation Disorder	Is characterized by pervasive irritability and intolerance of frustration. Given that most children and adolescents with Disruptive Mood Dysregulation Disorder also have symptoms that meet criteria for ADHD, an additional diagnosis may be made.

3.1.4 Differential Diagnosis for Attention-Deficit/Hyperactivity Disorder *(continued)*

Anxiety Disorders	May be characterized by symptoms of inattention due to fear, worry, and rumination. In ADHD, the inattention is because of attraction to external stimuli or new activities, or preoccupation with enjoyable activities.
Major Depressive Disorder	May be characterized by an inability to concentrate; however, the poor concentration is prominent only during Major Depressive Episodes.
Bipolar I and Bipolar II Disorder	May be characterized by increased activity, poor concentration, increased impulsivity, and distractibility, but these features are episodic, occurring several days to weeks at a time. Moreover, the symptoms are accompanied by elevated or irritable mood, grandiosity, and other specific bipolar features. Although individuals with ADHD may show significant changes in mood within the same day, such lability is distinct from a Manic or Hypomanic Episode, which must be sustained and last at least a week (or 4 days for a Hypomanic Episode) to be a clinical indicator of Bipolar I or Bipolar II Disorder.
Borderline, Antisocial, and Narcissistic Personality Disorders	Share the features of disorganization, social intrusiveness, emotional dysregulation, and cognitive dysregulation. These disorders are distinguished from ADHD by the presence of additional maladaptive features, such as self-injury, antisocial behavior, fear of abandonment, and lack of empathy. If criteria are met for both ADHD and a Personality Disorder, both may be diagnosed.

3.1.4 Differential Diagnosis for Attention-Deficit/Hyperactivity Disorder *(continued)*

Medication-induced symptoms of ADHD	Are characterized by symptoms of inattention, hyperactivity, or impulsivity caused by medications (e.g., bronchodilators, isoniazid, neuroleptics [resulting in akathisia], thyroid replacement medication) and remit when the medications are stopped. ADHD is not diagnosed if the symptoms occur only during medication use.
Neurocognitive Disorders	May be characterized by cognitive impairments similar to those in ADHD; they are distinguished by their typically later age at onset.

3.1.5 Differential Diagnosis for Specific Learning Disorder

Specific Learning Disorder, which is characterized by difficulties in learning and using academic skills (e.g., reading, spelling, written expression, performing arithmetic calculations, mathematical reasoning), must be differentiated from…	In contrast to Specific Learning Disorder…
Normal variations in academic attainment	Do not result in clinically significant interference with academic achievement, occupational performance, or activities of daily living that require these academic skills; the affected academic skills are not substantially and quantifiably below those expected for the individual's chronological age (based on appropriate standardized measures); or the difficulties abate with the provision of interventions that target the difficulties.
Poor academic performance due to lack of opportunity, poor teaching, or learning in a second language	Represents factors external to the individual and thus not indicative of an internal dysfunction. To justify a diagnosis of Specific Learning Disorder, the learning difficulties must persist in the presence of adequate educational opportunity, exposure to the same instruction as the peer group, and competency in the language of instruction.
Poor academic performance due to impaired vision or hearing or other neurological deficit	Is at a level that would be expected given the nature of the sensory or neurological deficit. Specific Learning Disorder can still be diagnosed if the academic difficulties are not adequately accounted for by the sensory or neurological deficit.
Intellectual Disability (Intellectual Developmental Disorder)	Consists of an overall impairment in intellectual functioning that is not confined to a particular academic skill. Specific Learning Disorder can be diagnosed along with Intellectual Disability as long as the learning difficulties are in excess of those usually associated with the Intellectual Disability.

3.1.5 Differential Diagnosis for Specific Learning Disorder *(continued)*

Autism Spectrum Disorder	Includes persistent deficits in social communication and social interaction, along with restricted, repetitive patterns of behaviors, interests, or activities; these deficits and patterns are not confined to a particular academic skill.
Communication Disorders	Involves impairment in speech or language skills that are not restricted to particular academic skills, such as reading or writing.
Major Neurocognitive Disorder	The difficulties are manifested as a marked decline from a former state, whereas in Specific Learning Disorder the difficulties occur during the developmental period and do not represent a loss of previously acquired skills.
Attention-Deficit/Hyperactivity Disorder	Is characterized by problems that reflect difficulties in performing academic skills due to inattention, hyperactivity, and/or impulsivity rather than specific difficulties learning academic skills.
Schizophrenia	Associated academic and cognitive processing difficulties may result in an often rapid decline in academic functioning that has its onset in adolescence or early adulthood, whereas the learning difficulties in Specific Learning Disorder become apparent during the elementary school years when children are required to learn to read, spell, write, and do mathematics.

3.1.6 Differential Diagnosis for Tic Disorders

Tic Disorders (i.e., Tourette's Disorder, Persistent [Chronic] Motor or Vocal Tic Disorder, Provisional Tic Disorder), which are characterized by sudden, rapid, recurrent, nonrhythmic motor movements or vocalizations, must be differentiated from…	In contrast to Tic Disorders…
Choreiform movements associated with neurological or other medical conditions	Are characterized by rapid, random, continual, abrupt, irregular, unpredictable, nonstereotyped actions that are usually bilateral and affect all parts of the body (i.e., face, trunk, and limbs).
Dystonic movements associated with neurological or other medical conditions	Are characterized by the simultaneous sustained contracture of both agonist and antagonist muscles, resulting in distorted posture or movement of parts of the body.
Myoclonus	Is characterized by sudden unidirectional movements that are often nonrhythmic and may be worsened by movement and occur during sleep. Myoclonus is differentiated from tics by its rapidity, lack of suppressibility, and absence of a premonitory urge.
Tics caused by substances or medications	Remit when the substance or medication (e.g., stimulant) is discontinued and are diagnosed as Unspecified Substance–Related Disorder or Other Medication-Induced Movement Disorder.
Stereotypic Movement Disorder, or stereotypies in Autism Spectrum Disorder	Are characterized by nonfunctional, usually rhythmic, seemingly driven behaviors that are generally more complex than tics.
Compulsions in Obsessive-Compulsive Disorder	Occur in response to an obsession or according to rigidly applied rules.
Schizophrenia	May be characterized by disorganized or bizarre vocalizations or behaviors that are accompanied by the other characteristic symptoms (e.g., delusions, negative symptoms) and have a characteristic course (e.g., marked decline in functioning).

Schizophrenia Spectrum and Other Psychotic Disorders

3.2.1 Differential Diagnosis for Schizophrenia or Schizophreniform Disorder[a]

Schizophrenia and Schizophreniform Disorder, which are characterized by a disturbance lasting for months (at least 6 months for Schizophrenia and between 1 and 6 months for Schizophreniform Disorder) that significantly impairs functioning and that includes at least 1 month of active-phase psychotic symptoms, must be differentiated from...	In contrast to Schizophrenia or Schizophreniform Disorder...
Psychotic Disorder Due to Another Medical Condition, Delirium, or Major Neurocognitive Disorder Due to Another Medical Condition	Requires the presence of an etiological general medical condition. Schizophrenia or Schizophreniform Disorder is not diagnosed if the psychotic symptoms are all due to the direct physiological effects of another medical condition.
Substance/Medication-Induced Psychotic Disorder, Substance/Medication-Induced Neurocognitive Disorder, Substance Intoxication Delirium, Substance Withdrawal Delirium, Medication-Induced Delirium, Substance Intoxication, or Substance Withdrawal	Requires that the psychotic symptoms be initiated and maintained by substance use (including medication side effects). Schizophrenia or Schizophreniform Disorder is not diagnosed if the psychotic symptoms are all due to the direct physiological effects of a substance (including medication).
Schizoaffective Disorder	Is characterized by symptoms that meet criteria for a Major Depressive Episode or Manic Episode, and the mood episodes are present for the majority of the total duration of the active and residual portion of the illness. In Schizophrenia or Schizophreniform Disorder, the mood episodes have been present for a minority of the total duration of the active and residual periods of the illness.
Major Depressive Disorder With Psychotic Features, Bipolar I or Bipolar II Disorder With Psychotic Features, Catatonia Associated With Major Depressive Disorder, or Catatonia Associated With Bipolar I or Bipolar II Disorder	Is characterized by psychotic or catatonic symptoms that occur exclusively during Manic or Major Depressive Episodes.

3.2.1 Differential Diagnosis for Schizophrenia or Schizophreniform Disorder[a] *(continued)*

Brief Psychotic Disorder	Is characterized by a total duration of psychotic symptoms of at least 1 day but less than 1 month.
Delusional Disorder	Is characterized by delusions occurring in the absence of the other characteristic symptoms of Schizophrenia (i.e., prominent auditory or visual hallucinations, disorganized speech, grossly disorganized or catatonic behavior, negative symptoms).
Posttraumatic Stress Disorder	May be characterized by flashbacks that have a hallucinatory quality and hypervigilance that may reach paranoid proportions, but it is distinguished by the requirement of exposure to a traumatic event with a characteristic cluster of intrusion, avoidance, and other symptoms.
Autism Spectrum Disorder	Is characterized by an early onset (e.g., before age 3 years) and an absence of prominent delusions or hallucinations. A diagnosis of Schizophrenia or Schizophreniform Disorder is warranted in individuals with a preexisting diagnosis of Autism Spectrum Disorder only if prominent hallucinations or delusions have been present for at least 1 month.
Schizotypal, Schizoid, and Paranoid Personality Disorders	Are characterized by personality features that are subthreshold versions of many of the symptoms of Schizophrenia (e.g., odd beliefs, perceptual distortions, odd thinking and speech, social anxiety).

[a] Schizophrenia and Schizophreniform Disorder have essentially the same differential diagnosis and thus have been combined for the purposes of this differential diagnosis table. They are differentiated primarily based on the duration of the disturbance. In Schizophreniform Disorder, the duration is between 1 and 6 months. In Schizophrenia, the duration is 6 months or longer.

3.2.2 Differential Diagnosis for Schizoaffective Disorder

Schizoaffective Disorder, which is characterized by times in which Major Depressive or Manic Episodes overlap with active-phase symptoms of Schizophrenia and times in which there are delusions or hallucinations without mood symptoms, must be differentiated from…	In contrast to Schizoaffective Disorder…
Psychotic Disorder Due to Another Medical Condition, Delirium, or Major Neurocognitive Disorder Due to Another Medical Condition	Requires the presence of an etiological general medical condition. Schizoaffective Disorder is not diagnosed if the psychotic or mood symptoms are all due to the direct physiological effects of another medical condition.
Substance/Medication-Induced Psychotic Disorder, Substance/Medication-Induced Neurocognitive Disorder, Substance Intoxication Delirium, Substance Withdrawal Delirium, Medication-Induced Delirium, Substance Intoxication, or Substance Withdrawal	Requires that the psychotic and mood symptoms be due to substance use (including medication side effects). Schizoaffective Disorder is not diagnosed if the psychotic or mood symptoms are all due to the direct physiological effects of a substance (including medication).
Schizophrenia	Is characterized either by no mood episodes or, if mood episodes have been present, by mood episodes that have been present for a minority of the total duration of the active and residual periods of the illness.
Bipolar I, Bipolar II, or Major Depressive Disorder With Psychotic Features	Is characterized by psychotic symptoms that occur exclusively during Manic or Major Depressive Episodes.
Delusional Disorder	Is characterized by delusions occurring in the absence of other symptoms that meet DSM-5 Criterion A for Schizophrenia (i.e., prominent auditory or visual hallucinations, disorganized speech, grossly disorganized or catatonic behavior, negative symptoms).

3.2.3 Differential Diagnosis for Delusional Disorder

Delusional Disorder, which is characterized by persistent delusions without other psychotic symptoms, must be differentiated from…	In contrast to Delusional Disorder…
Psychotic Disorder Due to Another Medical Condition, Delirium, or Major Neurocognitive Disorder Due to Another Medical Condition	Requires the presence of an etiological general medical condition. Delusional Disorder is not diagnosed if the delusions are all due to the direct physiological effects of another medical condition.
Substance/Medication-Induced Psychotic Disorder, Substance/Medication-Induced Neurocognitive Disorder, Substance Intoxication Delirium, Substance Withdrawal Delirium, Medication-Induced Delirium, Substance Intoxication, or Substance Withdrawal	Requires that the psychotic symptoms are due to substance use (including medication side effects). Delusional Disorder is not diagnosed if the delusions are all due to the direct physiological effects of a substance (including medication).
Schizophrenia or Schizophreniform Disorder	Is characterized by the presence of other symptoms (in addition to prominent delusions) that meet DSM-5 Criterion A for Schizophrenia (i.e., prominent auditory or visual hallucinations, delusions, disorganized speech, grossly disorganized or catatonic behavior, negative symptoms).
Bipolar or Major Depressive Disorder, With Psychotic Features	Is characterized by delusions that occur exclusively during Manic or Major Depressive Episodes. When there is a history of Manic or Major Depressive Episodes, Delusional Disorder can be diagnosed only if the total duration of all mood episodes remains brief relative to the total duration of the delusional disturbance. If not, then the appropriate diagnosis is Other Specified Psychotic Disorder.
Brief Psychotic Disorder	Is characterized by psychotic symptoms that last for less than 1 month. In Delusional Disorder, the minimum duration of the delusions is 1 month.

3.2.3 Differential Diagnosis for Delusional Disorder *(continued)*

Obsessive-Compulsive Disorder	If an individual with Obsessive-Compulsive Disorder is completely convinced that his or her Obsessive-Compulsive Disorder beliefs are true, then the diagnosis should be Obsessive-Compulsive Disorder With Absent Insight/Delusional Beliefs, rather than Delusional Disorder.
Body Dysmorphic Disorder	In situations in which an individual with Body Dysmorphic Disorder is completely convinced that his or her beliefs that his or her appearance is defective are true, then the diagnosis should be Body Dysmorphic Disorder With Absent Insight/Delusional Beliefs, rather than Delusional Disorder.
Paranoid Personality Disorder	Is characterized by paranoid ideation without clear-cut or persisting delusional beliefs.

3.2.4 Differential Diagnosis for Brief Psychotic Disorder

Brief Psychotic Disorder, which is characterized by psychotic symptoms lasting less than 1 month, must be differentiated from…	In contrast to Brief Psychotic Disorder…
Psychotic Disorder Due to Another Medical Condition, Delirium, or Major Neurocognitive Disorder Due to Another Medical Condition	Requires the presence of an etiological general medical condition. Brief Psychotic Disorder is not diagnosed if the psychotic symptoms are all due to the direct physiological effects of a general medical condition.
Substance/Medication-Induced Psychotic Disorder, Substance/Medication-Induced Neurocognitive Disorder, Substance Intoxication Delirium, Substance Withdrawal Delirium, Medication-Induced Delirium, Substance Intoxication, or Substance Withdrawal	Requires that the psychotic symptoms be due to substance use (including medication side effects). Brief Psychotic Disorder is not diagnosed if the psychotic symptoms are all due to the direct physiological effects of a substance (including medication).
Bipolar or Major Depressive Disorder, With Psychotic Features	Is characterized by psychotic symptoms occurring exclusively during mood episodes. Brief Psychotic Disorder is not diagnosed if the psychotic symptoms are better accounted for by Bipolar or Major Depressive Disorder With Psychotic Features.
Schizophreniform Disorder, Schizophrenia, or Delusional Disorder	Is characterized by psychotic symptoms that last 1 month or longer.
Psychotic symptoms occurring in the context of some Personality Disorders (e.g., Borderline Personality Disorder)	Are usually transient and last less than 1 day. If clinically significant, they may be diagnosed as Other Specified Schizophrenia Spectrum and Other Psychotic Disorder or as Unspecified Schizophrenia Spectrum and Other Psychotic Disorder. If psychotic symptoms persist for at least 1 day, the additional diagnosis of Brief Psychotic Disorder may be warranted.

3.2.5 Differential Diagnosis for Unspecified Catatonia

Unspecified Catatonia, which is for presentations in which there are clinically significant symptoms of Catatonia and either the nature of the underlying mental disorder or general medical condition is unclear or full criteria for the syndrome of Catatonia are not met, must be differentiated from...	In contrast to Unspecified Catatonia...
Catatonic Disorder Due to Another Medical Condition	Is characterized by the full syndrome of Catatonia that is due to the physiological effects of a medical condition, especially neurological conditions (e.g., neoplasms, head trauma, cerebrovascular disease, encephalitis) and metabolic conditions (e.g., hypercalcemia, hepatic encephalopathy, homocystinuria, diabetic ketoacidosis).
Mutism or posturing in Delirium Due to Another Medical Condition	Is characterized by catatonic symptoms occurring in the context of a disturbance in attention (i.e., reduced ability to direct, focus, sustain, and shift attention) and awareness (i.e., reduced orientation to the environment). Catatonic Disorder Due to Another Medical Condition is not diagnosed if the symptoms occur exclusively during the course of Delirium.
Akinesia, rigidity, or posturing in medication-induced movement disorders (including Neuroleptic Malignant Syndrome)	Is due to the direct physiological effects of a medication, including neuroleptics.
Catatonia Associated With Schizophrenia, Catatonia Associated With Schizoaffective Disorder, Catatonia Associated With Schizophreniform Disorder, or Catatonia Associated With Brief Psychotic Disorder	Is characterized by the full syndrome of Catatonia that is accompanied by other characteristic symptoms of the relevant psychotic disorder.
Catatonia Associated With Bipolar or Major Depressive Disorder	Is characterized by the full syndrome of Catatonia that occurs exclusively during a Manic or Major Depressive Episode.
Catatonia Associated With Autism Spectrum Disorder	Is characterized by the full syndrome of Catatonia that is accompanied by the characteristic symptoms of Autism Spectrum Disorder (e.g., social communication difficulties, restricted repertoire of interests and behaviors).

Bipolar and Related Disorders

3.3.1 Differential Diagnosis for Bipolar I Disorder

Bipolar I Disorder, which is characterized by at least one Manic Episode that may have been preceded by or followed by Hypomanic or Major Depressive Episodes, must be differentiated from…	In contrast to Bipolar I Disorder…
Bipolar and Related Disorder Due to Another Medical Condition	Requires the presence of an etiological medical condition. Bipolar I Disorder is not diagnosed if the mood episodes are all due to the direct physiological effects of another medical condition.
Substance/Medication-Induced Bipolar and Related Disorder	Is due to the direct physiological effects of a substance. A full Manic Episode that emerges during antidepressant treatment (e.g., with a selective serotonin reuptake inhibitor) but persists at a fully syndromal level beyond the physiological effect of that treatment meets criteria for a Manic Episode and, therefore, a Bipolar I Disorder diagnosis.
Major Depressive Disorder	Is characterized by the absence of both Manic Episodes and Hypomanic Episodes. Given that the presence of some manic or hypomanic symptoms (i.e., fewer symptoms or for a shorter duration than required for mania or hypomania) may still be compatible with a diagnosis of Major Depressive Disorder (and would warrant the use of the With Mixed Features specifier), it is important to ascertain whether the symptoms meet criteria for a Manic or Hypomanic Episode to determine whether it is more appropriate to make the diagnosis of a Bipolar Disorder.
Bipolar II Disorder	Is characterized by the presence of Hypomanic and Major Depressive Episodes and the absence of Manic Episodes. Bipolar II Disorder cannot be diagnosed if the criteria have ever been met for Bipolar I Disorder.

3.3.1 Differential Diagnosis for Bipolar I Disorder *(continued)*

Cyclothymic Disorder	Is characterized by numerous periods of hypomanic symptoms that do not meet criteria for a Manic or Hypomanic Episode and periods of depressive symptoms that do not meet criteria for a Major Depressive Episode. Moreover, the criteria can never have been met for any of these mood episodes in order for the diagnosis of Cyclothymic Disorder to apply.
Schizophrenia, Delusional Disorder, or Schizophreniform Disorder	Is characterized by psychotic symptoms, which may be accompanied by Manic or Major Depressive Episodes. The diagnosis is Schizophrenia, Delusional Disorder, or Schizophreniform Disorder if either no Manic or Major Depressive Episodes have occurred concurrently with the psychotic symptoms or, if they have occurred concurrently, the Manic and Major Depressive Episodes have been present for only a minority of the time. The diagnosis is Bipolar I Disorder With Psychotic Features if the psychotic symptoms have occurred exclusively during Manic and Major Depressive Episodes.
Schizoaffective Disorder	Is characterized by periods in which Manic and/or Major Depressive Episodes are concurrent with the active-phase symptoms of Schizophrenia, periods in which delusions or hallucinations occur for at least 2 weeks in the absence of a Manic or Major Depressive Episode, and Manic and Major Depressive Episodes are present for a majority of the total duration of the illness. The diagnosis is Bipolar I Disorder With Psychotic Features if the psychotic symptoms have occurred exclusively during Manic and Major Depressive Episodes.
Attention-Deficit/Hyperactivity Disorder	Is characterized by persistent symptoms of inattention, hyperactivity, and impulsivity, which may resemble the symptoms of a Manic Episode (e.g., distractibility, increased activity, impulsive behavior) and have their onset before age 12, whereas the symptoms of mania in Bipolar I Disorder occur in distinct episodes and typically begin in late adolescence or early adulthood.

3.3.1 Differential Diagnosis for Bipolar I Disorder *(continued)*

Disruptive Mood Dysregulation Disorder	Is characterized by severe recurrent temper outbursts manifested verbally and/or behaviorally, which are accompanied by persistently irritable or angry mood most of the day, nearly every day, in between the outbursts. In contrast, the irritability in Bipolar I Disorder occurs in distinct episodes that last at least 1 week, is clearly different from the individual's baseline, and is accompanied by the characteristic associated symptoms of mania (e.g., grandiosity, decreased need for sleep).
Personality Disorders (especially Borderline Personality Disorder)	May be characterized by symptoms such as mood lability and impulsivity that are persistent and have their onset by early adulthood. In contrast, the mood symptoms in Bipolar I Disorder occur in distinct episodes that represent a noticeable change from normal baseline functioning.

3.3.2 Differential Diagnosis for Bipolar II Disorder

Bipolar II Disorder, which is characterized by at least one Hypomanic Episode and one Major Depressive Episode, must be differentiated from…	In contrast to Bipolar II Disorder…
Bipolar and Related Disorder Due to Another Medical Condition	Requires the presence of an etiological medical condition. Bipolar II Disorder is not diagnosed if the mood episodes are all due to the direct physiological effects of another medical condition.
Substance/Medication-Induced Bipolar and Related Disorder	Is characterized by Hypomanic and Major Depressive Episodes that are due to the direct physiological effects of a substance (including medication). A full Hypomanic Episode that emerges during antidepressant treatment (e.g., with a selective serotonin reuptake inhibitor) but persists at a fully syndromal level beyond the physiological effect of that treatment meets criteria for a Hypomanic Episode, and therefore, potentially a Bipolar II Disorder diagnosis if there has also been a history of Major Depressive Episodes.
Major Depressive Disorder	Is characterized by the absence of both Manic Episodes and Hypomanic Episodes. Given that the presence of some manic or hypomanic symptoms (i.e., fewer symptoms or a shorter duration than required for mania or hypomania) may still be compatible with a diagnosis of Major Depressive Disorder (and would warrant the use of the With Mixed Features specifier), it is important to ascertain whether the symptoms meet criteria for a Hypomanic Episode to determine whether it is more appropriate to make the diagnosis of Bipolar II Disorder.
Bipolar I Disorder	Is characterized by the presence of at least one Manic Episode. Bipolar II Disorder cannot be diagnosed if the criteria have ever been met for Bipolar I Disorder.

3.3.2 Differential Diagnosis for Bipolar II Disorder *(continued)*

Cyclothymic Disorder	Is characterized by numerous periods of hypomanic symptoms that do not meet criteria for a Manic or Hypomanic Episode and periods of depressive symptoms that do not meet criteria for a Major Depressive Episode. Moreover, the criteria can never have been met for any of these mood episodes in order for the diagnosis of Cyclothymic Disorder to apply.
Schizophrenia	Is characterized by active-phase psychotic symptoms, which may be accompanied by Major Depressive Episodes. The diagnosis is Schizophrenia if either no Major Depressive Episodes have occurred concurrently with the active-phase symptoms, or if they have occurred concurrently, the Major Depressive Episodes have been present for only a minority of the time. The diagnosis is Bipolar II Disorder With Psychotic Features if the psychotic symptoms have occurred exclusively during Major Depressive Episodes.
Schizoaffective Disorder	Is characterized by periods in which Major Depressive Episodes are concurrent with the active-phase symptoms of Schizophrenia, periods in which delusions or hallucinations occur for at least 2 weeks in the absence of a Major Depressive Episode, and Major Depressive Episodes are present for a majority of the total duration of the illness. The diagnosis is Bipolar II Disorder With Psychotic Features if the psychotic symptoms have occurred exclusively during Major Depressive Episodes.
Attention-Deficit/Hyperactivity Disorder	Is characterized by persistent symptoms of inattention, hyperactivity, and impulsivity, which may resemble the symptoms of a Hypomanic Episode (e.g., distractibility, increased activity, impulsive behavior) and have their onset before age 12. In contrast, the symptoms of hypomania in Bipolar II Disorder occur in distinct episodes and typically begin in late adolescence or early adulthood.

3.3.2 Differential Diagnosis for Bipolar II Disorder *(continued)*

Disruptive Mood Dysregulation Disorder	Is characterized by severe recurrent temper outbursts manifested verbally and/or behaviorally, which are accompanied by persistently irritable or angry mood most of the day, nearly every day, in between the outbursts. In contrast, the irritability in Bipolar II Disorder occurs in distinct episodes that last at least 4 days, is clearly different from the individual's baseline, and is accompanied by the characteristic associated symptoms of hypomania (e.g., grandiosity, decreased need for sleep).
Personality Disorders (especially Borderline Personality Disorder)	May be characterized by symptoms such as mood lability and impulsivity that are persistent and have their onset by early adulthood. In contrast, the mood symptoms in Bipolar II Disorder occur in distinct episodes that represent a noticeable change from normal baseline functioning.

3.3.3 Differential Diagnosis for Cyclothymic Disorder

Cyclothymic Disorder, which is characterized by numerous periods with hypomanic symptoms that do not meet criteria for a Hypomanic Episode and numerous periods with depressive symptoms that do not meet criteria for a Major Depressive Episode, must be differentiated from...	In contrast to Cyclothymic Disorder...
Bipolar I or Bipolar II Disorder, With Rapid Cycling	Is characterized by four or more mood episodes (each of which meets full criteria for a Manic, Hypomanic, or Major Depressive Episode) occurring in a 12-month period. Cyclothymic Disorder is characterized by numerous periods of hypomanic and depressive symptoms that do not meet criteria for a Hypomanic or Major Depressive Episode. If criteria have ever been met for a Manic, Hypomanic, or Major Depressive Episode, Cyclothymic Disorder is not diagnosed.
Borderline Personality Disorder	Is characterized by additional personality features (e.g., identity disturbance, self-mutilating behavior) besides affective lability. If criteria are met for Cyclothymic Disorder and Borderline Personality Disorder, both can be diagnosed.
Bipolar and Related Disorder Due to Another Medical Condition	Requires the presence of an etiological general medical condition. Cyclothymic Disorder is not diagnosed if the mood symptoms are all due to the direct physiological effects of a general medical condition.
Substance/Medication-Induced Bipolar and Related Disorder	Is due to the direct physiological effects of a substance. Cyclothymic Disorder is not diagnosed if the mood symptoms are all due to the direct physiological effects of a substance (including medication).

Depressive Disorders

3.4.1 Differential Diagnosis for Major Depressive Disorder

Major Depressive Disorder, which is characterized by episodes of depressed mood or diminished interest or pleasure that last at least 2 weeks and that are accompanied by characteristic associated symptoms (e.g., changes in sleep, appetite, or activity level; fatigue; difficulty concentrating; feelings of worthlessness or excessive guilt; suicidal ideation or behavior), must be differentiated from…	In contrast to Major Depressive Disorder…
Bipolar I or Bipolar II Disorder	Includes one or more Manic or Hypomanic Episodes. Major Depressive Disorder cannot be diagnosed if a Manic or Hypomanic Episode has ever been present. A diagnosis of Major Depressive Disorder may be compatible with the presence of some manic or hypomanic symptoms (i.e., fewer symptoms or a shorter duration than required for mania or hypomania) and would warrant the use of the With Mixed Features specifier.
Depressive Disorder Due to Another Medical Condition	Requires the presence of an etiological medical condition. Major Depressive Disorder is not diagnosed if the major depressive–like episodes are all due to the direct physiological effects of a medical condition.
Substance/Medication-Induced Depressive Disorder	Is due to the direct physiological effects of a substance or medication. Major Depressive Disorder is not diagnosed if the major depressive–like episodes are all due to the direct physiological effects of a substance (including medication).
Persistent Depressive Disorder (Dysthymia)	Is characterized by depressed mood, more days than not, for at least 2 years. If criteria are met for both Major Depressive Disorder and Persistent Depressive Disorder, both can be diagnosed.

3.4.1 Differential Diagnosis for Major Depressive Disorder *(continued)*

Premenstrual Dysphoric Disorder	Is characterized by dysphoric mood that is present in the final week before the onset of menses and that starts to improve within a few days after the onset of menses, and becomes minimal or absent in the week postmenses. In contrast, the episodes in Major Depressive Disorder are not temporally connected to the menstrual cycle.
Disruptive Mood Dysregulation Disorder	Is characterized by severe, recurrent temper outbursts manifested verbally and/or behaviorally, accompanied by persistently irritable or angry mood most of the day, nearly every day, in between the outbursts. In contrast, in Major Depressive Disorder, irritability is confined to the Major Depressive Episodes.
Schizophrenia, Delusional Disorder, or Schizophreniform Disorder	Is characterized by psychotic symptoms, which may be accompanied by Major Depressive Episodes. The diagnosis is Schizophrenia, Delusional Disorder, or Schizophreniform Disorder if either no Major Depressive Episodes have occurred concurrently with the psychotic disorder or, if they have occurred concurrently, the Major Depressive Episodes have been present for only a minority of the time. The diagnosis is Major Depressive Disorder With Psychotic Features if the psychotic symptoms have occurred exclusively during Major Depressive Episodes.
Schizoaffective Disorder	Is characterized by periods in which Major Depressive Episodes are concurrent with the active-phase symptoms of Schizophrenia, periods in which delusions or hallucinations occur for at least 2 weeks in the absence of a Major Depressive Episode, and the Major Depressive Episodes are present for a majority of the total duration of the illness. The diagnosis is Major Depressive Disorder With Psychotic Features if the psychotic symptoms have occurred exclusively during Major Depressive Episodes.

3.4.1 Differential Diagnosis for Major Depressive Disorder *(continued)*

Major or Mild Neurocognitive Disorder Due to Another Medical Condition or Substance/Medication-Induced Major or Mild Neurocognitive Disorder	Is characterized by evidence of decline from a previous level of performance in one or more cognitive domains that is due to the physiological effects of a medical condition or the persisting effects of substance use.
Adjustment Disorder With Depressed Mood	Is characterized by depressive symptoms that occur in response to a stressor and do not meet criteria for a Major Depressive Episode.
Bereavement	Occurs in response to the loss of a loved one and is generally less severe than a Major Depressive Episode. The predominant affects in grief are feelings of emptiness and loss, whereas in Major Depressive Episode they are persistent depressed mood and a diminished ability to experience pleasure. Moreover, the dysphoric mood in grief is likely to decrease in intensity over days to weeks and occurs in waves that tend to be associated with thoughts or reminders of the deceased, whereas the depressed mood in a Major Depressive Episode is more persistent and not tied to specific thoughts or preoccupations.
Nonpathological periods of sadness	Is characterized by short duration, few associated symptoms, and lack of significant functional impairment or distress.

3.4.2 Differential Diagnosis for Persistent Depressive Disorder (Dysthymia)

Persistent Depressive Disorder, which is characterized by depressed mood for most of the day, for more days than not, for at least 2 years, must be differentiated from…	In contrast to Persistent Depressive Disorder…
Major Depressive Disorder	Includes one or more Major Depressive Episodes, which are characterized by a period of depressed mood or diminished interest or pleasure, most of the day nearly every day for at least 2 weeks, accompanied by at least five characteristic symptoms (e.g., sleep changes, appetite changes, changes in level of activity, fatigue, feelings of worthlessness or excessive guilt, difficulty concentrating, suicidal ideation or behavior). Persistent Depressive Disorder has a lower symptom threshold (i.e., only two symptoms plus depressed mood) and lower persistence threshold (i.e., more days than not) but requires at least a 2-year duration. Thus, a Major Depressive Episode lasting at least 2 years will meet criteria for Persistent Depressive Disorder. If criteria are met for both Major Depressive Disorder and Persistent Depressive Disorder, both should be diagnosed.
Chronic psychotic disorders (i.e., Schizophrenia, Delusional Disorder, Schizoaffective Disorder)	May be characterized by associated chronic depressed mood. A separate diagnosis of Persistent Depressive Disorder is not made if the symptoms occur only during the course of the psychotic disorder (including residual phases).
Depressive Disorder Due to Another Medical Condition	Requires the presence of an etiological medical condition. Persistent Depressive Disorder is not diagnosed if the depressive symptoms are all due to the direct physiological effects of a general medical condition. Chronic mild depression is a common associated feature of many chronic medical conditions (e.g., diabetes), and Persistent Depressive Disorder may be diagnosed if the medical condition is merely comorbid with and not the physiological cause of the depression.

3.4.2 Differential Diagnosis for Persistent Depressive Disorder (Dysthymia) *(continued)*

Substance/Medication-Induced Depressive Disorder	Is due to the direct physiological effects of a substance. Persistent Depressive Disorder is not diagnosed if the depressive symptoms are all due to the direct physiological effects of a substance (including medication).
Bipolar I and Bipolar II Disorders	Are characterized by Manic Episodes and Hypomanic Episodes, respectively. Persistent Depressive Disorder cannot be diagnosed if a Manic or Hypomanic Episode has ever been present.
Cyclothymic Disorder	Is characterized by hypomanic periods in addition to depressive periods. Persistent Depressive Disorder cannot be diagnosed if the criteria for Cyclothymic Disorder have ever been met.
Personality Disorder	Is characterized by an enduring pattern of inner experience and behavior that deviates markedly from the expectations of the individual's culture, with onset by adolescence or early adulthood. Personality disorders commonly co-occur with Persistent Depressive Disorder. If criteria are met for Persistent Depressive Disorder and a Personality Disorder, both may be diagnosed.

3.4.3 Differential Diagnosis for Premenstrual Dysphoric Disorder

Premenstrual Dysphoric Disorder—characterized by marked affective lability, irritability, anger, or increased interpersonal conflicts; marked depressed mood, feelings of hopelessness, or self-deprecating thoughts; or marked anxiety, tension, and/or feelings of being "keyed up" or "on edge"—which develops in the final week before the onset of menses, starts to improve within a few days after the onset of menses, and becomes minimal or absent in the week postmenses, must be differentiated from...	In contrast to Premenstrual Dysphoric Disorder...
Premenstrual syndrome	Is characterized by symptoms that occur during the premenstrual period of the menstrual cycle that fall short of the required threshold of five symptoms for Premenstrual Dysphoric Disorder. Moreover, there is no requirement for affective symptoms during the premenstrual period.
Dysmenorrhea	Is characterized by painful menses that begin with the onset of menses. In contrast, Premenstrual Dysphoric Disorder begins before the onset of menses and is characterized by affective changes.
Depressive Disorder Due to Another Medical Condition	Is characterized by dysphoric symptoms that are due to the direct physiological effects of an identified medical condition (e.g., hyperthyroidism).
Substance/Medication-Induced Depressive Disorder (including hormonal treatments)	Is characterized by dysphoric symptoms that are due to the direct physiological effects of a substance or medication. Moderate to severe premenstrual symptoms may develop after initiation of exogenous hormone use. If the woman stops taking hormones and the symptoms disappear, this is consistent with Substance/Medication-Induced Depressive Disorder.

3.4.3 Differential Diagnosis for Premenstrual Dysphoric Disorder *(continued)*

Bipolar I Disorder	Is characterized by Manic and Major Depressive Episodes that are temporally unrelated to the menstrual cycle. However, because the onset of menses constitutes a memorable event, some women may report that mood symptoms occur only during the premenstrual period or that symptoms worsen premenstrually. Prospective daily symptom ratings during at least two symptomatic cycles are therefore important for documenting the time of onset and offset of mood symptoms.
Major Depressive Disorder or Persistent Depressive Disorder (Dysthymia)	Is characterized by Major Depressive Episodes or depressive symptoms that are temporally unrelated to the menstrual cycle. However, because the onset of menses constitutes a memorable event, some women may report that mood symptoms occur only during the premenstrual period or that symptoms worsen premenstrually. Prospective daily symptom ratings during at least two symptomatic cycles are therefore important for documenting the time of onset and offset of mood symptoms.

3.4.4 Differential Diagnosis for Disruptive Mood Dysregulation Disorder

Disruptive Mood Dysregulation Disorder, which is characterized by severe recurrent temper outbursts manifested verbally and/or behaviorally that are grossly out of proportion in intensity to the provocation and that are accompanied by a persistently irritable or angry mood most of the day, nearly every day, in between the outbursts, must be differentiated from…	In contrast to Disruptive Mood Dysregulation Disorder…
Depressive Disorder Due to Another Medical Condition	Is characterized by dysphoric symptoms that are due to the direct physiological effects of an identified medical condition.
Substance/Medication-Induced Depressive Disorder	Is characterized by dysphoric symptoms that are due to the direct physiological effects of a substance or medication.
Bipolar I and Bipolar II Disorders	Are characterized by episodic illnesses with discrete episodes of mood perturbation that are distinguishable from the child's baseline. In addition, the change in mood during Manic or Hypomanic Episodes is accompanied by increased energy and activity as well as associated cognitive, behavioral, and physical symptoms (e.g., distractibility, rapid speech, decreased need for sleep). In contrast, the irritability of Disruptive Mood Dysregulation Disorder is persistent and present chronically over many months.
Oppositional Defiant Disorder	Is characterized by a pattern of angry/irritable mood, argumentative/defiant behavior, or vindictiveness. In contrast, Disruptive Mood Dysregulation Disorder is also characterized by the presence of severe and frequently recurrent outbursts and a persistent disruption in mood between outbursts. If criteria are met for both disorders, only Disruptive Mood Dysregulation Disorder is diagnosed.

3.4.4 Differential Diagnosis for Disruptive Mood Dysregulation Disorder *(continued)*

Major Depressive Disorder	May be characterized by irritable mood accompanying the episodes of depressed mood or diminished interest or pleasure. Children whose irritability is present only in the context of a Major Depressive Episode should receive a diagnosis of Major Depressive Disorder rather than Disruptive Mood Dysregulation Disorder. If the irritability extends outside the depressed episodes, both diagnoses may be appropriate.
Anxiety Disorders	May be characterized by irritable mood occurring in anxiety-provoking situations. Children whose irritability is manifest only in anxiety-provoking contexts should receive the relevant Anxiety Disorder diagnosis rather than a diagnosis of Disruptive Mood Dysregulation Disorder. If the irritability extends outside the anxiety-provoking situations, diagnoses of both Disruptive Mood Dysregulation Disorder and the Anxiety Disorder may be appropriate.
Autism Spectrum Disorder	May be characterized by temper outbursts, especially when routines are disturbed. If temper outbursts are better explained by Autism Spectrum Disorder, then Disruptive Mood Dysregulation Disorder is not diagnosed.
Intermittent Explosive Disorder	Is characterized by aggressive outbursts that can resemble the severe temper tantrums in Disruptive Mood Dysregulation Disorder; however, there is no persistent irritable or angry mood between outbursts as in Disruptive Mood Dysregulation Disorder. In addition, Intermittent Explosive Disorder requires only 3 months of active symptoms, in contrast to the 12-month requirement for Disruptive Mood Dysregulation Disorder. Intermittent Explosive Disorder is not diagnosed if criteria are met for Disruptive Mood Dysregulation Disorder.

Anxiety Disorders

3.5.1 Differential Diagnosis for Separation Anxiety Disorder

Separation Anxiety Disorder, which is characterized by developmentally inappropriate and excessive anxiety concerning separation from major attachment figures, must be differentiated from...	In contrast to Separation Anxiety Disorder...
Generalized Anxiety Disorder	Is characterized by anxiety and worry in a multitude of different areas and is not limited to issues of separation from family.
Panic Disorder	Is characterized by recurrent unexpected Panic Attacks. In contrast, individuals with Separation Anxiety Disorder may experience Panic Attacks but only when threatened with separation from major attachment figures.
Agoraphobia	Is characterized by anxiety about being trapped or incapacitated in places or situations from which escape is perceived as difficult in the event of panic-like symptoms or other incapacitating symptoms. In Separation Anxiety Disorder, the focus of the fear is on separation from major attachment figures.
Posttraumatic Stress Disorder	May be characterized by fear of separation from loved ones after traumatic events such as disasters, particularly when periods of separation from loved ones were experienced during the traumatic event. However, the main symptoms involve reexperiencing memories or avoiding situations associated with the traumatic event itself, whereas in Separation Anxiety Disorder, the worries and avoidance concern the well-being of attachment figures and fears of being separated from them.
Social Anxiety Disorder (Social Phobia)	May be characterized by school refusal that is due to the fear of being judged negatively by peers or teachers. In contrast, school refusal in Separation Anxiety Disorder is due to worries about being separated from major attachment figures.

3.5.1 Differential Diagnosis for Separation Anxiety Disorder *(continued)*

Illness Anxiety Disorder	May be characterized by the individual's worry about specific illnesses he or she may have, but the main concern is the medical diagnosis itself. In Separation Anxiety Disorder, the focus of illness concern is on the possibility that the illness might result in the person's being separated from major attachment figures.
Conduct Disorder	May be characterized by school avoidance (truancy), but anxiety about separation is not responsible for the school absences, and the child or adolescent usually stays away from, rather than returns to, the home.
Oppositional Defiant Disorder	Is characterized by persistent oppositional behavior unrelated to the anticipation or occurrence of separation. In contrast, some children and adolescents with Separation Anxiety Disorder may be oppositional in the context of being forced to separate from attachment figures.
Depressive disorders	May be associated with reluctance to leave home that is due to loss of interest, fatigue, or concern about crying in public rather than worry or fear of untoward events befalling attachment figures.
Dependent Personality Disorder	Is characterized by an indiscriminate tendency to rely on others. In contrast, in Separation Anxiety Disorder, the concern is about the proximity and safety of main attachment figures.
Borderline Personality Disorder	Is characterized by fear of abandonment by loved ones, but there are also problems with identity, self-direction, interpersonal functioning, and impulsivity. If criteria are met for both Separation Anxiety Disorder and Borderline Personality Disorder, both may be diagnosed.

3.5.1 Differential Diagnosis for Separation Anxiety Disorder *(continued)*

Developmentally appropriate separation anxiety	Is part of normal early development and may indicate the development of secure attachment relationships, such as when infants around age 1 year experience stranger anxiety.

3.5.2 Differential Diagnosis for Selective Mutism

Selective Mutism, which is characterized by consistent failure to speak in specific social situations in which there is an expectation for speaking, must be differentiated from…	In contrast to Selective Mutism…
Communication Disorders	Are characterized by speech disturbances (e.g., dysfluencies, speech sound problems) that occur consistently regardless of the situation that the individual is in. In contrast, in Selective Mutism the speech difficulties occur only in certain situations (e.g., social situations with children and adults) but not others (e.g., with immediate family).
Autism Spectrum Disorder and Schizophrenia Spectrum and Other Psychotic Disorders	May also be characterized by difficulty speaking in social situations, but unlike Selective Mutism, these difficulties are evident even when the individual is speaking with immediate family members.
Social Anxiety Disorder (Social Phobia)	Is characterized by fear and anxiety occurring in social situations in which the person is exposed to possible scrutiny by others, whereas a diagnosis of Selective Mutism specifically describes a pattern of inability to speak in certain situations, which are typically social. In situations where the failure to speak is associated with feelings of social anxiety, both diagnoses of Selective Mutism and Social Anxiety Disorder may be made.

3.5.3 Differential Diagnosis for Specific Phobia

Specific Phobia, which is characterized by marked fear or anxiety about a specific object or situation, must be differentiated from…	In contrast to Specific Phobia…
Agoraphobia	Is characterized by fear and avoidance of situations from two or more agoraphobic clusters (i.e., public transportation, open spaces, enclosed places, standing in line or being in a crowd, being outside of the home alone). In Specific Phobia, Situational Type, the fear and avoidance is confined to only one situation (e.g., heights) or several situations, all of which fall within the same cluster (e.g., elevators and airplanes, both within the public transportation cluster).
Social Anxiety Disorder (Social Phobia)	Is characterized by fear and avoidance restricted to social situations.
Posttraumatic Stress Disorder or Acute Stress Disorder	Is characterized by fear and avoidance confined to stimuli that remind the individual of a previously experienced life-threatening event.
Obsessive-Compulsive Disorder	May be characterized by fear and avoidance associated with the content of the obsessions (e.g., avoidance of dirt by an individual with a contamination obsession).
Separation Anxiety Disorder	Is characterized by fear or avoidance of situations in which the individual would be separated from major attachment figures.
Psychotic Disorders	May be characterized by avoidance that occurs as a consequence of a delusional belief (e.g., avoidance of flying by an individual with a persecutory delusional system who is convinced that he or she is going to be the target of a terrorist attack).
Anorexia Nervosa, Avoidant/Restrictive Food Intake Disorder, Bulimia Nervosa, and Binge-Eating Disorder	May be characterized by avoidance behavior, but it is exclusively related to avoiding food and food-related cues.

3.5.3 Differential Diagnosis for Specific Phobia *(continued)*

Nonpathological avoidance of circumscribed objects or situations	Either represents a realistic level of avoidance given the actual danger (e.g., avoidance of skydiving from an airplane) or is not severe enough to cause clinically significant impairment or distress, often because of the ease of avoiding the phobic stimulus (e.g., a person who fears snakes but rarely would encounter one because he or she lives in Manhattan).
Transient fears in childhood	Are common and short-lived, lasting for less than 6 months.

3.5.4 Differential Diagnosis for Social Anxiety Disorder (Social Phobia)

Social Anxiety Disorder, which is characterized by marked fear or anxiety about social situations in which the individual is exposed to possible scrutiny by others, must be differentiated from…	In contrast to Social Anxiety Disorder…
Panic Disorder	Is typically not limited to social situations and is characterized by the initial onset of unexpected Panic Attacks.
Agoraphobia	May be characterized by fear and avoidance of social situations (e.g., going to a movie), but the individual's fear is that escape might be difficult or help might not be available in the event of incapacitation or panic-like symptoms. In Social Anxiety Disorder, the focus of the fear is scrutiny by others.
Generalized Anxiety Disorder	May be characterized by social worries, but the focus is more on the nature of ongoing relationships than on fear of negative evaluation. For example, individuals with Generalized Anxiety Disorder, particularly children, may be excessively worried about the quality of their social performance, but they also worry about the quality of their performance in nonsocial situations where social evaluation by others is not the issue (e.g., getting a good grade on a test). In Social Anxiety Disorder, the worries are exclusively focused on social performance and the scrutiny of others.
Specific Phobia	May be characterized by fear of embarrassment or humiliation related to the individual's intense reaction to exposure to phobic stimuli (e.g., embarrassment about fainting when having blood drawn), but there is not a general fear of negative evaluation in other social situations.

3.5.4 Differential Diagnosis for Social Anxiety Disorder (Social Phobia) *(continued)*

Separation Anxiety Disorder	May be characterized by avoidance of social settings (including school refusal), but the avoidance is due to concerns about being separated from attachment figures or concerns about being embarrassed by needing to leave prematurely to return to attachment figures. Individuals with Social Anxiety Disorder tend to be uncomfortable even in social situations in which attachment figures are present.
Selective Mutism	Is characterized by a failure to speak in some situations due to a fear of negative evaluation, but unlike Social Anxiety Disorder, there is no fear of negative evaluation in social situations where no speaking is required (e.g., nonverbal play).
Oppositional Defiant Disorder	May be characterized by a refusal to speak due to opposition to authority figures. Individuals with Social Anxiety Disorder may be afraid to speak due to fear of negative evaluation.
Autism Spectrum Disorder	Is characterized by social anxiety and social communication deficits that typically result in a lack of age-appropriate social relationships. Although individuals with Social Anxiety Disorder may appear impaired when first interacting with unfamiliar peers or adults, they typically have adequate age-appropriate social relationships and social communication capacity.
Avoidant Personality Disorder	Is conceptualized as a Personality Disorder but describes many of the same individuals who have Social Anxiety Disorder. If criteria are met for Social Anxiety Disorder and Avoidant Personality Disorder, both diagnoses may be given.

3.5.4 Differential Diagnosis for Social Anxiety Disorder (Social Phobia) *(continued)*

Major Depressive Disorder	Is characterized by negative self-esteem that may be accompanied by concerns about being negatively evaluated by others, but these concerns extend beyond social situations. Individuals with Social Anxiety Disorder are worried about being negatively evaluated because of certain social behaviors, physical symptoms, or appearance, and generally do not experience negative self-esteem outside of social situations.
Body Dysmorphic Disorder	Is characterized by the relatively fixed belief that particular features render the individual misshapen or ugly, which may result in social anxiety and avoidance of social situations. A separate diagnosis of Social Anxiety Disorder is generally not warranted if the social fears and avoidance are restricted to body dysmorphic concerns.
Delusional Disorder	May be characterized by delusions and/or hallucinations that focus on being rejected or offending others. In contrast, the concerns in Social Anxiety Disorder are not held with delusional intensity.
Medical conditions	May produce symptoms that may be socially embarrassing (e.g., trembling in Parkinson's disease, reddening in rosacea). An additional diagnosis of Social Anxiety Disorder is given only when the fear of negative evaluation by others because of those symptoms is disproportionate.

3.5.4 Differential Diagnosis for Social Anxiety Disorder (Social Phobia) *(continued)*

Social anxiety and avoidance associated with other mental disorders, such as Eating Disorders or Schizophrenia	Are characterized by anxiety that occurs only during the course of the other mental disorder. If the anxiety is judged to be better accounted for by the other mental disorder, an additional diagnosis of Social Anxiety Disorder is not given. For example, social fears and discomfort can occur as part of Schizophrenia, but other evidence for psychotic symptoms will also be present. Social anxiety may co-occur with Eating Disorders, but if the fear of negative evaluation about symptoms (e.g., purging and vomiting) is the sole source of social anxiety, an additional diagnosis of Social Anxiety Disorder is not warranted.
Normal shyness	Is a common personality trait that for most shy people does not lead to clinically significant adverse impact on functioning.

3.5.5 Differential Diagnosis for Panic Disorder

Panic Disorder, which is characterized by recurrent unexpected Panic Attacks followed by a month of worry or a change in behavior related to the attacks, must be differentiated from…	In contrast to Panic Disorder…
Anxiety Disorder Due to Another Medical Condition	Requires the presence of an etiological medical condition (e.g., hyperthyroidism). Panic Disorder is not diagnosed if the Panic Attacks are all due to the direct physiological effects of a general medical condition on the central nervous system.
Substance/Medication-Induced Anxiety Disorder	Is due to the direct physiological effects of a substance or medication. Panic Disorder is not diagnosed if the Panic Attacks are all due to the direct physiological effects of a substance (including medication).
Panic Attacks occurring as part of another mental disorder	Many mental disorders (e.g., Social Anxiety Disorder [Social Phobia], Specific Phobia, Separation Anxiety Disorder, Obsessive-Compulsive Disorder, Hoarding Disorder, Posttraumatic Stress Disorder, Major Depressive Disorder) may be characterized by Panic Attacks occurring in situations in which the individual is already experiencing some level of anxiety related to that disorder. For example, a person with Social Anxiety Disorder may become so anxious in a social situation that it triggers a Panic Attack, or an individual with contamination concerns in Obsessive-Compulsive Disorder may develop extreme distress when exposed to germs or dirt, which culminates in a Panic Attack. In such cases, the specifier "With Panic Attacks" may be noted. In contrast, the Panic Attacks in individuals with Panic Disorder are unexpected (i.e., the Panic Attacks come on "out of the blue"), at least during the initial phase of the disorder.

3.5.5 Differential Diagnosis for Panic Disorder *(continued)*

Exposure to an extremely anxiety-provoking experience	May be characterized by the development of a Panic Attack (e.g., an individual having a Panic Attack while being held up at gunpoint). In contrast, the Panic Attacks in individuals with Panic Disorder are unexpected (i.e., come on out of the blue), at least during the initial phase of the disorder.
Isolated Panic Attack	Is characterized by a single Panic Attack, which may or may not have come on out of the blue and by itself is not indicative of psychopathology. A diagnosis of Panic Disorder requires at least two unexpected Panic Attacks.
Limited-symptom attacks	Are characterized by panic-like attacks that have fewer than the minimum of four symptoms required for a Panic Attack.

3.5.6 Differential Diagnosis for Agoraphobia

Agoraphobia, which is characterized by fear or avoidance of multiple situations due to thoughts that escape might be difficult or help might not be available in the event of developing panic-like symptoms, must be differentiated from…	In contrast to Agoraphobia…
Social Anxiety Disorder (Social Phobia)	Is characterized by avoidance specifically of social situations in which the person will be exposed to the scrutiny of others.
Specific Phobia, Situational Type	Is characterized by avoidance of a specific feared situation, such as closed spaces, as opposed to fear and avoidance of multiple situations across two or more of the agoraphobic clusters (i.e., public transportation, open spaces, enclosed places, standing in line or being in a crowd, being outside of the home alone).
Posttraumatic Stress Disorder or Acute Stress Disorder	May be characterized by avoidance of people, places, activities, or situations that arouse upsetting memories, thoughts, or feelings about the traumatic event.
Major Depressive Disorder	Some individuals with Major Depressive Disorder may be housebound due to feelings of apathy, fatigue, loss of capacity to experience pleasure, or concerns about crying in public. In contrast, the lack of willingness of some individuals with Agoraphobia to leave their homes is a result of extreme fears that help might not be available in the event of developing panic-like symptoms.
Psychotic Disorder featuring delusions (e.g., Delusional Disorder, Schizophrenia, Major Depressive Disorder With Psychotic Features)	May be characterized by avoidance that results from delusional concerns (e.g., avoidance of going outside one's house because of the conviction that one is being followed).

3.5.6 Differential Diagnosis for Agoraphobia *(continued)*

Obsessive-Compulsive Disorder	May be characterized by avoidance behavior that is intended to prevent triggering an obsession or compulsion (e.g., avoidance of "dirty" objects related to fears of contamination or avoidance of kitchen knives by someone who is having obsessive thoughts of stabbing his or her spouse).
Separation Anxiety Disorder	Is characterized by avoidance of situations that involve being away from major attachment figures, including refusing to go out of one's house because of a fear of separation.
Avoidance related to potentially disabling medical conditions	May be characterized by avoidance that results from realistic concerns (e.g., about fainting for an individual with an arrhythmia). However, in contrast to Agoraphobia, the avoidance is at a level that is appropriate and realistic given the nature of the medical condition.

3.5.7 Differential Diagnosis for Generalized Anxiety Disorder

Generalized Anxiety Disorder, which is characterized by excessive anxiety and worry lasting at least 6 months, must be differentiated from…	In contrast to Generalized Anxiety Disorder…
Anxiety Disorder Due to Another Medical Condition	Requires the presence of an etiological medical condition (e.g., pheochromocytoma). Generalized Anxiety Disorder is not diagnosed if the generalized anxiety is due to the direct physiological effects of a general medical condition.
Substance/Medication-Induced Anxiety Disorder	Is due to the direct physiological effects of a substance or medication and may have its onset during intoxication with or withdrawal from an abused substance, or occur as a side effect of a medication. Generalized Anxiety Disorder is not diagnosed if the generalized anxiety is due to the direct physiological effects of a substance on the central nervous system, such as during Cocaine Intoxication or Opioid Withdrawal.
Panic Disorder	Is characterized by anxiety and worry about having additional Panic Attacks. An additional diagnosis of Generalized Anxiety Disorder should be made only if there is additional anxiety and worry unrelated to the Panic Attacks.
Social Anxiety Disorder (Social Phobia)	Is characterized by excessive anxiety and worry focused exclusively on social situations. An additional diagnosis of Generalized Anxiety Disorder should be made only if there is anxiety and worry focused on nonsocial situations (e.g., work or school performance).
Somatic Symptom Disorder or Illness Anxiety Disorder	May be characterized by excessive anxiety and worry focused exclusively on health, becoming ill, or the seriousness of somatic symptoms (e.g., worry that a headache is indicative of a brain tumor). An additional diagnosis of Generalized Anxiety Disorder should be made only if there is anxiety and worry focused on non-health-related situations.

3.5.7 Differential Diagnosis for Generalized Anxiety Disorder *(continued)*

Separation Anxiety Disorder	Is characterized by excessive anxiety and worry focused exclusively on concerns about separation from major attachment figures. An additional diagnosis of Generalized Anxiety Disorder should be made only if there is anxiety and worry focused on situations that are unrelated to separation concerns.
Posttraumatic Stress Disorder or Acute Stress Disorder	Is characterized by anxiety occurring in relation to exposure to internal or external cues that symbolize or resemble an aspect of the traumatic event or as part of the generalized hyperarousal and reactivity associated with having been exposed to the traumatic event. An additional diagnosis of Generalized Anxiety Disorder should be made only if there is anxiety and worry focused on situations that are unrelated to the traumatic event.
Anorexia Nervosa or Bulimia Nervosa	May be characterized by anxiety or worry associated with the fear of gaining weight. An additional diagnosis of Generalized Anxiety Disorder should be made only if there is anxiety and worry unrelated to issues about weight.
Obsessive-Compulsive Disorder	Is usually characterized by repetitive anxiety-provoking thoughts that are experienced as intrusive, unwanted, inappropriate, and ego-dystonic, and that are usually accompanied by compulsions that serve to reduce the anxiety. In contrast, the worries in Generalized Anxiety Disorder typically arise from everyday routine life, such as possible job responsibilities, the health of family members, finances, or minor matters such as household chores or being late for appointments.

3.5.7 Differential Diagnosis for Generalized Anxiety Disorder *(continued)*

Adjustment Disorder With Anxiety	Is characterized by clinically significant anxiety symptoms that do not meet the criteria for any specific anxiety disorder (including Generalized Anxiety Disorder) and that occur in response to a stressor.
Bipolar Disorders, Depressive Disorders, and Schizophrenia Spectrum and Other Psychotic Disorders	Are commonly characterized by anxiety occurring as an associated feature, but include other specific symptoms characteristic of the particular mood or Psychotic Disorder. Generalized Anxiety Disorder should not be diagnosed separately if it has occurred only during the course of a Bipolar, Depressive, or Psychotic Disorder.
Nonpathological anxiety	Is characterized by worries that are more controllable or are not severe enough to cause clinically significant distress or impairment in functioning.

Obsessive-Compulsive and Related Disorders

3.6.1 Differential Diagnosis for Obsessive-Compulsive Disorder

Obsessive-Compulsive Disorder (OCD), which is characterized by obsessions (i.e., recurrent thoughts, urges, or images that are experienced as intrusive and unwanted that the person attempts to ignore or suppress) and/or compulsions (i.e., repetitive behaviors or mental acts that the person feels driven to perform in response to an obsession or according to rules that must be applied rigidly), must be differentiated from…	In contrast to Obsessive-Compulsive Disorder…
Obsessive-Compulsive and Related Disorder Due to Another Medical Condition	Requires the presence of an etiological medical condition. OCD is not diagnosed if the obsessions and compulsions are all due to the direct physiological effects of a general medical condition.
Substance/Medication-Induced Obsessive-Compulsive and Related Disorder	Is due to the direct physiological effects of a substance or medication. OCD is not diagnosed if the obsessions and compulsions are all due to the direct physiological effects of a substance (including medication).
Hoarding Disorder	Is characterized by a persistent difficulty discarding or parting with possessions and an excessive accumulation of objects. However, for an individual with certain obsessions (e.g., concerns about incompleteness or harm) with associated hoarding compulsions (e.g., acquiring all objects in a set to attain a sense of completeness), a diagnosis of OCD should be given instead.
Body Dysmorphic Disorder or Eating Disorder	Is characterized by recurrent thoughts exclusively related to a preoccupation with appearance or body weight.

3.6.1 Differential Diagnosis for Obsessive-Compulsive Disorder *(continued)*

Specific Phobia	Is characterized by fear and avoidance cued to specific circumscribed objects or situations. In OCD, the fear and avoidance of a specific object or situation is related to avoiding the triggering of an obsession or compulsion (e.g., avoidance of dirt in an individual with a contamination obsession).
Social Anxiety Disorder (Social Phobia)	Is characterized by fear and avoidance cued to social situations, and repetitive reassurance behavior is focused on reducing the social fear.
Trichotillomania (Hair-Pulling Disorder) or Excoriation (Skin-Picking) Disorder	Is characterized by recurrent thoughts and actions limited to hair pulling or skin picking.
Illness Anxiety Disorder	Is characterized by recurrent thoughts exclusively related to the idea that one has a serious disease.
Major Depressive Episode	May be characterized by recurrent ruminations that are usually mood congruent and not necessarily experienced as intrusive or distressing. Moreover, depressive ruminations are not linked to compulsions, as is typical of OCD.
Generalized Anxiety Disorder	Is characterized by recurrent thoughts (i.e., worries) about real-life concerns, and the thoughts are not accompanied by compulsions.
Delusional Disorder	Is characterized by recurrent thoughts that are held with delusional conviction.
Schizophrenia	Is characterized by ruminative delusional thoughts and stereotyped behaviors that are accompanied by other characteristic symptoms of Schizophrenia (e.g., hallucinations, disorganized speech, negative symptoms).

3.6.1 Differential Diagnosis for Obsessive-Compulsive Disorder *(continued)*

Tic Disorders	Are characterized by sudden, rapid, recurrent, nonrhythmic motor movements or vocalizations (e.g., eye blinking, throat clearing) that are less complex than compulsions and are not aimed at neutralizing obsessions.
Stereotypic Movement Disorder	Is characterized by repetitive, seemingly driven, nonfunctional motor behaviors (e.g., head banging, body rocking, self-biting) that are less complex than compulsions and are not aimed at neutralizing obsessions.
Driven ("compulsive") behaviors associated with other mental disorders	Are associated with disorders such as Gambling Disorder, Paraphilic Disorders, and Substance Use Disorders, and are characterized by the person's deriving pleasure from the activity and wanting to resist it only because of its deleterious consequences. In contrast, the obsessions and compulsions in OCD are a source of intense anxiety and are not experienced as pleasurable.
Obsessive-Compulsive Personality Disorder	Involves an enduring and pervasive maladaptive pattern of excessive perfectionism and rigid control and is not characterized by the presence of obsessions or compulsions.
Nonpathological superstitions and repetitive behaviors	Are not time-consuming and do not result in clinically significant impairment or distress.

3.6.2 Differential Diagnosis for Body Dysmorphic Disorder

Body Dysmorphic Disorder, which is characterized by a preoccupation with perceived defects or flaws in physical appearance, must be differentiated from…	In contrast to Body Dysmorphic Disorder…
Normal appearance concerns and concerns about clearly noticeable physical defects	Do not involve excessive appearance-related preoccupations and repetitive behaviors that are time-consuming, are usually difficult to resist or control, and cause marked distress or impairment.
Anorexia Nervosa and Bulimia Nervosa	Are characterized by concerns that are limited to body shape and weight. A comorbid diagnosis of Body Dysmorphic Disorder may be appropriate if appearance preoccupations go beyond overall body shape and weight (e.g., preoccupation with a perceived facial defect).
Gender Dysphoria	Is characterized by bodily concerns that are limited to wanting to get rid of primary or secondary sexual characteristics. Body Dysmorphic Disorder should be diagnosed only if appearance preoccupations go beyond physical manifestations of gender.
Major Depressive Episode, Avoidant Personality Disorder, and Social Anxiety Disorder (Social Phobia)	Are often characterized by feelings of low self-esteem and defectiveness that may include concerns about body appearance. In contrast, in Body Dysmorphic Disorder, the individual is preoccupied by his or her perceived defects in appearance and performs repetitive behaviors (e.g., mirror checking, excessive grooming, skin picking, reassurance seeking) or mental acts (e.g., comparing his or her appearance with that of others) in response to the appearance concerns.
Obsessive-Compulsive Disorder	Includes intrusive thoughts and repetitive behaviors that are not limited to concerns about appearance.

3.6.2 Differential Diagnosis for Body Dysmorphic Disorder *(continued)*

Trichotillomania (Hair-Pulling Disorder)	Is characterized by recurrent pulling out of one's hair resulting in hair loss, accompanied by repeated attempts to stop that are not motivated by a desire to improve defects in appearance related to excessive body hair. However, if the hair-pulling behavior occurs in conjunction with a preoccupation with a defect in appearance involving excessive body hair, then a diagnosis of Body Dysmorphic Disorder may be more appropriate.
Excoriation (Skin-Picking) Disorder	Is characterized by recurrent skin picking resulting in skin lesions, accompanied by repeated attempts to stop that are not motivated by a desire to improve the appearance of a perceived skin defect. If the skin-picking behavior occurs in conjunction with a preoccupation with a perceived skin defect, then a diagnosis of Body Dysmorphic Disorder may be more appropriate.
Delusional Disorder, Somatic Type	Is characterized by prominent delusions involving bodily functions or sensations. For some individuals with Body Dysmorphic Disorder, their beliefs about a defect in appearance are held with delusional conviction (i.e., they are completely convinced that their view of their perceived defects is accurate). These individuals are diagnosed as having Body Dysmorphic Disorder With Absent Insight, as opposed to having Delusional Disorder.
Histrionic Personality Disorder or Narcissistic Personality Disorder	May be characterized by concerns with appearance that do not involve specific defects.
Body integrity identity disorder (preoccupation with the desire to become disabled, with onset in childhood)	May be characterized by a preoccupation with the desire to have a limb amputated to correct a perceived mismatch between the person's sense of bodily identity and his or her anatomical configuration. However, unlike with Body Dysmorphic Disorder, the preoccupation does not focus on the limb's appearance.

3.6.3 Differential Diagnosis for Hoarding Disorder

Hoarding Disorder, which is characterized by persistent difficulty discarding or parting with possessions because of a perceived need to save the items, must be differentiated from…	In contrast to Hoarding Disorder…
Obsessive-Compulsive and Related Disorder Due to Another Medical Condition	Requires the presence of an etiological medical condition (e.g., traumatic brain injury, surgical resection for seizure control, cerebrovascular disease). Hoarding Disorder is not diagnosed if the hoarding behavior is due to the direct physiological effects of a general medical condition.
Major Neurocognitive Disorder Due to a neurodegenerative condition, such as frontotemporal lobar degeneration or Alzheimer's disease	The onset of the accumulating behavior is gradual and follows the course of the neurocognitive disorder and may be accompanied with self-neglect and severe domestic squalor, alongside other neuropsychiatric symptoms. Hoarding Disorder is not diagnosed if the accumulation of objects is judged to be a direct consequence of a degenerative brain disorder.
Autism Spectrum Disorder	May include the excessive accumulation of objects related to a fixated interest that is abnormal in intensity (e.g., collecting matchbox covers), in which case a diagnosis of Hoarding Disorder is not made.

3.6.3 Differential Diagnosis for Hoarding Disorder *(continued)*

Obsessive-Compulsive Disorder	Is characterized by repetitive behaviors that the individual feels driven to perform in response to an obsession or according to rules that must be applied rigidly, and that are generally experienced by the individual as ego-dystonic. This is in contrast to the ego-syntonic accumulation of items in Hoarding Disorder. When an accumulation of objects occurs as a direct consequence of Obsessive-Compulsive Disorder (e.g., not discarding objects to avoid endless checking rituals), a diagnosis of Hoarding Disorder is not made. However, when severe hoarding appears concurrently with other typical symptoms of Obsessive-Compulsive Disorder but are judged to be independent from these symptoms, both Hoarding Disorder and Obsessive-Compulsive Disorder may be diagnosed.
Psychotic Disorder (e.g., Schizophrenia)	May be characterized by an accumulation of objects as a consequence of a delusional belief (e.g., collecting discarded pieces of aluminum foil to protect oneself from radiation) or a command hallucination, in which case a diagnosis of Hoarding Disorder is not made.
Major Depressive Episode	May be associated with a cluttered environment that occurs as a direct consequence of depressive symptoms such as fatigue, inertia, and psychomotor retardation, in which case a diagnosis of Hoarding Disorder is not made.
Normal collecting behavior	Is organized and systematic, even if in some cases the actual amount of possessions may be similar to an individual with Hoarding Disorder. Moreover, it does not produce the clutter, distress, or impairment typical of Hoarding Disorder.

3.6.4 Differential Diagnosis for Trichotillomania (Hair-Pulling Disorder)

Trichotillomania, which is characterized by recurrent pulling out of one's hair accompanied by repeated attempts to stop hair pulling, must be differentiated from…	In contrast to Trichotillomania…
Medical conditions that cause hair loss	Certain conditions such as scarring alopecia (e.g., alopecia areata) and nonscarring alopecia (e.g., chronic discoid lupus erythematosus) can fully account for the hair loss. Trichotillomania is not diagnosed if the hair pulling is attributable to one of these medical conditions.
Obsessive-Compulsive Disorder	Is characterized by behavior that is performed in response to an obsession or according to rules that must be applied rigidly. Trichotillomania is not diagnosed if the hair pulling is a direct consequence of an obsession or compulsion (e.g., individuals with symmetry concerns may pull out hairs as part of their symmetry rituals).
Body Dysmorphic Disorder	Is characterized by a preoccupation with an imagined defect in physical appearance that in some cases may result in a preoccupation with removing body hair that the individual perceives as ugly or abnormal. Trichotillomania is not diagnosed if the hair pulling is a direct consequence of the preoccupation with a perceived defect in appearance.
Psychotic Disorder (e.g., Schizophrenia)	May be characterized by hair pulling in response to delusions or hallucinations. Trichotillomania is not diagnosed if the hair pulling is better accounted for by a Psychotic Disorder.

3.6.4 Differential Diagnosis for Trichotillomania (Hair-Pulling Disorder) *(continued)*

Stereotypic Movement Disorder	Involves repetitive behaviors other than (or in addition to) hair pulling (e.g., hand shaking or waving, body rocking, head banging).
Normative hair removal or manipulation	Is characterized by hair removal that is performed solely for cosmetic reasons (i.e., to improve one's physical appearance) or by behavior that is confined to twisting, playing with, or biting one's hair. In such cases, distress or impairment in functioning is not significant and thus such presentations would not qualify for a diagnosis of Trichotillomania.

3.6.5 Differential Diagnosis for Excoriation (Skin-Picking) Disorder

Excoriation Disorder, which is characterized by recurrent skin picking resulting in skin lesions accompanied by repeated attempts to stop, must be differentiated from…	In contrast to Excoriation Disorder…
Obsessive-Compulsive and Related Disorder Due to Another Medical Condition	The skin picking is due to the direct physiological effects of a general medical condition. Excoriation Disorder is not diagnosed if the skin picking is attributable to the direct physiological effects of a dermatological condition (e.g., scabies).
Substance/Medication-Induced Obsessive-Compulsive and Related Disorder	The skin picking is due to the direct physiological effects of a substance (e.g., cocaine). Excoriation Disorder is not diagnosed if the skin picking is fully attributable to the substance.
Obsessive-Compulsive Disorder	May include skin lesions occurring as a consequence of severe washing compulsions. Excoriation Disorder is not diagnosed if the skin lesions are better explained by Obsessive-Compulsive Disorder.
Body Dysmorphic Disorder	May include skin-picking behavior to improve a perceived defect in appearance. Excoriation Disorder is not diagnosed if the skin picking is better explained by Body Dysmorphic Disorder.
Psychotic Disorder (e.g., Schizophrenia)	May include skin picking in response to a delusion (i.e., parasitosis) or tactile hallucination (i.e., formication). In such cases, Excoriation Disorder should not be diagnosed.
Stereotypic Movement Disorder	Involves repetitive behaviors other than (or in addition to) skin picking (e.g., hand shaking or waving, body rocking, head banging).

Trauma- and Stressor-Related Disorders

3.7.1 Differential Diagnosis for Posttraumatic Stress Disorder or Acute Stress Disorder[a]

Posttraumatic Stress Disorder (PTSD) and Acute Stress Disorder (ASD), which are characterized by exposure to actual or threatened death, serious injury, or sexual violence, followed by the development of intrusion symptoms, persistent avoidance of stimuli associated with the trauma, negative alterations of cognitions and mood, and marked alterations in arousal and reactivity, must be differentiated from…	In contrast to Posttraumatic Stress Disorder or Acute Stress Disorder…
Adjustment Disorder	Is characterized by a stressor of any level of severity and does not have a specific response pattern (e.g., intrusion symptoms). The diagnosis of Adjustment Disorder is used when the response to an extreme stressor does not meet the criteria for PTSD or ASD (or another specific mental disorder) when the symptom pattern of PTSD or ASD occurs in response to a nontraumatic stressor (e.g., spouse leaving, being fired).
Persistent complex bereavement disorder (in DSM-5 Section III)	Is characterized by intrusive thoughts and memories of the deceased that persist for at least 12 months after the loss. In contrast to PTSD, where the intrusions revolve around traumatic events related to the loss, in persistent complex bereavement disorder the intrusions focus on many aspects of the deceased including positive aspects of the relationship and distress over the separation.
Other mental disorders that may occur after exposure to an extreme stressor	Are characterized by a response pattern that meets criteria for another mental disorder in DSM-5 (e.g., Brief Psychotic Disorder, Major Depressive Disorder).
Obsessive-Compulsive Disorder	Is usually characterized by recurrent intrusive thoughts, but these are experienced as inappropriate and are not related to an experienced traumatic event.

3.7.1 Differential Diagnosis for Posttraumatic Stress Disorder or Acute Stress Disorder[a] *(continued)*

Panic Disorder	May be characterized by arousal and dissociative symptoms, but these occur during Panic Attacks and are not associated with a traumatic stressor.
Generalized Anxiety Disorder	May be characterized by persistent symptoms of irritability and anxiety, but unlike PTSD or ASD, these symptoms are not associated with a traumatic stressor.
Dissociative Disorders	Are characterized by dissociative symptoms that are not necessarily related to exposure to a traumatic stressor (but often are). Dissociative symptoms occurring in the context of the full syndrome of PTSD might justify the use of the With Dissociative Symptoms specifier.
Psychotic Disorders (e.g., Schizophrenia)	May be characterized by perceptual symptoms such as illusions or hallucinations. These should be differentiated from flashbacks in PSTD or ASD, which are characterized by sensory intrusions comprising part of the traumatic event that can occur with complete loss of awareness of present surroundings. These episodes are typically brief but can be associated with prolonged distress and heightened arousal. They are generally not considered to be psychotic phenomena.
Traumatic brain injury	Is characterized by neurocognitive symptoms (e.g., persistent disorientation and confusion) that develop after a traumatic brain injury (e.g., traumatic accident, bomb blast, acceleration/deceleration trauma). Because this traumatic event can also lead to the development of ASD and PTSD, both diagnoses should be considered.
Malingering	Is characterized by feigning of symptoms and must always be ruled out when legal, financial, and other benefits play a role.

[a]PTSD and ASD are differentiated based on duration. The duration of the response pattern in ASD is from 3 days to 1 month after exposure to the traumatic stressor. The duration of the response pattern in PTSD is more than 1 month.

3.7.2 Differential Diagnosis for Adjustment Disorder

Adjustment Disorder, which is characterized by the development of clinically significant emotional or behavioral symptoms that do not meet the criteria for another mental disorder, must be differentiated from...	In contrast to Adjustment Disorder...
All other specified mental disorders	Are characterized by a specific symptom pattern and do not require that the symptoms occur in response to a stressor (except Posttraumatic Stress Disorder, Acute Stress Disorder, Reactive Attachment Disorder, and Disinhibited Social Engagement Disorder). Adjustment Disorder is not diagnosed if the symptoms meet criteria for a specific mental disorder or represent an exacerbation of an existing disorder. Adjustment Disorder can be diagnosed in addition to another mental disorder if the latter does not explain the particular symptoms that occur in reaction to the stressor. For example, an individual may develop an Adjustment Disorder With Depressed Mood after losing a job while at the same time having a diagnosis of Obsessive-Compulsive Disorder.
Posttraumatic Stress Disorder or Acute Stress Disorder	Each requires that the stressor be extreme and requires characteristic intrusion symptoms, persistent avoidance of stimuli associated with the trauma, negative alterations of cognitions and mood, and marked alterations in arousal and reactivity.
Other Specified or Unspecified categories (e.g., Other Specified Depressive Disorder)	Are diagnosed only when the criteria are not met for any specified DSM-5 disorder (including Adjustment Disorder).

3.7.2 Differential Diagnosis for Adjustment Disorder *(continued)*

Psychological Factors Affecting Other Medical Conditions	Are characterized by specific psychological entities (e.g., psychological symptoms, behaviors, other factors) that precipitate, exacerbate, or put an individual at risk for medical illness, or worsen an existing condition. In contrast, when a medical condition acts as a psychosocial stressor leading to a psychological reaction, Adjustment Disorder is diagnosed.
Bereavement	Is characterized by a reaction to the loss of a loved one that is in keeping with what would be expected. Adjustment Disorder can be diagnosed only if the symptoms are in excess of what is expected.
Persistent complex bereavement disorder (in DSM-5 Section III)	Is characterized by a persistent maladaptive and pathological reaction to the death of a loved one. In contrast to Adjustment Disorder, which has a maximum duration of 6 months, persistent complex bereavement disorder requires a minimum of 12 months of symptoms.
Nonpathological reactions to stress	Are characterized by symptoms that are within what would be expected given the nature of the stressor and that do not lead to clinically significant distress or impairment.

Dissociative Disorders

3.8.1 Differential Diagnosis for Dissociative Amnesia

Dissociative Amnesia, which is characterized by an inability to recall important autobiographical information, usually of a traumatic or stressful nature, must be differentiated from...	In contrast to Dissociative Amnesia...
Memory impairment in a Major or Mild Neurocognitive Disorder Due to Another Medical Condition	Is characterized by memory loss for personal information that is usually embedded in cognitive, linguistic, affective, attentional, and behavioral disturbances. In Dissociative Amnesia, memory deficits are primarily for autobiographical information, and intellectual and other cognitive abilities are preserved.
Alcohol or other substance-induced memory loss	Is characterized by the ability to recall events immediately (i.e., intact working memory), but not after a few minutes, given the failure of memory storage secondary to the direct effects of the substance on the central nervous system. Substance-induced "blackouts" usually cannot be reversed.
Posttraumatic amnesia due to brain injury	Is characterized by a history of a clear-cut physical trauma, a period of unconsciousness or amnesia, objective evidence of brain injury, and a brief retrograde amnesia for the time before the head injury. If the retrograde posttraumatic amnesia is so extensive that it is out of proportion to the brain injury, a comorbid diagnosis of Dissociative Amnesia may be appropriate.
Dissociative Identity Disorder	Is characterized by pervasive discontinuities in sense of self and agency, accompanied by many other dissociative symptoms. In individuals with Dissociative Amnesia, the amnesia tends to be localized, selective, and relatively stable. Dissociative Amnesia is not diagnosed if the memory gaps are better explained by Dissociative Identity Disorder.

3.8.1 Differential Diagnosis for Dissociative Amnesia *(continued)*

Posttraumatic Stress Disorder or Acute Stress Disorder	May be characterized by an inability to recall part or all of a specific traumatic event. Amnesia confined to the traumatic event occurring in the context of Posttraumatic Stress Disorder would generally not warrant an additional diagnosis of Dissociative Amnesia. However, if the amnesia extends beyond the immediate time of the trauma, a comorbid diagnosis of Dissociative Amnesia may be warranted (e.g., for a rape victim who cannot recall most events for the entire day of the rape).
Malingering or Factitious Disorder	Is characterized by amnesia that is feigned. No test, battery of tests, or set of procedures, however, can invariably distinguish Dissociative Amnesia from feigned amnesia, and the same contextual factors associated with feigned amnesia (e.g., financial, sexual, or legal problems; or a wish to escape stressful circumstances) are also associated with Dissociative Amnesia.
Everyday memory loss, amnesia for dreams, amnesia for childhood experiences, posthypnotic amnesia, or age-related memory loss	Is characterized by difficulties in memory that are normative given the context.

3.8.2 Differential Diagnosis for Depersonalization/Derealization Disorder

Depersonalization/Derealization Disorder, which is characterized by persistent or recurrent experiences of depersonalization, must be differentiated from...	In contrast to Depersonalization/Derealization Disorder...
Dissociative symptoms due to a general medical condition	Require the presence of an etiological medical condition, such as a seizure disorder, and would be diagnosed as Other Specified Mental Disorder Due to Another Medical Condition, With Dissociative Symptoms. Depersonalization/Derealization Disorder is not diagnosed if the symptoms are all due to the direct physiological effects of a general medical condition on the central nervous system.
Substance Intoxication or Substance Withdrawal	May be characterized by dissociative symptoms along with the other symptoms of Substance Intoxication or Substance Withdrawal. The most common precipitating substances are cannabis, hallucinogens, ketamine, ecstasy, and salvia. Depersonalization/derealization symptoms attributable to the physiological effects of substances during acute intoxication or withdrawal are not diagnosed as Depersonalization/Derealization Disorder. However, substances can intensify the symptoms of a preexisting Depersonalization/Derealization Disorder. The differential diagnosis thus depends on a careful assessment of the temporal relationship between substance use and depersonalization/derealization symptoms.
Dissociative Identity Disorder	May be characterized by symptoms of depersonalization or derealization accompanying the pervasive discontinuities in sense of self and agency. Depersonalization/Derealization Disorder is not diagnosed if the symptoms are better explained by Dissociative Identity Disorder.

3.8.2 Differential Diagnosis for Depersonalization/Derealization Disorder *(continued)*

Panic Attacks	May be characterized by symptoms of depersonalization or derealization accompanying the other symptoms of the Panic Attack. Panic Attack symptoms have an abrupt onset and reach a peak within minutes. In contrast, episodes of depersonalization or derealization in Depersonalization/Derealization Disorder typically last for hours, weeks, or months. Depersonalization/Derealization Disorder is not diagnosed if the symptoms occur only during a Panic Attack.
Posttraumatic Stress Disorder or Acute Stress Disorder	May be characterized by dissociative symptoms that develop in response to exposure to a traumatic stressor (and for Posttraumatic Stress Disorder, would be indicated by using the specifier With Dissociative Symptoms). Depersonalization/Derealization Disorder is not diagnosed if the symptoms are better explained by Posttraumatic Stress Disorder or Acute Stress Disorder.
Psychotic Disorders (e.g., Schizophrenia)	May be characterized by delusions in which the individual believes that he or she is dead or that the world is not real. In contrast, reality testing about the depersonalization/derealization is intact in Depersonalization/Derealization Disorder (i.e., the person knows that he or she is not really dead and that the world is real).
Major Depressive Disorder	May be characterized by feelings of numbness, deadness, apathy, and being in a dream along with the other characteristic symptoms of depression during Major Depressive Episodes. In Depersonalization/Derealization Disorder, feelings of numbness are associated with other symptoms of the disorder (e.g., a sense of detachment from one's self) and occur when the individual is not depressed.

3.8.2 Differential Diagnosis for Depersonalization/Derealization Disorder *(continued)*

"Normal" symptoms of depersonalization or derealization	Are transient and lack clinically significant impairment or distress. Approximately one-half of all adults have experienced at least one lifetime episode of depersonalization/derealization. Depersonalization/derealization symptoms meeting full criteria for this disorder are much less common, with a lifetime prevalence of approximately 2%.

Somatic Symptom and Related Disorders

3.9.1 Differential Diagnosis for Somatic Symptom Disorder

Somatic Symptom Disorder, which is characterized by somatic symptoms that are distressing or result in significant disruption of daily life and are accompanied by excessive thoughts, feelings, or behaviors related to the somatic symptoms or associated health concerns, must be differentiated from…	In contrast to Somatic Symptom Disorder…
Distressing somatic symptoms characteristic of a medical condition	Are characterized by a lack of disproportionate and persistent thoughts about the seriousness of one's somatic symptoms, the absence of a persistently high level of anxiety about health or the somatic symptoms, and not devoting excessive time and energy to the somatic symptoms or health concerns. Having somatic symptoms of unclear etiology is not by itself sufficient for the diagnosis of Somatic Symptom Disorder, and having somatic symptoms of an established medical condition (e.g., diabetes or heart disease) does not exclude the diagnosis of Somatic Symptom Disorder if the criteria are otherwise met.
Illness Anxiety Disorder	Is characterized by extensive worries about health, but no or minimal somatic symptoms. In Somatic Symptom Disorder, the predominant focus is on the distressing somatic complaints.
Body Dysmorphic Disorder	Is characterized by a preoccupation with a perceived defect in physical appearance. In Somatic Symptom Disorder, the concern about somatic symptoms reflects concerns about underlying illness, not of a defect in appearance.

3.9.1 Differential Diagnosis for Somatic Symptom Disorder *(continued)*

Conversion Disorder (Functional Neurological Symptom Disorder)	Requires the loss of function (e.g., of a limb) as the presenting symptom, whereas in Somatic Symptom Disorder the focus is on the distress that particular symptoms cause. Moreover, a diagnosis of Somatic Symptom Disorder requires the presence of accompanying excessive thoughts, feelings, or behaviors related to the somatic symptoms or associated health concerns.
Generalized Anxiety Disorder	Is characterized by worry about multiple events, situations, or activities, which may include concerns about the individual's health. The main focus of worry in Somatic Symptom Disorder is on somatic symptoms and health concerns.
Panic Disorder	Is characterized by somatic symptoms occurring in the context of Panic Attacks and consequent worries about the health significance of the Panic Attacks. In Somatic Symptom Disorder, the anxiety and somatic symptoms are relatively persistent.
Obsessive-Compulsive Disorder	Is characterized by recurrent thoughts that are experienced as intrusive and unwanted and that the person attempts to ignore or suppress, and that are accompanied by repetitive behaviors that the individual feels driven to perform. In Somatic Symptom Disorder, the recurrent concerns about somatic symptoms or illness are less intrusive and there are no associated repetitive behaviors that the person feels driven to perform.
Depressive Disorders	Are commonly accompanied by somatic symptoms, but these are usually limited to episodes of depressed mood. Moreover, the somatic symptoms in the Depressive Disorders are accompanied by dysphoric mood and their characteristic associated symptoms.
Psychotic Disorders (e.g., Schizophrenia)	May have somatic concerns that are of a delusional nature.
Factitious Disorder or Malingering	Is characterized by physical symptoms that are intentionally produced or feigned.

3.9.2 Differential Diagnosis for Illness Anxiety Disorder

Illness Anxiety Disorder, which is characterized by a preoccupation with having or acquiring a serious illness without accompanying somatic symptoms, must be differentiated from...	In contrast to Illness Anxiety Disorder...
Expectable concerns regarding a medical condition	Concerns and distress about the medical condition are proportionate to its severity. A comorbid diagnosis of Illness Anxiety Disorder is appropriate only if the health-related anxiety and disease concerns are clearly disproportionate to the seriousness of the medical condition. Transient preoccupations related to a medical condition generally do not justify a diagnosis of Illness Anxiety Disorder.
Somatic Symptom Disorder	Is characterized by the presence of significant somatic symptoms. In contrast, individuals with Illness Anxiety Disorder have no or minimal somatic symptoms and are primarily concerned with the idea that they have a serious illness.
Specific Phobia of contracting a disease	Is characterized by a fear that one might contract a disease rather than a fear that one already has the disease as in Illness Anxiety Disorder.
Generalized Anxiety Disorder	Is characterized by anxiety and worry about multiple events, situations, or activities, only one of which may involve health.
Panic Disorder	May be characterized by anxiety or worry specifically regarding the idea that the Panic Attacks reflect the presence of a serious medical illness such as heart disease. Although individuals with Panic Disorder may have health anxiety, their anxiety is typically very acute and episodic. In contrast, the health anxiety and fears in Illness Anxiety Disorder are more chronic and enduring. Some individuals with Illness Anxiety Disorder experience Panic Attacks that are triggered by their illness concerns.

3.9.2 Differential Diagnosis for Illness Anxiety Disorder *(continued)*

Obsessive-Compulsive Disorder	May be characterized by intrusive thoughts that focus on fears of getting a disease in the future, and there usually are additional obsessions or compulsions involving other concerns. The intrusive thoughts of individuals with Illness Anxiety Disorder are about having a disease and may be accompanied by associated compulsive behaviors (e.g., seeking reassurance).
Body Dysmorphic Disorder	Is characterized by concerns that are limited to the individual's physical appearance, which is viewed as defective or flawed.
Adjustment Disorder	Is characterized by marked distress or impairment in functioning that develops in response to a psychosocial stressor (e.g., being diagnosed with a medical condition) and is time-limited (i.e., persisting for no longer than 6 months after the termination of the stressor). A diagnosis of Illness Anxiety Disorder requires the continuous persistence of disproportionate health-related anxiety for more than 6 months.
Major Depressive Disorder	May be characterized by ruminations about health and excessive worry about illness, along with the characteristic symptoms of a Major Depressive Episode (e.g., depressed mood, diminished interest or pleasure). A separate diagnosis of Illness Anxiety Disorder is not made if these concerns occur only during the Major Depressive Episodes. However, if excessive illness worry persists after remission of an episode of Major Depressive Disorder, the diagnosis of Illness Anxiety Disorder should be considered.

3.9.2 Differential Diagnosis for Illness Anxiety Disorder *(continued)*

Psychotic Disorders (e.g., Delusional Disorder)	May be characterized by somatic delusions (e.g., that an organ is rotting or dead) or delusional beliefs of having an illness. Concerns about illness in individuals with Illness Anxiety Disorder do not attain the rigidity and intensity seen in the somatic delusions occurring in Psychotic Disorders, and the person can acknowledge the possibility that the feared disease is not present.

3.9.3 Differential Diagnosis for Conversion Disorder (Functional Neurological Symptom Disorder)

Conversion Disorder, which is characterized by symptoms of altered voluntary motor or sensory function that are incompatible with recognized neurological or medical conditions, must be differentiated from...	In contrast to Conversion Disorder...
Occult neurological or other medical conditions, or substance/medication-induced disorders	Fully account for the deficits involving voluntary motor or sensory functioning. Conversion Disorder can be diagnosed only if, after appropriate investigation, the symptom or deficit cannot be fully explained by a neurological or general medical condition or by the direct effects of a substance or medication.
Somatic Symptom Disorder	Is characterized by distressing somatic symptoms accompanied by excessive thoughts, feelings, or behaviors related to the somatic symptoms or associated health concerns without regard to whether the somatic symptoms are adequately explained by a medical condition. In contrast, in Conversion Disorder, clinical and/or laboratory findings must provide evidence that the neurological symptoms are incompatible with recognized neurological or general medical conditions.
Illness Anxiety Disorder	Is characterized by a focus on the "serious disease" underlying the pseudoneurological symptoms.
Depressive Disorders	May be characterized by feelings of general "heaviness" of the limbs accompanied by core depressive symptoms, whereas the weakness of Conversion Disorder is more focal and prominent.

3.9.3 Differential Diagnosis for Conversion Disorder (Functional Neurological Symptom Disorder) ***(continued)***

Dissociative Disorders	Involve neurological functions (e.g., memory, consciousness) other than voluntary motor or sensory functioning.
Factitious Disorder or Malingering	Is characterized by symptoms that are intentionally produced or feigned. In Conversion Disorder, even though the presenting neurological symptoms are inconsistent with a bona fide neurological condition, they are not being intentionally feigned by the individual. Conversion Disorder is not diagnosed if the symptoms are intentionally produced or feigned.

3.9.4 Differential Diagnosis for Psychological Factors Affecting Other Medical Conditions

Psychological Factors Affecting Other Medical Conditions, which are characterized by psychological factors that adversely affect the course or treatment of a medical condition, that constitute health risks for the individual, or that influence the underlying pathophysiology, must be differentiated from…	In contrast to Psychological Factors Affecting Other Medical Conditions…
Mental disorder due to a general medical condition	Is characterized by a temporal association between symptoms of a mental disorder and a general medical condition, but the causal relationship is in the opposite direction. In a mental disorder due to a general medical condition, the medical condition is judged to be causing the mental disorder through a direct physiological mechanism, whereas in Psychological Factors Affecting Other Medical Conditions, the psychological or behavioral factors are judged to affect the course of the medical condition.
Adjustment Disorder	May be characterized by a clinically significant psychological response to a general medical condition that is the identifiable stressor. For example, an individual with angina who develops maladaptive anticipatory anxiety would be diagnosed as having an Adjustment Disorder With Anxiety, whereas an individual with angina that is precipitated whenever he or she becomes enraged would be diagnosed as having Psychological Factors Affecting Other Medical Conditions.

3.9.4 Differential Diagnosis for Psychological Factors Affecting Other Medical Conditions *(continued)*

Mental disorder causing or exacerbating another medical condition	Symptoms meeting full criteria for a mental disorder frequently result in medical complications, most notably Substance Use Disorders (e.g., Severe Alcohol Use Disorder, Severe Tobacco Use Disorder). If an individual has a mental disorder that adversely affects or causes a general medical condition, both the mental disorder and the medical condition are diagnosed; however, Psychological Factors Affecting Other Medical Conditions is diagnosed when the psychological traits or behaviors do not meet criteria for a mental disorder.
Somatic Symptom Disorder	Is characterized by a combination of distressing somatic symptoms and excessive or maladaptive thoughts, feelings, and behaviors occurring in response to these symptoms, with the emphasis being on the maladaptive thoughts, feelings, and behaviors (e.g., an individual with angina who worries constantly that he will have a heart attack takes his blood pressure multiple times per day and restricts his activities). In Psychological Factors Affecting Other Medical Conditions, the emphasis is on the exacerbation of the general medical condition (e.g., an individual with angina that is precipitated whenever he becomes anxious).
Illness Anxiety Disorder	Is characterized by high illness anxiety that is distressing or disruptive to daily life with no or minimal somatic symptoms. In Psychological Factors Affecting Other Medical Conditions, anxiety may be a relevant psychological factor affecting a medical condition, but the clinical concern is the adverse effects on the medical condition.

3.9.5 Differential Diagnosis for Factitious Disorder[a]

Factitious Disorder, which is characterized by falsification of physical or psychological signs or symptoms or induction of injury or disease in oneself or another person, associated with identified deception, must be differentiated from…	In contrast to Factitious Disorder…
Somatic Symptom Disorder	May be characterized by excessive attention and treatment seeking for perceived medical concerns, but there is no evidence that the individual is providing false information or behaving deceptively.
Malingering	Is characterized by the intentional reporting or feigning of symptoms for personal gain (e.g., money, time off work), whereas the diagnosis of Factitious Disorder requires that the feigning behaviors persists even in the absence of obvious external incentives.
Conversion Disorder (Functional Neurological Symptom Disorder)	Is characterized by neurological symptoms that are inconsistent with neurological pathophysiology. Factitious Disorder with neurological symptoms is distinguished from Conversion Disorder by evidence of deceptive falsification of symptoms.
Borderline Personality Disorder	May be characterized by deliberate physical self-harm in the absence of suicidal intent. Factitious Disorder requires that the induction of injury occurs in association with deception.
Child or elder abuse (as distinguished from Factitious Disorder Imposed on Another)	Is characterized by lying about abuse injuries in dependents solely to protect oneself from liability. Such individuals are not diagnosed with Factitious Disorder Imposed on Another because the deceptive behavior is motivated by an obvious external incentive (i.e., protection from criminal liability). Caregivers who are found to lie more extensively than needed for immediate self-protection may be diagnosed with Factitious Disorder Imposed on Another.

[a]Factitious Disorder comes in two forms: Factitious Disorder Imposed on Self, in which an individual feigns medical or psychiatric symptoms, and Factitious Disorder Imposed on Another, in which an individual deceptively induces a disease or injury in another, usually a dependent child or elder.

Feeding and Eating Disorders

3.10.1 Differential Diagnosis for Avoidant/Restrictive Food Intake Disorder

Avoidant/Restrictive Food Intake Disorder (ARFID), which is characterized by a persistent failure to meet appropriate nutritional and/or energy needs related to an eating or feeding disturbance, must be differentiated from...	In contrast to Avoidant/Restrictive Food Intake Disorder...
Other medical conditions	Restriction of food intake may occur in other medical conditions (e.g., gastrointestinal disease, food allergies and intolerances, occult malignancies), especially with ongoing symptoms such as vomiting, loss of appetite, nausea, abdominal pain, or diarrhea. A diagnosis of ARFID may be appropriate if the disturbance of intake exceeds that routinely associated with the medical condition and warrants additional clinical attention or if it persists after resolution of the medical condition.
Specific neurological, structural, or congenital disorders and conditions associated with feeding difficulties	Feeding difficulties are common in a number of congenital and neurological conditions often related to problems with oral/esophageal/pharyngeal structure and function. A diagnosis of ARFID may be appropriate if the disturbance of food intake exceeds that routinely associated with the medical condition and warrants additional clinical attention.
Reactive Attachment Disorder	The disturbance in the caregiver-child relationship typically affects feeding and the child's intake. A diagnosis of ARFID may be appropriate if the feeding disturbance is a primary focus for intervention.
Autism Spectrum Disorder	May be characterized by rigid eating behaviors and heightened sensory sensitivities. However, this often does not result in the level of impairment (e.g., weight loss, nutritional deficiency) that would be required for a diagnosis of ARFID. ARFID should be diagnosed only if the eating disturbance requires specific treatment.

3.10.1 Differential Diagnosis for Avoidant/Restrictive Food Intake Disorder *(continued)*

Specific Phobia, Other Type, with a fear of vomiting	Is characterized by avoidance of situations that may lead to choking or vomiting and may result in food avoidance and some restriction of food intake. When the eating problem itself becomes the primary focus on clinical attention, a diagnosis of ARFID is warranted.
Anorexia Nervosa	Although both ARFID and Anorexia Nervosa are characterized by food restrictions and low weight, individuals with Anorexia Nervosa also have a fear of gaining weight or becoming fat, or persistent behavior that interferes with weight gain, as well as specific disturbances in their perception and experience of body weight and shape.
Major Depressive Disorder	May be characterized by appetite loss to such an extent that individuals present with significantly restricted food intake and weight loss, which usually abates with resolution of the depression. A diagnosis of ARFID may be appropriate if the eating disturbance requires specific treatment.
Schizophrenia Spectrum and Other Psychotic Disorders	May be characterized by odd eating behaviors, avoidance of specific foods due to delusional beliefs, or other manifestations of avoidant or restrictive intake. A diagnosis of ARFID may be appropriate if the eating disturbance requires specific treatment.

3.10.2 Differential Diagnosis for Anorexia Nervosa

Anorexia Nervosa, which is characterized by a restriction of energy intake relative to requirements, leading to a significantly low body weight; an intense fear of gaining weight; and a disturbance in the way in which one's body weight or shape is experienced, must be differentiated from…	In contrast to Anorexia Nervosa…
Other medical conditions	A number of other medical conditions (e.g., neoplasms, infections, metabolic or endocrine conditions) are characterized by weight loss. However, with such conditions, unlike Anorexia Nervosa, there is no disturbance in the way the person's body weight or shape is experienced, no intense fear of weight gain, and no persisting in behaviors that interfere with appropriate weight gain. The weight loss is often accompanied by loss of appetite and includes signs, symptoms, or laboratory findings characteristic of the underlying medical condition.
Substance Use Disorders	May be characterized by low weight due to poor nutritional intake, but individuals abusing substances generally do not fear gaining weight and do not have disturbances in body image. Some individuals abusing stimulants for the purpose of appetite suppression may be motivated by a desire to interfere with weight gain; if the other symptoms of Anorexia Nervosa are also present, the diagnosis would be warranted.
Bulimia Nervosa	In both conditions, the person may engage in recurrent episodes of binge eating, engage in inappropriate behavior to avoid weight gain (e.g., self-induced vomiting), and be overly concerned with body shape and weight. The conditions are differentiated based on body weight. Individuals with Bulimia Nervosa maintain body weight at or above a minimally normal level, whereas those with Anorexia Nervosa maintain a significantly low body weight.

3.10.2 Differential Diagnosis for Anorexia Nervosa *(continued)*

Avoidant/Restrictive Food Intake Disorder	Is characterized by significant weight loss and nutritional deficiency and restriction of food intake, but unlike Anorexia Nervosa the weight loss and food restrictions are not motivated by a fear of gaining weight or becoming fat.
Weight loss in Depressive Disorders	Is not accompanied by a desire for excessive weight loss or an intense fear of gaining weight or getting fat, and includes the presence of characteristic features of a Depressive Disorder (e.g., depressed mood, loss of interest).
Schizophrenia	May be characterized by unusual eating behavior, but it is not accompanied by a desire for excessive weight loss or an intense fear of gaining weight or getting fat, and it is accompanied by the characteristic features of Schizophrenia (e.g., delusions, hallucinations, disorganized speech).
Obsessive-Compulsive Disorder	In both conditions, there may be repetitive intrusive thoughts and compulsive behaviors. In Anorexia Nervosa, however, these thoughts and behaviors are limited to weight, eating, or food. An additional diagnosis of Obsessive-Compulsive Disorder should be considered only if there are additional obsessions or compulsions unrelated to weight, eating, or food (e.g., contamination).
Social Anxiety Disorder (Social Phobia)	In Anorexia Nervosa and Social Anxiety Disorder, individuals may feel humiliated or embarrassed to be seen eating in public. In Anorexia Nervosa, social fears are limited to eating behaviors. An additional diagnosis of Social Anxiety Disorder is warranted only if there are fears of other social situations (e.g., speaking in public).

3.10.2 Differential Diagnosis for Anorexia Nervosa *(continued)*

Body Dysmorphic Disorder	In Anorexia Nervosa and Body Dysmorphic Disorder, individuals may be preoccupied with an imagined defect in bodily appearance. In Anorexia Nervosa, the preoccupation is limited to body shape and weight. An additional diagnosis of Body Dysmorphic Disorder is warranted only if there are distortions about the body that are unrelated to weight or being fat (e.g., preoccupation with the shape of one's nose).

3.10.3 Differential Diagnosis for Bulimia Nervosa

Bulimia Nervosa, which is characterized by recurrent episodes of binge eating accompanied by inappropriate compensatory behaviors to prevent weight gain, must be differentiated from…	In contrast to Bulimia Nervosa…
Vomiting or diarrhea in general medical conditions or with excessive substance use	Is due to the direct physiological effects of the general medical condition or substance use.
Anorexia Nervosa	May be characterized by episodes of binge eating and purging. In contrast to Bulimia Nervosa, the diagnosis of Anorexia Nervosa requires significantly low body weight (i.e., weight that is less than minimally normal). Individuals whose binge-eating behavior occurs only during episodes of Anorexia Nervosa are given the diagnosis Anorexia Nervosa, Binge-Eating/Purging Type. If the full criteria for Anorexia Nervosa, Binge-Eating/Purging Type, are no longer met because for example, weight becomes normal, a diagnosis of Bulimia Nervosa should be given only if criteria for Bulimia Nervosa are met for at least 3 months.
Binge-Eating Disorder	Is characterized by binge eating in the absence of the regular use of inappropriate compensatory mechanisms to counteract the effects of binge eating. In contrast, Bulimia Nervosa requires binge eating and inappropriate compensatory behaviors at least once a week for 3 months.
Kleine-Levin syndrome	Is characterized by overeating, but the characteristic psychological features of Bulimia Nervosa, such as overconcern with body shape and weight, are not present.

3.10.3 Differential Diagnosis for Bulimia Nervosa *(continued)*

Major Depressive Episode With Atypical Features in Major Depressive Disorder or Bipolar I Disorder	May be characterized by overeating along with the other symptoms of depression, but the overeating does not necessarily occur in the form of binge eating and individuals do not engage in inappropriate compensatory behaviors and do not exhibit the characteristic excessive concern with body shape and weight. If criteria are met for Bulimia Nervosa and a Major Depressive Episode With Atypical Features, then both should be diagnosed.
Borderline Personality Disorder	May be characterized by binge eating along with the characteristic features of Borderline Personality Disorder (e.g., self-mutilation, unstable relationships). In contrast, the diagnosis of Bulimia Nervosa requires inappropriate compensatory behaviors after the binge eating as well as overconcern with body shape and weight. If criteria are met for Bulimia Nervosa and Borderline Personality Disorder, both can be diagnosed.

3.10.4 Differential Diagnosis for Binge-Eating Disorder

Binge-Eating Disorder, which is characterized by recurrent episodes of binge eating accompanied by marked distress, must be differentiated from…	In contrast to Binge-Eating Disorder…
Bulimia Nervosa	Both conditions are characterized by recurrent binge eating, but in Bulimia Nervosa there are recurrent inappropriate compensatory behaviors (e.g., purging, driven exercise).
Obesity	Although many individuals with Binge-Eating Disorder are obese, those with Binge-Eating Disorder are more likely to have higher levels of overvaluation of body weight and shape, have significantly higher rates of psychiatric comorbidity, and have a higher likelihood of long-term successful outcome of evidence-based psychological treatment.
Major Depressive Episode With Atypical Features in Major Depressive Disorder or Bipolar I Disorder	May be characterized by overeating along with the other symptoms of depression, but the overeating does not necessarily occur in the form of binge eating and the eating may or may not be associated with a loss of control. If criteria are met for Binge-Eating Disorder and a Major Depressive Episode With Atypical Features, then both should be diagnosed.
Borderline Personality Disorder	Includes binge eating in the impulsive behavior criterion that is part of the definition of Borderline Personality Disorder. If the full criteria for Binge-Eating Disorder and Borderline Personality Disorder are met, both diagnoses can be given.

Sleep-Wake Disorders

3.11.1 Differential Diagnosis for Insomnia Disorder

Insomnia Disorder, which is characterized by dissatisfaction with sleep quantity or quality associated with difficulty initiating or maintaining sleep, or early-morning awakening with inability to return to sleep, must be differentiated from…	In contrast to Insomnia Disorder…
Short sleepers (individuals who require little sleep)	Short sleepers do not have any difficulty falling or staying asleep and lack symptoms of daytime sleepiness (e.g., fatigue, concentration problems, irritability). By attempting to sleep for a longer period of time by prolonging time in bed, some short sleepers may create an insomnia-like sleep pattern.
Sleep deprivation	Is characterized by an inadequate opportunity or circumstance for sleep and is typically temporary (e.g., professional or family obligations forcing a person to stay awake). Insomnia Disorder would not be diagnosed in such circumstances.
Delayed Sleep Phase and Shift Work Types of Circadian Rhythm Sleep-Wake Disorder	In Circadian Rhythm Sleep-Wake Disorder, Shift Work Type, there is a history of recent shift work with consequent disturbance in sleep. Individuals with Circadian Rhythm Sleep-Wake Disorder, Delayed Sleep Phase Type (i.e., "night owls"), report sleep-onset insomnia only when they try to sleep at socially normal times, but do not report difficulty falling asleep or staying asleep when their bed and rising times are delayed coinciding with their endogenous circadian rhythm. Insomnia Disorder is not diagnosed if the difficulties initiating and maintaining sleep are better explained by, and occur exclusively during the course of, a Circadian Rhythm Sleep-Wake Disorder.

3.11.1 Differential Diagnosis for Insomnia Disorder *(continued)*

Restless Legs Syndrome	Is characterized by urges to move the legs and accompanying unpleasant leg sensations, and often produces difficulties initiating and maintaining sleep. Insomnia Disorder is not diagnosed if the difficulties initiating and maintaining sleep are better explained by, and occur exclusively during the course of, Restless Legs Syndrome.
Breathing-Related Sleep Disorders	Are characterized by loud snoring, breathing pauses during sleep, and excessive daytime sleepiness, with up to half of these individuals reporting insomnia symptoms. Insomnia Disorder is not diagnosed if the difficulties initiating and maintaining sleep are better explained by, and occur exclusively during the course of, Breathing-Related Sleep Disorders.
Narcolepsy	Is characterized by excessive daytime sleepiness, cataplexy, sleep paralysis, and sleep-related hallucinations, along with complaints of insomnia. Insomnia Disorder is not diagnosed if the difficulties initiating and maintaining sleep are better explained by, and occur exclusively during the course of, Narcolepsy.
Parasomnias (i.e., Non–Rapid Eye Movement Sleep Arousal Disorders, Nightmare Disorder, Rapid Eye Movement Sleep Behavior Disorder)	Are characterized by unusual behaviors or events during sleep that may lead to intermittent awakenings and difficulty resuming sleep; however, it is these behavioral events, rather than the insomnia per se, that dominate the clinical picture. Insomnia Disorder is not diagnosed if the difficulties initiating and maintaining sleep are better explained by, and occur exclusively during the course of, the Parasomnia.

3.11.1 Differential Diagnosis for Insomnia Disorder *(continued)*

Insomnia associated with another mental disorder or general medical condition	The diagnosis of Insomnia Disorder is given whether it occurs as an independent condition or is comorbid with another mental disorder (e.g., Major Depressive Disorder) or general medical condition (e.g., pain). A specifier is used to indicate if it is with a non–sleep disorder mental comorbidity or with other medical comorbidity.
Substance/Medication-Induced Sleep Disorder, Insomnia Type	Is due to the direct physiological effects of a substance or medication. Insomnia Disorder is not diagnosed if the symptoms are attributable to the direct physiological effects of a substance (including medication).

3.11.2 Differential Diagnosis for Hypersomnolence Disorder

Hypersomnolence Disorder, which is characterized by excessive sleepiness associated with lapses into sleep, unrefreshing prolonged main sleep episodes, or difficulty being fully awake after abrupt awakening, must be differentiated from…	In contrast to Hypersomnolence Disorder…
Normal long sleepers	Require a greater than average amount of sleep. Long sleepers do not have excessive sleepiness, sleep inertia, or automatic behavior when they obtain their required amount of nocturnal sleep, and they report their sleep to be refreshing. If social or occupational demands lead to shorter nocturnal sleep, daytime symptoms may appear. In individuals with Hypersomnolence Disorder, symptoms of excessive sleepiness occur regardless of nocturnal sleep duration.
Inadequate amount of nocturnal sleep	Can produce symptoms of daytime sleepiness very similar to those of Hypersomnolence Disorder. An average sleep duration of fewer than 7 hours per night strongly suggests inadequate nocturnal sleep, and an average of more than 9–10 hours of unrefreshing sleep per 24-hour period suggests a diagnosis of Hypersomnolence Disorder. Unlike Hypersomnolence Disorder, insufficient nocturnal sleep is unlikely to persist unabated for decades.
Daytime fatigue resulting from Insomnia Disorder	Is characterized by excessive sleepiness related to insufficient sleep quantity or quality. Hypersomnolence Disorder is not diagnosed if the excessive sleepiness is better explained by, and occurs exclusively during the course of, Insomnia Disorder.

3.11.2 Differential Diagnosis for Hypersomnolence Disorder *(continued)*

Narcolepsy	Is characterized by recurrent periods of irrepressible need to sleep, lapsing into sleep, or napping occurring within the same day, which are accompanied by other characteristic features such as cataplexy, hypocretin deficiency, and specific polysomnographic findings (i.e., rapid eye movement [REM] sleep latency of 15 minutes or less, or a multiple sleep latency test showing a mean sleep latency of 8 minutes or less and two or more sleep-onset REM periods). Hypersomnolence Disorder is not diagnosed if the excessive sleepiness is better explained by, and occurs exclusively during the course of, Narcolepsy.
Breathing-Related Sleep Disorders	Are characterized by daytime sleepiness accompanied by specific polysomnographic findings (e.g., a minimum number of apneas or hypopneas per hour) and often nighttime symptoms (e.g., loud snoring, breathing pauses). Hypersomnolence Disorder is not diagnosed if the excessive sleepiness is better explained by, and occurs exclusively during the course of, a Breathing-Related Sleep Disorder.
Circadian Rhythm Sleep-Wake Disorders	Are often characterized by daytime sleepiness, accompanied by a history of an abnormal sleep-wake schedule (with shifted or regular hours). Hypersomnolence Disorder is not diagnosed if the excessive sleepiness is better explained by, and occurs exclusively during the course of, a Circadian Rhythm Sleep-Wake Disorder.
Parasomnias (i.e., Non–Rapid Eye Movement Sleep Arousal Disorders, Nightmare Disorder, Rapid Eye Movement Sleep Behavior Disorder)	May be characterized by daytime sleepiness related to nightmares, sleep terrors, sleepwalking, or episodes of arousal during REM sleep associated with vocalization and/or complex motor behaviors. Hypersomnolence Disorder is not diagnosed if the excessive sleepiness is better explained by, and occurs exclusively during the course of, a Parasomnia.

3.11.2 Differential Diagnosis for Hypersomnolence Disorder *(continued)*

Hypersomnolence associated with another mental disorder or general medical condition	The diagnosis of Hypersomnolence Disorder is given whether it occurs as an independent condition or is comorbid with another mental disorder (e.g., hypersomnia in Major Depressive Disorder) or a general medical condition (e.g., Parkinson's disease). A specifier is used to indicate if it is with a non–sleep disorder mental comorbidity or with other medical comorbidity.
Substance/Medication-Induced Sleep Disorder, Daytime Sleepiness Type	Is due to the direct physiological effects of a substance. Hypersomnolence Disorder is not diagnosed if the symptoms are attributable to the direct physiological effects of a substance (including medication).

Sexual Dysfunctions

3.12.1 Differential Diagnosis for Sexual Dysfunctions

A Sexual Dysfunction, which is characterized by the presence of sexual symptoms (i.e., hypoactive desire, arousal problems, early ejaculation, delayed orgasm, pain during intercourse) that are experienced in all, or almost all, occasions of sexual activity, must be differentiated from…	In contrast to a Sexual Dysfunction…
Medical condition that accounts for the sexual dysfunction	If the dysfunction is entirely attributable to the direct physiological effects of a general medical condition (e.g., autonomic neuropathy), a DSM-5 Sexual Dysfunction diagnosis is not made.
Substance/Medication-Induced Sexual Dysfunction	Involves a sexual dysfunction that is better explained by the use, misuse, or discontinuation of a substance or medication. A Sexual Dysfunction diagnosis is not given if the dysfunction is entirely attributable to the direct physiological effects of a substance or medication.
Sexual problems associated with a nonsexual mental disorder (e.g., Major Depressive or Bipolar Disorder, Posttraumatic Stress Disorder, Psychotic Disorder)	Are characterized by a sexual dysfunction that occurs only in the context of the symptoms of the other mental disorder (e.g., low sexual desire in the context of a Major Depressive Episode). If the sexual dysfunction was present before the onset of the nonsexual mental disorder or persists once the nonsexual mental disorder has resolved, a separate diagnosis of Sexual Dysfunction may be warranted.
Sexual problems associated with severe relationship distress or partner violence	If severe relationship distress or partner violence better explains the sexual difficulties, then a Sexual Dysfunction diagnosis is not made and an appropriate V or Z code for the relationship problem should be used instead.

3.12.1 Differential Diagnosis for Sexual Dysfunctions *(continued)*

Sexual problems associated with a relational problem	Are often limited to a specific partner (situational) and are characterized by an exacerbation when the relational problem gets worse. In some situations, both a Sexual Dysfunction and relational problem may be diagnosed together.
Sexual problems not due to a Sexual Dysfunction	May be the result of inadequate sexual stimulation, which can prevent the experience of arousal or orgasm. Although there may still be a need for care, a diagnosis of a Sexual Dysfunction is not made.

Gender Dysphoria

3.13.1 Differential Diagnosis for Gender Dysphoria

Gender Dysphoria, which is characterized by a marked incongruence between one's experienced or expressed gender and assigned gender, is accompanied by a strong desire to be the experienced gender, and causes clinically significant distress or impairment, must be differentiated from…	In contrast to Gender Dysphoria…
Nonconformity of gender roles	Is characterized by nonconformity to stereotypical gender role behavior (e.g., "tomboyish" behavior in girls, occasional cross-dressing in adult men) that occurs in the absence of clinically significant distress or impairment in social, occupational, or other areas of functioning. Gender Dysphoria is characterized by the strong desire to be of the expressed gender rather than the assigned one and by the extent and pervasiveness of gender-variant activities and interests.
Transvestic Disorder	Is characterized by cross-dressing behavior that generates sexual excitement and causes distress and/or impairment without the individual's primary gender being called into question. An individual who is aroused by cross-dressing and who also has Gender Dysphoria can be given both diagnoses.
Body Dysmorphic Disorder	May be characterized by the persistent desire to alter or remove a specific body part or feature because it is perceived as abnormally formed and ugly and not because it represents a repudiated assigned gender. When an individual's presentation meets criteria for both Gender Dysphoria and Body Dysmorphic Disorder, both diagnoses can be given.

3.13.1 Differential Diagnosis for Gender Dysphoria *(continued)*

Psychotic Disorder (e.g., Schizophrenia)	May rarely be characterized by delusions of belonging to the other gender. In the absence of other symptoms characteristic of a Psychotic Disorder (e.g., hallucinations, other delusions), insistence by an individual with Gender Dysphoria that he or she is of the other gender is not considered a delusion.

Disruptive, Impulse-Control, and Conduct Disorders

3.14.1 Differential Diagnosis for Oppositional Defiant Disorder

Oppositional Defiant Disorder (ODD), which is characterized by a pattern of angry/irritable mood, argumentative/defiant behavior, or vindictiveness, must be differentiated from…	In contrast to Oppositional Defiant Disorder…
Nonpathological oppositional behavior typical of certain developmental stages	Is not clinically significant or is not a persistent pattern.
Adjustment Disorder With Disturbance of Conduct	Is a time-limited maladaptive response to a stressor and does not meet criteria for ODD.
Conduct Disorder	Is characterized by conduct problems that are of a more severe nature than those of ODD and include aggression toward people or animals, destruction of property, or a pattern of theft or deceit. Moreover, Conduct Disorder does not include problems of emotional dysregulation (i.e., angry and irritable mood). If criteria are met for ODD and Conduct Disorder, both may be diagnosed.
Attention-Deficit/Hyperactivity Disorder	May be characterized by oppositional behavior that occurs solely in situations related to the individual's failure to conform to requests that demand sustained effort and attention or requests to sit still. If oppositional behavior occurs in other situations, then an additional diagnosis of ODD may be appropriate.
Disruptive Mood Dysregulation Disorder	Is characterized by temper outbursts that are much more frequent (three or more times per week), chronic (12 months or more), persistent (no periods lasting more than 3 months without symptoms), and severe (verbal rages or physical aggression toward people or property) than those in ODD. ODD is not diagnosed if criteria are met for Disruptive Mood Dysregulation Disorder.

3.14.1 Differential Diagnosis for Oppositional Defiant Disorder *(continued)*

Intermittent Explosive Disorder	Is characterized by recurrent behavioral outbursts that involve serious physical or verbal aggression toward others, which is not part of the definition of ODD. An additional diagnosis of Intermittent Explosive Disorder can be made if the recurrent impulsive aggressive outbursts are in excess of those usually seen in ODD and warrant independent clinical attention.
Bipolar Disorders, Depressive Disorders, or Psychotic Disorders	Are associated with oppositional behavior that occurs only in the context of a mood disturbance or in relation to delusions or hallucinations.
Intellectual Disability (Intellectual Developmental Disorder)	May be characterized by oppositional behavior that accompanies the intellectual deficits. A diagnosis of ODD is given only if the oppositional behavior is markedly greater than is commonly observed among individuals of comparable mental age and with comparable severity of Intellectual Disability.
Language Disorder	May be associated with oppositional behavior related to a failure to follow directions that is the result of impaired language comprehension.
Selective Mutism	Is characterized by a failure to speak due to fear of negative evaluation rather than by a motivation to be oppositional.

3.14.2 Differential Diagnosis for Intermittent Explosive Disorder

Intermittent Explosive Disorder, which is characterized by recurrent behavioral outbursts that are grossly out of proportion to the provocation or any precipitating psychosocial stressors, must be differentiated from…	In contrast to Intermittent Explosive Disorder…
Substance Intoxication or Substance Withdrawal	May be characterized by aggressive behavior that is due to the direct physiological effects of intoxication with, or withdrawal from, a substance. Intermittent Explosive Disorder is not diagnosed if the aggressive outbursts occur only during episodes of Substance Intoxication or Substance Withdrawal.
Delirium Due to Another Medical Condition, Major or Mild Neurocognitive Disorder Due to Another Medical Condition, Substance Intoxication Delirium, Substance Withdrawal Delirium, Medication-Induced Delirium, or Substance/Medication-Induced Major or Mild Neurocognitive Disorder	Includes characteristic symptoms (e.g., impaired attention and orientation and fluctuating course in Delirium) accompanying the aggressive outbursts and requires the presence of an etiological medical condition or substance/medication use. Nonspecific abnormalities on neurological examination (e.g., "soft signs") and nonspecific electroencephalographic changes do not constitute an etiological medical condition and instead are compatible with a diagnosis of Intermittent Explosive Disorder.
Personality Change Due to Another Medical Condition, Aggressive Type	The change from the person's previous characteristic personality pattern involves aggressive outbursts and requires the presence of an etiological medical condition. Nonspecific abnormalities on neurological examination (e.g., "soft signs") and nonspecific electroencephalographic changes do not constitute an etiological medical condition and instead are compatible with a diagnosis of Intermittent Explosive Disorder.

3.14.2 Differential Diagnosis for Intermittent Explosive Disorder *(continued)*

Disruptive Mood Dysregulation Disorder	Is characterized by aggressive outbursts accompanied by a persistently negative mood state (i.e., irritability, anger) most of the day, nearly every day, between the impulsive aggressive outbursts with onset before age 10 years. Intermittent Explosive Disorder is not diagnosed if the aggressive outbursts are better explained by a diagnosis of Disruptive Mood Dysregulation Disorder.
Antisocial Personality Disorder or Borderline Personality Disorder	May be characterized by recurrent problematic impulsive aggressive outbursts occurring in the context of a long-standing Personality Disorder. Intermittent Explosive Disorder is not diagnosed if the aggressive outbursts are better explained by one of these Personality Disorders.
Attention-Deficit/Hyperactivity Disorder (ADHD), Conduct Disorder, or Oppositional Defiant Disorder	May be associated with aggressive outbursts. In ADHD, the characteristic impulsivity may be manifested by impulsive aggressive outbursts; in Conduct Disorder, aggression is characteristically proactive and predatory; in Oppositional Defiant Disorder, the aggression typically takes the form of temper tantrums and verbal arguments with authority figures. An additional diagnosis of Intermittent Explosive Disorder can be made if the recurrent impulsive aggressive outbursts are in excess of those usually seen in these disorders and warrant independent clinical attention.
Other mental disorders (e.g., Schizophrenia, Manic Episode)	May include impulsive aggression as an associated feature along with their characteristic features. Intermittent Explosive Disorder is not diagnosed if the aggressive behavior occurs only during episodes of one of these disorders (e.g., during Manic Episodes, during delusional periods).
Aggressive behavior not attributable to a mental disorder	Is motivated by political or religious belief, revenge, monetary gain, thrill seeking, or another reason not related to a mental disorder.

3.14.3 Differential Diagnosis for Conduct Disorder

Conduct Disorder, which is characterized by a repetitive and persistent pattern of behavior in which the basic rights of others or major age-appropriate societal norms or rules are violated, must be differentiated from…	In contrast to Conduct Disorder…
Oppositional Defiant Disorder	Is characterized by disruptive behaviors that are typically of a less severe nature than those in Conduct Disorder and do not include aggression toward individuals or animals, destruction of property, or a pattern of theft or deceit. Moreover, Oppositional Defiant Disorder includes problems of emotional dysregulation (i.e., angry and irritable mood) that are not part of the definition of Conduct Disorder. If criteria are met for both conditions, both may be diagnosed.
Attention-Deficit/Hyperactivity Disorder	Is characterized by hyperactive and impulsive behavior that may be disruptive but does not by itself violate societal norms or the rights of others. If criteria are met for both disorders, both may be diagnosed.
Bipolar I or Bipolar II Disorder, Major Depressive Disorder, Persistent Depressive Disorder (Dysthymia), or Disruptive Mood Dysregulation Disorder	May be characterized by behavioral problems associated with irritability and aggression and can be distinguished from Conduct Disorder by the absence of substantial levels of aggressive or nonaggressive conduct problems during periods in which there is no mood disturbance.
Intermittent Explosive Disorder	Is characterized by aggression that is limited to impulsive aggression, is not premeditated, and is not committed to achieve some tangible objective. If criteria for both disorders are met, the diagnosis of Intermittent Explosive Disorder should be given only when the recurrent impulsive aggressive outbursts warrant independent clinical attention.
Antisocial behavior related to a Psychotic Disorder (e.g., Schizophrenia)	Occurs only in response to delusions or hallucinations.

3.14.3 Differential Diagnosis for Conduct Disorder *(continued)*

Adjustment Disorder With Disturbance of Conduct	Is characterized by time-limited conduct problems that are below the severity threshold for Conduct Disorder and that clearly occur in response to a psychosocial stressor as opposed to being part of a long-standing pattern.
Child or Adolescent Antisocial Behavior	Is below the severity threshold for Conduct Disorder or is not part of a long-standing pattern (i.e., isolated antisocial acts).
Antisocial Personality Disorder	Can be diagnosed only in individuals age 18 years or older. Conduct Disorder is not diagnosed if the individual is age 18 or older and if criteria are met for Antisocial Personality Disorder.

Substance-Related and Addictive Disorders

3.15.1 Differential Diagnosis for Substance Use Disorders

Substance Use Disorder, which is characterized by a problematic pattern of substance use leading to clinically significant impairment or distress, must be differentiated from...	In contrast to Substance Use Disorder...
Nonpathological use of the substance	Is characterized by repeated use at relatively low doses and may involve occasional periods of intoxication not associated with negative consequences (e.g., intoxication restricted to occasional weekends so that it does not impair work or school functioning). Substance Use Disorders are characterized by heavy use leading to significant distress or impaired functioning. Differentiating between nonpathological substance use and a Substance Use Disorder may be complicated by the fact that denial of heavy substance use and substance-related problems is common with individuals who are referred to treatment by others (e.g., school, family, employer, criminal justice system).
Substance/Medication-Induced Mental Disorders (including Substance Intoxication and Substance Withdrawal)	Are characterized by central nervous system syndromes that develop in the context of the effects of substances of abuse, medications, or toxin exposure. They are distinguished from Substance Use Disorders, which are pathological patterns of behaviors related to pattern of use of a substance. Given that the heavy substance use characteristic of a Substance Use Disorder often leads to the development of a Substance-Induced Disorder, they commonly co-occur and both should be diagnosed (e.g., Severe Cocaine Use Disorder with comorbid Cocaine-Induced Psychotic Disorder, With Onset During Intoxication).

3.15.1 Differential Diagnosis for Substance Use Disorders *(continued)*

Conduct Disorder in childhood and Antisocial Personality Disorder in adulthood	Substance Use (including Alcohol Use) Disorders are seen in the majority of individuals with Antisocial Personality Disorder and preexisting Conduct Disorder and are associated with the early onset of the Substance Use Disorder.
Substance use during Manic Episodes	Involves episodes of characteristic symptoms (e.g., elevated mood, irritability, distractibility, decreased need for sleep, flight of ideas) that persist at times when the individual is not using substances. If substance use during a Manic Episode meets criteria for a Substance Use Disorder, both may be diagnosed.

3.15.2 Differential Diagnosis for Gambling Disorder

Gambling Disorder, which is characterized by persistent and recurrent problematic gambling behavior leading to clinically significant impairment or distress, must be differentiated from…	In contrast to Gambling Disorder…
Professional gambling	Is characterized by discipline and limited risk taking and is intended to be a source of income.
Social gambling	Usually occurs among friends and is characterized by limited time spent on gambling and limited risk taking.
Manic Episode	Is characterized by symptoms (e.g., euphoric mood, rapid speech, increased self-esteem, flight of ideas) that persist at times when the individual is not gambling. Gambling Disorder is not diagnosed if the gambling behavior is better accounted for by a Manic Episode.
Internet Gaming Disorder (in DSM-5 Section III)	Is characterized by a preoccupation with the use of the Internet to play games, often with other players, leading to clinically significant distress or impairment. In contrast to Gambling Disorder, the wager of money is not involved.

Neurocognitive Disorders

3.16.1 Differential Diagnosis for Delirium

Delirium, which is characterized by a disturbance in attention (i.e., reduced ability to direct, focus, sustain, and shift attention) and awareness (reduced orientation to the environment) that tends to fluctuate during the course of the day and that is due to the physiological effects of a substance or medical condition, must be differentiated from…	In contrast to Delirium…
Major or Mild Neurocognitive Disorder	Is characterized by a relatively stable or gradually progressive course, typically a much longer duration, and despite a number of cognitive deficits, a lack of impairment of the ability to maintain attention and be aware of one's environment. Episodes of Delirium, however, can occur in a preexisting neurocognitive disorder. Major or Mild Neurocognitive Disorder is not diagnosed if the deficits occur exclusively in the context of Delirium. When Delirium occurs in the context of a preexisting neurocognitive disorder, it should be separately diagnosed.
Substance Intoxication or Substance Withdrawal	May be characterized by deficits in attention and awareness, but these disturbances do not predominate in the clinical picture and are not sufficiently severe to warrant clinical attention. Substance Intoxication Delirium or Substance Withdrawal Delirium is diagnosed instead of Substance Intoxication or Substance Withdrawal only when the disturbance in consciousness predominates and warrants clinical attention.

3.16.1 Differential Diagnosis for Delirium *(continued)*

Substance/Medication-Induced Psychotic Disorder or Psychotic Disorder Due to Another Medical Condition	Is characterized by delusions or hallucinations due to the physiological effects of a substance, medication, or general medical condition, but these symptoms are not accompanied by a disturbance in attention and awareness and the additional disturbances in cognition, language, or visuospatial ability characteristic of a Delirium are not present. Substance/Medication-Induced Psychotic Disorder and Psychotic Disorder Due to Another Medical Condition are not diagnosed if the psychotic symptoms occur exclusively during the course of the Delirium.
Schizophrenia Spectrum and Other Psychotic Disorders, Bipolar Disorders, or Depressive Disorders	May be characterized by delusions, hallucinations, or agitation, but they are not due to the direct physiological effects of a general medical condition or substance/medication use; they are not accompanied by a disturbance in attention and awareness and the additional disturbances in cognition, language, or visuospatial ability characteristic of a Delirium.

3.16.2 Differential Diagnosis for Major or Mild Neurocognitive Disorder[a]

Major or Mild Neurocognitive Disorder, which is characterized by evidence of cognitive decline from a previous level of performance in one or more cognitive domains (complex attention, executive function, learning and memory, language, perceptual-motor, or social cognition) that is due to a medical condition or the persisting effects of a substance, must be differentiated from...	In contrast to Major or Mild Neurocognitive Disorder...
Delirium	Is characterized by a disturbance in attention (i.e., reduced ability to direct, focus, sustain, and shift attention) and awareness (reduced orientation to the environment) that develops over a short period of time, usually hours to a few days, and tends to fluctuate during the course of the day. In contrast, most types of Major or Mild Neurocognitive Disorder (e.g., due to Alzheimer's disease) have a gradual onset and a gradually deteriorating course. Major or Mild Neurocognitive Disorder is not diagnosed if the cognitive deficits occur exclusively in the context of Delirium. However, periods of Delirium can be superimposed on a neurocognitive disorder and should be diagnosed if present.
Substance Intoxication or Substance Withdrawal	May be characterized by cognitive impairment that remits when the acute effects of intoxication or withdrawal subside. In contrast, Substance/Medication-Induced Major or Mild Neurocognitive Disorder is diagnosed only if the cognitive impairments persist long beyond the period of acute intoxication or withdrawal.

3.16.2 Differential Diagnosis for Major or Mild Neurocognitive Disorder[a] *(continued)*

Intellectual Disability (Intellectual Developmental Disorder)	Is characterized by intellectual and adaptive functioning deficits in conceptual, social, and practical domains that have their onset during the developmental period. In contrast, Major or Mild Neurocognitive Disorder represents a decline in cognitive functioning. Individuals with Intellectual Disability can also be diagnosed with a neurocognitive disorder if they undergo a decline in cognitive functioning due to the direct effects of a comorbid medical condition (e.g., an individual with Down syndrome who loses further cognitive capacity following a head injury).
Schizophrenia	May be characterized by cognitive impairment and deterioration in functioning, In contrast to Major or Mild Neurocognitive Disorder, Schizophrenia has a generally earlier age at onset, less severe cognitive impairment, and a characteristic symptom pattern (e.g., delusions and hallucinations), and is not due to the direct effects of a general medical condition or substance/medication use.
Dissociative Amnesia or amnesia occurring in other dissociative disorders	Usually involves a circumscribed loss of memory related to traumatic events and is not due to the direct effects of a general medical condition or substance/medication use.
Major Depressive Disorder	May be characterized by memory deficits, difficulty concentrating, and other cognitive impairments, but in contrast to Major or Mild Neurocognitive Disorder, these deficits improve when the depression remits, are associated with other characteristic depressive symptoms, and are not due to the direct effects of a general medical condition or substance/medication use.

3.16.2 Differential Diagnosis for Major or Mild Neurocognitive Disorder[a] *(continued)*

Bipolar I Disorder	May be characterized by chronic cognitive impairment that impacts long-term functioning. In contrast to Major or Mild Neurocognitive Disorder, Bipolar I Disorder generally has an earlier age at onset, less severe cognitive impairment, and the presence of Manic and Major Depressive Episodes, and is not due to the direct effects of a general medical condition or substance/medication use.
Age-related cognitive decline	Is characterized by cognitive impairment that is in keeping with what would be expected for the individual's age and is not due to the direct effects of a general medical condition or substance/medication use.

[a]The two types of neurocognitive disorder in DSM-5, Major and Mild, are differentiated based on the severity of the neurocognitive deficits. Major Neurocognitive Disorder is characterized by a significant cognitive decline that is severe enough to interfere with independence, whereas Mild Neurocognitive Disorder is characterized by a modest cognitive decline that is not severe enough to interfere with everyday activities, although greater effort, compensatory strategies, or accommodation may be required.

Personality Disorders

3.17.1 Differential Diagnosis for Paranoid Personality Disorder

Paranoid Personality Disorder, which is characterized by pervasive distrust and suspiciousness of others such that their motives are interpreted as malevolent, must be differentiated from…	In contrast to Paranoid Personality Disorder…
Delusional Disorder, Persecutory Type; Schizophrenia; Bipolar I or Bipolar II Disorder With Psychotic Features; and Depressive Disorder With Psychotic Features	Are characterized by a period of persistent psychotic symptoms. To give an additional diagnosis of Paranoid Personality Disorder, the personality disorder must have been present before the onset of psychotic symptoms and must persist when the psychotic symptoms are in remission.
Personality Change Due to Another Medical Condition, Paranoid Type	Is characterized by a change in personality related to the direct effects of a general medical condition.
Social discomfort and paranoid ideation in Schizotypal Personality Disorder	Also include symptoms such as magical thinking, unusual perceptual disturbances, and odd speech or behavior.
Aloof behavior in Schizoid Personality Disorder	Is not characterized by paranoid ideation.
Reacting to minor stimuli in Borderline Personality Disorder or Histrionic Personality Disorder	Is not necessarily associated with pervasive suspiciousness.
Reluctance to confide in others in Avoidant Personality Disorder	Is due to a fear of being embarrassed or found inadequate.
Suspiciousness or alienation in Narcissistic Personality Disorder	Is characterized by fears of having imperfections or flaws revealed.

3.17.2 Differential Diagnosis for Schizoid Personality Disorder

Schizoid Personality Disorder, which is characterized by a pervasive pattern of detachment from social relationships and a restricted range of expression of emotions in interpersonal settings, must be differentiated from...	In contrast to Schizoid Personality Disorder...
Schizophrenia	May be characterized by a period of persistent psychotic symptoms, diminished emotional expression, and social withdrawal accompanied by other symptoms of Schizophrenia, such as hallucinations or disorganized speech. To give an additional diagnosis of Schizoid Personality Disorder, the personality disorder must have been present before the onset of Schizophrenia symptoms and must persist when the symptoms are in remission.
Autism Spectrum Disorder	Is characterized by more severely impaired social interactions and stereotyped behaviors and interests.
Personality Change Due to Another Medical Condition, Apathetic Type	Is characterized by a change in personality related to the direct effects of a general medical condition.
Schizotypal Personality Disorder	Is characterized by cognitive and perceptual disturbances in addition to the social isolation.
Paranoid Personality Disorder	Is characterized by suspiciousness and paranoid ideation.
Avoidant Personality Disorder	Is characterized by an active desire for relationships that is constrained by a fear of embarrassment or rejection.
Obsessive-Compulsive Personality Disorder	May be characterized by social detachment related to devotion to work and discomfort with emotions rather than lack of capacity to form intimate relationships.

3.17.3 Differential Diagnosis for Schizotypal Personality Disorder

Schizotypal Personality Disorder, which is characterized by a pervasive pattern of social and interpersonal deficits marked by acute discomfort with, and reduced capacity for, close relationships as well as by cognitive or perceptual distortions and eccentricities of behavior, must be differentiated from…	In contrast to Schizotypal Personality Disorder…
Delusional Disorder, Schizophrenia, Bipolar I or Bipolar II Disorder With Psychotic Features, and Depressive Disorder With Psychotic Features	Are characterized by a period of persistent psychotic symptoms. To give an additional diagnosis of Schizotypal Personality Disorder, the personality disorder must have been present before the onset of psychotic symptoms and must persist when the psychotic symptoms are in remission.
Autism Spectrum Disorder	Is characterized by more severely impaired social interactions and stereotyped behaviors and interests.
Language Disorders	Are characterized by greater severity of disturbance in language accompanied by compensatory efforts to communicate by other means (e.g., gestures).
Personality Change Due to Another Medical Condition, Paranoid Type	Is characterized by a change in personality related to the direct effects of a general medical condition.
Social detachment in Paranoid Personality Disorder and Schizoid Personality Disorder	Is characterized by the lack of cognitive or perceptual distortions and lack of marked eccentricity or oddness.
Avoidant Personality Disorder	Is characterized by an active desire for relationships that is constrained by a fear of embarrassment or rejection.
Suspiciousness or social withdrawal in Narcissistic Personality Disorder	Is related to fears of having imperfections revealed.
Borderline Personality Disorder	Is characterized by impulsive and manipulative behavior.
Transient schizotypal traits in adolescents	Reflect transient emotional turmoil rather than an enduring personality disorder.

3.17.4 Differential Diagnosis for Antisocial Personality Disorder

Antisocial Personality Disorder, which is characterized by a pervasive pattern of disregard for and violation of the rights of others occurring since age 15 years, must be differentiated from...	In contrast to Antisocial Personality Disorder...
Isolated antisocial behavior due to substance use	Is exclusively related to drug taking and is not part of a pattern of antisocial behavior that began in childhood.
Antisocial behavior occurring in Schizophrenia or a Manic Episode	Is associated with the characteristic symptoms of these disorders and is not associated with preexisting Conduct Disorder. Antisocial Personality Disorder should not be diagnosed if the antisocial behavior occurs exclusively during the course of Schizophrenia or a Manic Episode.
Conduct Disorder	Is characterized by a repetitive and persistent pattern of behavior in which the basic rights of others or major age-appropriate societal norms or rules are violated; Conduct Disorder can be diagnosed at any age. The diagnosis of Antisocial Personality Disorder is not given to individuals under age 18 years and is given only if there is a history of some symptoms of Conduct Disorder before age 15 years. For individuals over age 18 years, a diagnosis of Conduct Disorder is given only if the criteria for Antisocial Personality Disorder are not met.
Glibness, exploitativeness, and lack of empathy in Narcissistic Personality Disorder	Are not characterized by impulsivity, aggressiveness, and a previous pattern of Conduct Disorder.
Superficial emotionality in Histrionic Personality Disorder	Is not characterized by impulsivity, aggressiveness, and a previous pattern of Conduct Disorder.
Manipulative behavior in Borderline Personality Disorder	Is not characterized by impulsivity, aggressiveness, and a previous pattern of Conduct Disorder.

3.17.4 Differential Diagnosis for Antisocial Personality Disorder *(continued)*

Antisocial behavior in Paranoid Personality Disorder	Is motivated by revenge rather than desire for gain.
Adult antisocial behavior	Is not characterized by a long-standing pattern of antisocial behavior with onset in childhood or adolescence and other personality features of Antisocial Personality Disorder.

3.17.5 Differential Diagnosis for Borderline Personality Disorder

Borderline Personality Disorder, which is characterized by a pervasive pattern of instability of interpersonal relationships, self-image, and affects, and marked impulsivity, must be differentiated from…	In contrast to Borderline Personality Disorder…
Histrionic Personality Disorder	Is not characterized by self-destructiveness, angry disruptions in close relationships, and chronic feelings of deep emptiness and loneliness.
Paranoid ideation or illusions in Schizotypal Personality Disorder	Are characterized by paranoid ideation that is less interpersonally reactive and less amenable to the provision of external structure and support.
Paranoid ideation or angry reactions to minor stimuli in Paranoid Personality Disorder and Narcissistic Personality Disorder	Are characterized by relative stability of self-image and relative lack of self-destructiveness, impulsivity, and abandonment concerns.
Manipulative behavior in Antisocial Personality Disorder	Is motivated by a desire for power, profit, or material gain rather than a desire for nurturance.
Abandonment concerns in Dependent Personality Disorder	Are characterized by a reaction to the threat of abandonment with increasing appeasement and submission and attempts to seek a replacement relationship to provide caregiving and support.
Personality Change Due to Another Medical Condition, Labile Type	Is characterized by a change in personality related to the direct effects of a general medical condition.

3.17.6 Differential Diagnosis for Histrionic Personality Disorder

Histrionic Personality Disorder, which is characterized by a pervasive pattern of excessive emotionality and attention seeking, must be differentiated from...	In contrast to Histrionic Personality Disorder...
Borderline Personality Disorder	Is characterized by self-destructiveness, angry disruptions in close relationships, and identity disturbance.
Manipulative behavior in Antisocial Personality Disorder	Is motivated by a desire for profit, power, or material gain rather than a desire for attention and approval.
Attention seeking in Narcissistic Personality Disorder	Is characterized by a need for praise for being superior.
Dependent Personality Disorder	Is characterized by excessive dependence on others for praise and guidance without the flamboyant emotions characteristic of Histrionic Personality Disorder.
Personality Change Due to Another Medical Condition, Disinhibited Type	Is characterized by a change in personality related to the direct effects of a general medical condition.

3.17.7 Differential Diagnosis for Narcissistic Personality Disorder

Narcissistic Personality Disorder, which is characterized by a pervasive pattern of grandiosity (in fantasy or behavior), need for admiration, and lack of empathy, must be differentiated from...	In contrast to Narcissistic Personality Disorder...
Need for attention in Histrionic Personality Disorder	Is related to a need for approval as opposed to a need for admiration.
Lack of empathy in Antisocial Personality Disorder	Is characterized by impulsivity, aggression, and deceit, and is less characterized by a need for admiration by others.
Need for attention in Borderline Personality Disorder	Is characterized by instability in self-image, self-destructiveness, impulsivity, and abandonment concerns.
Perfectionism in Obsessive-Compulsive Personality Disorder	Is characterized by striving to attain perfection and a belief that others cannot do things as well, as opposed to a belief that perfection has already been achieved.
Suspiciousness and social withdrawal in Schizotypal Personality Disorder and Paranoid Personality Disorder	Are related to paranoid ideation as opposed to fears that imperfections or flaws will be revealed.
Grandiosity in Manic or Hypomanic Episodes	Occurs only during episodes of elevated or irritable mood.
Personality Change Due to Another Medical Condition, Labile Type	Is characterized by a change in personality related to the direct effects of a general medical condition.

3.17.8 Differential Diagnosis for Avoidant Personality Disorder

Avoidant Personality Disorder, which is characterized by a pervasive pattern of social inhibition, feelings of inadequacy, and hypersensitivity to negative evaluation, must be differentiated from…	In contrast to Avoidant Personality Disorder…
Avoidance in Agoraphobia	Typically starts after the onset of Panic Attacks and may vary based on their frequency and intensity.
Feelings of inadequacy, hypersensitivity to criticism, and need for reassurance in Dependent Personality Disorder	Are characterized by concerns about being taken care of as opposed to avoidance of humiliation or rejection.
Social isolation in Schizoid Personality Disorder and Schizotypal Personality Disorder	Is characterized by contentment with (or even a preference for) the social isolation.
Reluctance to confide in others in Paranoid Personality Disorder	Is motivated by fears that personal information will be used with malicious intent as opposed to fears of being embarrassed.
Personality Change Due to Another Medical Condition	Is characterized by a change in personality related to the direct effects of a general medical condition.

3.17.9 Differential Diagnosis for Dependent Personality Disorder

Dependent Personality Disorder, which is characterized by a pervasive and excessive need to be taken care of that leads to submissive and clinging behavior and fears of separation, must be differentiated from...	In contrast to Dependent Personality Disorder...
Separation Anxiety Disorder	Is characterized by a persistent and excessive fear or anxiety concerning being physically separated from major attachment figures. In Dependent Personality Disorder, the focus on concern is specifically on the need to be taken care of, rather than separated per se. If criteria are met for both disorders, both can be diagnosed.
Dependency consequent to a mental disorder or a general medical condition	Occurs exclusively during the mental disorder or general medical condition and varies according to its severity.
Fear of abandonment in Borderline Personality Disorder	Is characterized by a reaction to anticipated abandonment with feelings of emotional emptiness, rage, and demands.
Need for reassurance and approval in Histrionic Personality Disorder	Is characterized by gregarious flamboyance with active demands for attention.
Avoidant Personality Disorder	Is characterized by such a strong fear of humiliation and rejection that there is social withdrawal until the person is certain of being accepted.
Personality Change Due to Another Medical Condition	Is characterized by a change in personality related to the direct effects of a general medical condition.

3.17.10 Differential Diagnosis for Obsessive-Compulsive Personality Disorder

Obsessive-Compulsive Personality Disorder, which is characterized by a pervasive pattern of preoccupation with orderliness, perfectionism, and mental and interpersonal control, at the expense of flexibility, openness, and efficiency, must be differentiated from…	In contrast to Obsessive-Compulsive Personality Disorder…
Obsessive-Compulsive Disorder	Is characterized by the presence of true obsessions and/or compulsions.
Hoarding Disorder	Is characterized by persistent difficulty discarding or parting with possessions regardless of their actual value, which is only one of the criteria for Obsessive-Compulsive Personality Disorder. In Hoarding Disorder, in contrast to Obsessive-Compulsive Personality Disorder, this symptom predominates in the clinical picture and results in the accumulation of possessions that clutter active living areas and substantially compromise their intended use. If criteria are met for both conditions, both can be diagnosed.
Perfectionism in Narcissistic Personality Disorder	Is characterized by a belief that perfection has already been achieved.
Lack of generosity in Antisocial Personality Disorder	Is characterized by an indulgence of self as opposed to a miserly spending style toward both self and others.
Social detachment in Schizoid Personality Disorder	Occurs in the context of a lack of capacity for intimacy as opposed to discomfort with emotion and excessive devotion to work.
Personality Change Due to Another Medical Condition	Is characterized by a change in personality related to the direct effects of a general medical condition.

3.17.11 Differential Diagnosis for Personality Change Due to Another Medical Condition

Personality Change Due to Another Medical Condition, which is characterized by persistent personality disturbance due to the direct physiological effects of a general medical condition that represents a change from the individual's characteristic personality pattern, must be differentiated from…	In contrast to Personality Change Due to Another Medical Condition…
Personality change as an associated feature in Delirium	Includes fluctuating cognitive deficits in addition to personality changes. Personality Change Due to Another Medical Condition is not diagnosed if the personality disturbance occurs exclusively during the course of Delirium.
Personality change as an associated feature in Major or Mild Neurocognitive Disorder	Includes memory impairment and other cognitive deficits in addition to personality changes. Personality Change Due to Another Medical Condition may be diagnosed in addition to the Major or Mild Neurocognitive Disorder if the personality disturbance is a prominent feature.
Personality change associated with another Mental Disorder Due to Another Medical Condition (e.g., Depressive Disorder Due to Another Medical Condition)	Includes additional prominent psychiatric symptoms due to the direct physiological effects of a general medical condition (e.g., depressed mood). Personality Change Due to Another Medical Condition is not diagnosed if the disturbance is better accounted for by the other Mental Disorder Due to Another Medical Condition.
Personality change as a result of a Substance Use Disorder	Is not due to the direct effects of a general medical condition and abates when the Substance Use Disorder is in remission.
Personality change associated with another mental disorder (e.g., social withdrawal in Schizophrenia)	Is not due to the direct effects of a general medical condition.
Personality Disorders	Have a different age at onset (i.e., by adolescence or early adulthood), course, and characteristic features and are not due to the direct effects of a general medical condition.

Paraphilic Disorders

3.18.1 Differential Diagnosis for Paraphilic Disorders

Paraphilic disorders—characterized by an intense and persistent sexual interest in spying on others in private activities (Voyeuristic Disorder); exposing one's genitals (Exhibitionistic Disorder); touching or rubbing against a nonconsenting individual (Frotteuristic Disorder); undergoing humiliation, bondage, or suffering (Sexual Masochism Disorder); inflicting humiliation, bondage, or suffering (Sexual Sadism Disorder); sexual focus on children (Pedophilic Disorder); focusing on nonliving objects or body parts (Fetishistic Disorder); or cross-dressing (Transvestic Disorder) that causes clinically significant distress or impairment—must be differentiated from…	In contrast to a paraphilic disorder…
Nonpathological use of sexual fantasies, behaviors, or objects	Does not cause clinically significant distress or impairment, is typically not obligatory for sexual functioning, and involves only consenting partners.
Sexual behavior resulting from a decrease in judgment, social skills, or impulse control related to another mental disorder (e.g., Manic Episode, Major or Mild Neurocognitive Disorder, Schizophrenia)	Is typically not an individual's preferred or obligatory pattern, occurs exclusively during the course of the mental disorder, often has a later age at onset, and is accompanied by the characteristic features of the mental disorder (e.g., cognitive impairment, delusions).
Spying on others engaged in private activities in Conduct Disorder and Antisocial Personality Disorder (as distinguished from Voyeuristic Disorder)	Are characterized by additional norm-breaking and antisocial behaviors. They are differentiated from the antisocial behavior in Voyeuristic Disorder by the lack of the specific sexual interest in secretly watching unsuspecting others who are naked or engaging in sexual activity.

3.18.1 Differential Diagnosis for Paraphilic Disorders *(continued)*

Child molestation in Conduct Disorder and Antisocial Personality Disorder (as distinguished from Pedophilic Disorder)	Are characterized by a pattern of lack of empathy and disregard for the rights of others, which may include opportunistic child molestation. This is differentiated from Pedophilic Disorder, in which there is an established pattern of sexual arousal to children.
Substance Intoxication	Is characterized by disinhibited behaviors that might involve committing certain sexual offenses (e.g., peeking, exhibiting one's genitals, rubbing against an unsuspecting person). It is differentiated from a Paraphilic Disorder by the absence of a persistent pattern of sexual interest in spying on others, exposing one's genitals, or rubbing against an unsuspecting person.
Medication side effect (e.g., dopamine agonist medication)	Is characterized by paraphilia-like sexual behavior that is a side effect of a medication (particularly dopamine agonist medications used to treat Parkinson's disease) that is uncharacteristic of the individual's sexual behavior when not taking the medication.
Obsessive-Compulsive Disorder (as distinguished from Pedophilic Disorder)	May be characterized by ego-dystonic thoughts and worries about possible attraction to children as well as other ego-dystonic, intrusive sexual ideas (e.g., concerns about homosexuality). In contrast to Pedophilic Disorder, there is an absence of sexual thoughts about children during high states of sexual arousal (e.g., approaching orgasm during masturbation).

Appendix

DSM-5 Classification

Before each disorder name, ICD-9-CM codes are provided, followed by ICD-10-CM codes in parentheses. Blank lines indicate that either the ICD-9-CM or the ICD-10-CM code is not applicable. For some disorders, the code can be indicated only according to the subtype or specifier.

ICD-9-CM codes are to be used for coding purposes in the United States through September 30, 2015. ICD-10-CM codes are to be used starting October 1, 2015. For DSM-5 coding and other updates, see the DSM-5® Update on www.PsychiatryOnline.org.

Note for all mental disorders due to another medical condition: Indicate the name of the other medical condition in the name of the mental disorder due to [the medical condition]. The code and name for the other medical condition should be listed first immediately before the mental disorder due to the medical condition.

Neurodevelopmental Disorders

Intellectual Disabilities

___.__	(___.__)	Intellectual Disability (Intellectual Developmental Disorder) *Specify* current severity:
317	(F70)	Mild
318.0	(F71)	Moderate
318.1	(F72)	Severe
318.2	(F73)	Profound
315.8	(F88)	Global Developmental Delay
319	(F79)	Unspecified Intellectual Disability (Intellectual Developmental Disorder)

Communication Disorders

315.32 (F80.2) Language Disorder

315.39 (F80.0) Speech Sound Disorder

315.35 (F80.81) Childhood-Onset Fluency Disorder (Stuttering)

Note: Later-onset cases are diagnosed as 307.0 (F98.5) adult-onset fluency disorder.

315.39 (F80.89) Social (Pragmatic) Communication Disorder

307.9 (F80.9) Unspecified Communication Disorder

Autism Spectrum Disorder

299.00 (F84.0) Autism Spectrum Disorder

Specify if: Associated with a known medical or genetic condition or environmental factor; Associated with another neurodevelopmental, mental, or behavioral disorder

Specify current severity for Criterion A and Criterion B: Requiring very substantial support, Requiring substantial support, Requiring support

Specify if: With or without accompanying intellectual impairment, With or without accompanying language impairment, With catatonia (use additional code 293.89 [F06.1])

Attention-Deficit/Hyperactivity Disorder

___.__ (___.__) Attention-Deficit/Hyperactivity Disorder

Specify whether:

314.01 (F90.2) Combined presentation

314.00 (F90.0) Predominantly inattentive presentation

314.01 (F90.1) Predominantly hyperactive/impulsive presentation

Specify if: In partial remission

Specify current severity: Mild, Moderate, Severe

314.01 (F90.8) Other Specified Attention-Deficit/Hyperactivity Disorder

314.01 (F90.9) Unspecified Attention-Deficit/Hyperactivity Disorder

Specific Learning Disorder

___.__ (___.__) Specific Learning Disorder

Specify if:

315.00 (F81.0) With impairment in reading (*specify* if with word reading accuracy, reading rate or fluency, reading comprehension)

315.2 (F81.81) With impairment in written expression (*specify* if with spelling accuracy, grammar and punctuation accuracy, clarity or organization of written expression)

315.1 (F81.2) With impairment in mathematics (*specify* if with number sense, memorization of arithmetic facts, accurate or fluent calculation, accurate math reasoning)

Specify current severity: Mild, Moderate, Severe

Motor Disorders

315.4 (F82) Developmental Coordination Disorder

307.3 (F98.4) Stereotypic Movement Disorder

Specify if: With self-injurious behavior, Without self-injurious behavior
Specify if: Associated with a known medical or genetic condition, neurodevelopmental disorder, or environmental factor
Specify current severity: Mild, Moderate, Severe

Tic Disorders

307.23 (F95.2) Tourette's Disorder

307.22 (F95.1) Persistent (Chronic) Motor or Vocal Tic Disorder

Specify if: With motor tics only, With vocal tics only

307.21 (F95.0) Provisional Tic Disorder

307.20 (F95.8) Other Specified Tic Disorder

307.20 (F95.9) Unspecified Tic Disorder

Other Neurodevelopmental Disorders

315.8 (F88) Other Specified Neurodevelopmental Disorder

315.9 (F89) Unspecified Neurodevelopmental Disorder

Schizophrenia Spectrum and Other Psychotic Disorders

The following specifiers apply to Schizophrenia Spectrum and Other Psychotic Disorders where indicated:

[a]*Specify* if: The following course specifiers are only to be used after a 1-year duration of the disorder: First episode, currently in acute episode; First episode, currently in partial remission; First episode, currently in full remission; Multiple episodes, currently in acute episode; Multiple episodes, currently in partial remission; Multiple episodes, currently in full remission; Continuous; Unspecified

[b]*Specify* if: With catatonia (use additional code 293.89 [F06.1])

[c]*Specify* current severity of delusions, hallucinations, disorganized speech, abnormal psychomotor behavior, negative symptoms, impaired cognition, depression, and mania symptoms

301.22 (F21) Schizotypal (Personality) Disorder

297.1 (F22) Delusional Disorder[a, c]

Specify whether: Erotomanic type, Grandiose type, Jealous type, Persecutory type, Somatic type, Mixed type, Unspecified type
Specify if: With bizarre content

298.8 (F23) Brief Psychotic Disorder[b, c]

Specify if: With marked stressor(s), Without marked stressor(s), With peripartum onset

295.40 (F20.81) Schizophreniform Disorder[b, c]

Specify if: With good prognostic features, Without good prognostic features

295.90 (F20.9) Schizophrenia[a, b, c]

___.___	(___.___)	Schizoaffective Disorder[a, b, c]
		Specify whether:
295.70	(F25.0)	Bipolar type
295.70	(F25.1)	Depressive type
___.___	(___.___)	Substance/Medication-Induced Psychotic Disorder[c]
		Note: See the criteria set and corresponding recording procedures for substance-specific codes and ICD-9-CM and ICD-10-CM coding.
		Specify if: With onset during intoxication, With onset during withdrawal
___.___	(___.___)	Psychotic Disorder Due to Another Medical Condition[c]
		Specify whether:
293.81	(F06.2)	With delusions
293.82	(F06.0)	With hallucinations
293.89	(F06.1)	Catatonia Associated With Another Mental Disorder (Catatonia Specifier)
293.89	(F06.1)	Catatonic Disorder Due to Another Medical Condition
293.89	(F06.1)	Unspecified Catatonia
		Note: Code first **781.99 (R29.818)** other symptoms involving nervous and musculoskeletal systems.
298.8	(F28)	Other Specified Schizophrenia Spectrum and Other Psychotic Disorder
298.9	(F29)	Unspecified Schizophrenia Spectrum and Other Psychotic Disorder

Bipolar and Related Disorders

The following specifiers apply to Bipolar and Related Disorders where indicated:

[a]*Specify:* With anxious distress (*specify* current severity: mild, moderate, moderate-severe, severe); With mixed features; With rapid cycling; With melancholic features; With atypical features; With mood-congruent psychotic features; With mood-incongruent psychotic features; With catatonia (use additional code 293.89 [F06.1]); With peripartum onset; With seasonal pattern

___.___	(___.___)	Bipolar I Disorder[a]
___.___	(___.___)	Current or most recent episode manic
296.41	(F31.11)	Mild
296.42	(F31.12)	Moderate
296.43	(F31.13)	Severe
296.44	(F31.2)	With psychotic features
296.45	(F31.73)	In partial remission
296.46	(F31.74)	In full remission
296.40	(F31.9)	Unspecified
296.40	(F31.0)	Current or most recent episode hypomanic
296.45	(F31.71)	In partial remission
296.46	(F31.72)	In full remission
296.40	(F31.9)	Unspecified
___.___	(___.___)	Current or most recent episode depressed

296.51 (F31.31)		Mild
296.52 (F31.32)		Moderate
296.53 (F31.4)		Severe
296.54 (F31.5)		With psychotic features
296.55 (F31.75)		In partial remission
296.56 (F31.76)		In full remission
296.50 (F31.9)		Unspecified
296.7 (F31.9)	Current or most recent episode unspecified	

296.89 (F31.81) Bipolar II Disorder[a]

Specify current or most recent episode: Hypomanic, Depressed
Specify course if full criteria for a mood episode are not currently met: In partial remission, In full remission
Specify severity if full criteria for a major depressive episode are currently met: Mild, Moderate, Severe

301.13 (F34.0) Cyclothymic Disorder

Specify if: With anxious distress

___.__ (___.__) Substance/Medication-Induced Bipolar and Related Disorder

Note: See the criteria set and corresponding recording procedures for substance-specific codes and ICD-9-CM and ICD-10-CM coding.
Specify if: With onset during intoxication, With onset during withdrawal

293.83 (___.__) Bipolar and Related Disorder Due to Another Medical Condition

Specify if:

(F06.33) With manic features
(F06.33) With manic- or hypomanic-like episode
(F06.34) With mixed features

296.89 (F31.89) Other Specified Bipolar and Related Disorder

296.80 (F31.9) Unspecified Bipolar and Related Disorder

Depressive Disorders

The following specifiers apply to Depressive Disorders where indicated:

[a]*Specify:* With anxious distress (*specify* current severity: mild, moderate, moderate-severe, severe); With mixed features; With melancholic features; With atypical features; With mood-congruent psychotic features; With mood-incongruent psychotic features; With catatonia (use additional code 293.89 [F06.1]); With peripartum onset; With seasonal pattern

296.99 (F34.8) Disruptive Mood Dysregulation Disorder

___.__ (___.__) Major Depressive Disorder[a]

___.__ (___.__)	Single episode	
296.21 (F32.0)		Mild
296.22 (F32.1)		Moderate
296.23 (F32.2)		Severe
296.24 (F32.3)		With psychotic features
296.25 (F32.4)		In partial remission
296.26 (F32.5)		In full remission
296.20 (F32.9)		Unspecified

___.__	(___.__)	Recurrent episode
296.31	(F33.0)	Mild
296.32	(F33.1)	Moderate
296.33	(F33.2)	Severe
296.34	(F33.3)	With psychotic features
296.35	(F33.41)	In partial remission
296.36	(F33.42)	In full remission
296.30	(F33.9)	Unspecified

300.4 (F34.1) Persistent Depressive Disorder (Dysthymia)[a]

Specify if: In partial remission, In full remission

Specify if: Early onset, Late onset

Specify if: With pure dysthymic syndrome; With persistent major depressive episode; With intermittent major depressive episodes, with current episode; With intermittent major depressive episodes, without current episode

Specify current severity: Mild, Moderate, Severe

625.4 (N94.3) Premenstrual Dysphoric Disorder

___.__ (___.__) Substance/Medication-Induced Depressive Disorder

Note: See the criteria set and corresponding recording procedures for substance-specific codes and ICD-9-CM and ICD-10-CM coding.

Specify if: With onset during intoxication, With onset during withdrawal

293.83 (___.__) Depressive Disorder Due to Another Medical Condition

Specify if:

(F06.31)	With depressive features
(F06.32)	With major depressive–like episode
(F06.34)	With mixed features

311 (F32.8) Other Specified Depressive Disorder

311 (F32.9) Unspecified Depressive Disorder

Anxiety Disorders

309.21 (F93.0) Separation Anxiety Disorder

313.23 (F94.0) Selective Mutism

300.29 (___.__) Specific Phobia

Specify if:

(F40.218)	Animal
(F40.228)	Natural environment
(___.__)	Blood-injection-injury
(F40.230)	Fear of blood
(F40.231)	Fear of injections and transfusions
(F40.232)	Fear of other medical care
(F40.233)	Fear of injury
(F40.248)	Situational
(F40.298)	Other

300.23	**(F40.10)**	Social Anxiety Disorder (Social Phobia) *Specify* if: Performance only
300.01	**(F41.0)**	Panic Disorder
___.__	(___.__)	Panic Attack Specifier
300.22	**(F40.00)**	Agoraphobia
300.02	**(F41.1)**	Generalized Anxiety Disorder
___.__	(___.__)	Substance/Medication-Induced Anxiety Disorder **Note:** See the criteria set and corresponding recording procedures for substance-specific codes and ICD-9-CM and ICD-10-CM coding. *Specify* if: With onset during intoxication, With onset during withdrawal, With onset after medication use
293.84	**(F06.4)**	Anxiety Disorder Due to Another Medical Condition
300.09	**(F41.8)**	Other Specified Anxiety Disorder
300.00	**(F41.9)**	Unspecified Anxiety Disorder

Obsessive-Compulsive and Related Disorders

The following specifier applies to Obsessive-Compulsive and Related Disorders where indicated:
[a]*Specify* if: With good or fair insight, With poor insight, With absent insight/delusional beliefs

300.3	**(F42)**	Obsessive-Compulsive Disorder[a] *Specify* if: Tic-related
300.7	**(F45.22)**	Body Dysmorphic Disorder[a] *Specify* if: With muscle dysmorphia
300.3	**(F42)**	Hoarding Disorder[a] *Specify* if: With excessive acquisition
312.39	**(F63.3)**	Trichotillomania (Hair-Pulling Disorder)
698.4	**(L98.1)**	Excoriation (Skin-Picking) Disorder
___.__	(___.__)	Substance/Medication-Induced Obsessive-Compulsive and Related Disorder **Note:** See the criteria set and corresponding recording procedures for substance-specific codes and ICD-9-CM and ICD-10-CM coding. *Specify* if: With onset during intoxication, With onset during withdrawal, With onset after medication use
294.8	**(F06.8)**	Obsessive-Compulsive and Related Disorder Due to Another Medical Condition *Specify* if: With obsessive-compulsive disorder–like symptoms, With appearance preoccupations, With hoarding symptoms, With hair-pulling symptoms, With skin-picking symptoms
300.3	**(F42)**	Other Specified Obsessive-Compulsive and Related Disorder
300.3	**(F42)**	Unspecified Obsessive-Compulsive and Related Disorder

Trauma- and Stressor-Related Disorders

313.89	(F94.1)	Reactive Attachment Disorder *Specify* if: Persistent *Specify* current severity: Severe
313.89	(F94.2)	Disinhibited Social Engagement Disorder *Specify* if: Persistent *Specify* current severity: Severe
309.81	(F43.10)	Posttraumatic Stress Disorder (includes Posttraumatic Stress Disorder for Children 6 Years and Younger) *Specify* whether: With dissociative symptoms *Specify* if: With delayed expression
308.3	(F43.0)	Acute Stress Disorder
___.__	(___.__)	Adjustment Disorders *Specify* whether:
309.0	(F43.21)	With depressed mood
309.24	(F43.22)	With anxiety
309.28	(F43.23)	With mixed anxiety and depressed mood
309.3	(F43.24)	With disturbance of conduct
309.4	(F43.25)	With mixed disturbance of emotions and conduct
309.9	(F43.20)	Unspecified
309.89	(F43.8)	Other Specified Trauma- and Stressor-Related Disorder
309.9	(F43.9)	Unspecified Trauma- and Stressor-Related Disorder

Dissociative Disorders

300.14	(F44.81)	Dissociative Identity Disorder
300.12	(F44.0)	Dissociative Amnesia *Specify* if:
300.13	(F44.1)	With dissociative fugue
300.6	(F48.1)	Depersonalization/Derealization Disorder
300.15	(F44.89)	Other Specified Dissociative Disorder
300.15	(F44.9)	Unspecified Dissociative Disorder

Somatic Symptom and Related Disorders

300.82	(F45.1)	Somatic Symptom Disorder *Specify* if: With predominant pain *Specify* if: Persistent *Specify* current severity: Mild, Moderate, Severe

300.7	(F45.21)	Illness Anxiety Disorder *Specify* whether: Care seeking type, Care avoidant type
300.11	(___.__)	Conversion Disorder (Functional Neurological Symptom Disorder) *Specify* symptom type:
	(F44.4)	With weakness or paralysis
	(F44.4)	With abnormal movement
	(F44.4)	With swallowing symptoms
	(F44.4)	With speech symptom
	(F44.5)	With attacks or seizures
	(F44.6)	With anesthesia or sensory loss
	(F44.6)	With special sensory symptom
	(F44.7)	With mixed symptoms *Specify* if: Acute episode, Persistent *Specify* if: With psychological stressor (specify stressor), Without psychological stressor
316	(F54)	Psychological Factors Affecting Other Medical Conditions *Specify* current severity: Mild, Moderate, Severe, Extreme
300.19	(F68.10)	Factitious Disorder (includes Factitious Disorder Imposed on Self, Factitious Disorder Imposed on Another) *Specify*: Single episode, Recurrent episodes
300.89	(F45.8)	Other Specified Somatic Symptom and Related Disorder
300.82	(F45.9)	Unspecified Somatic Symptom and Related Disorder

Feeding and Eating Disorders

The following specifiers apply to Feeding and Eating Disorders where indicated:
[a]*Specify* if: In remission
[b]*Specify* if: In partial remission, In full remission
[c]*Specify* current severity: Mild, Moderate, Severe, Extreme

307.52	(___.__)	Pica[a]
	(F98.3)	In children
	(F50.8)	In adults
307.53	(F98.21)	Rumination Disorder[a]
307.59	(F50.8)	Avoidant/Restrictive Food Intake Disorder[a]
307.1	(___.__)	Anorexia Nervosa[b, c] *Specify* whether:
	(F50.01)	Restricting type
	(F50.02)	Binge-eating/purging type
307.51	(F50.2)	Bulimia Nervosa[b, c]
307.51	(F50.8)	Binge-Eating Disorder[b, c]
307.59	(F50.8)	Other Specified Feeding or Eating Disorder
307.50	(F50.9)	Unspecified Feeding or Eating Disorder

Elimination Disorders

307.6 (F98.0) Enuresis
Specify whether: Nocturnal only, Diurnal only, Nocturnal and diurnal

307.7 (F98.1) Encopresis
Specify whether: With constipation and overflow incontinence, Without constipation and overflow incontinence

___.__ (___.__) Other Specified Elimination Disorder
788.39 (N39.498) With urinary symptoms
787.60 (R15.9) With fecal symptoms

___.__ (___.__) Unspecified Elimination Disorder
788.30 (R32) With urinary symptoms
787.60 (R15.9) With fecal symptoms

Sleep-Wake Disorders

The following specifiers apply to Sleep-Wake Disorders where indicated:
[a]*Specify* if: Episodic, Persistent, Recurrent
[b]*Specify* if: Acute, Subacute, Persistent
[c]*Specify* current severity: Mild, Moderate, Severe

307.42 (F51.01) Insomnia Disorder[a]
Specify if: With non–sleep disorder mental comorbidity, With other medical comorbidity, With other sleep disorder

307.44 (F51.11) Hypersomnolence Disorder[b, c]
Specify if: With mental disorder, With medical condition, With another sleep disorder

___.__ (___.__) Narcolepsy[c]
Specify whether:
347.00 (G47.419) Narcolepsy without cataplexy but with hypocretin deficiency
347.01 (G47.411) Narcolepsy with cataplexy but without hypocretin deficiency
347.00 (G47.419) Autosomal dominant cerebellar ataxia, deafness, and narcolepsy
347.00 (G47.419) Autosomal dominant narcolepsy, obesity, and type 2 diabetes
347.10 (G47.429) Narcolepsy secondary to another medical condition

Breathing-Related Sleep Disorders

327.23 (G47.33) Obstructive Sleep Apnea Hypopnea[c]

___.__ (___.__) Central Sleep Apnea
Specify whether:
327.21 (G47.31) Idiopathic central sleep apnea
786.04 (R06.3) Cheyne-Stokes breathing
780.57 (G47.37) Central sleep apnea comorbid with opioid use
Note: First code opioid use disorder, if present.
Specify current severity

___.__	(___.__)	Sleep-Related Hypoventilation *Specify* whether:
327.24	(G47.34)	Idiopathic hypoventilation
327.25	(G47.35)	Congenital central alveolar hypoventilation
327.26	(G47.36)	Comorbid sleep-related hypoventilation *Specify* current severity
___.__	(___.__)	Circadian Rhythm Sleep-Wake Disorders[a] *Specify* whether:
307.45	(G47.21)	Delayed sleep phase type *Specify* if: Familial, Overlapping with non-24-hour sleep-wake type
307.45	(G47.22)	Advanced sleep phase type *Specify* if: Familial
307.45	(G47.23)	Irregular sleep-wake type
307.45	(G47.24)	Non-24-hour sleep-wake type
307.45	(G47.26)	Shift work type
307.45	(G47.20)	Unspecified type

Parasomnias

___.__	(___.__)	Non–Rapid Eye Movement Sleep Arousal Disorders *Specify* whether:
307.46	(F51.3)	Sleepwalking type *Specify* if: With sleep-related eating, With sleep-related sexual behavior (sexsomnia)
307.46	(F51.4)	Sleep terror type
307.47	(F51.5)	Nightmare Disorder[b, c] *Specify* if: During sleep onset *Specify* if: With associated non–sleep disorder, With associated other medical condition, With associated other sleep disorder
327.42	(G47.52)	Rapid Eye Movement Sleep Behavior Disorder
333.94	(G25.81)	Restless Legs Syndrome
___.__	(___.__)	Substance/Medication-Induced Sleep Disorder **Note:** See the criteria set and corresponding recording procedures for substance-specific codes and ICD-9-CM and ICD-10-CM coding. *Specify* whether: Insomnia type, Daytime sleepiness type, Parasomnia type, Mixed type *Specify* if: With onset during intoxication, With onset during discontinuation/withdrawal
780.52	(G47.09)	Other Specified Insomnia Disorder
780.52	(G47.00)	Unspecified Insomnia Disorder
780.54	(G47.19)	Other Specified Hypersomnolence Disorder
780.54	(G47.10)	Unspecified Hypersomnolence Disorder
780.59	(G47.8)	Other Specified Sleep-Wake Disorder
780.59	(G47.9)	Unspecified Sleep-Wake Disorder

Sexual Dysfunctions

The following specifiers apply to Sexual Dysfunctions where indicated:
[a]*Specify* whether: Lifelong, Acquired
[b]*Specify* whether: Generalized, Situational
[c]*Specify* current severity: Mild, Moderate, Severe

302.74 (F52.32) Delayed Ejaculation[a, b, c]

302.72 (F52.21) Erectile Disorder[a, b, c]

302.73 (F52.31) Female Orgasmic Disorder[a, b, c]
Specify if: Never experienced an orgasm under any situation

302.72 (F52.22) Female Sexual Interest/Arousal Disorder[a, b, c]

302.76 (F52.6) Genito-Pelvic Pain/Penetration Disorder[a, c]

302.71 (F52.0) Male Hypoactive Sexual Desire Disorder[a, b, c]

302.75 (F52.4) Premature (Early) Ejaculation[a, b, c]

___.__ (___.__) Substance/Medication-Induced Sexual Dysfunction[c]
Note: See the criteria set and corresponding recording procedures for substance-specific codes and ICD-9-CM and ICD-10-CM coding.
Specify if: With onset during intoxication, With onset during withdrawal, With onset after medication use

302.79 (F52.8) Other Specified Sexual Dysfunction

302.70 (F52.9) Unspecified Sexual Dysfunction

Gender Dysphoria

___.__ (___.__) Gender Dysphoria

302.6 (F64.2) Gender Dysphoria in Children
Specify if: With a disorder of sex development

302.85 (F64.1) Gender Dysphoria in Adolescents and Adults
Specify if: With a disorder of sex development
Specify if: Posttransition
Note: Code the disorder of sex development if present, in addition to gender dysphoria.

302.6 (F64.8) Other Specified Gender Dysphoria

302.6 (F64.9) Unspecified Gender Dysphoria

Disruptive, Impulse-Control, and Conduct Disorders

313.81 (F91.3) Oppositional Defiant Disorder
Specify current severity: Mild, Moderate, Severe

312.34 (F63.81) Intermittent Explosive Disorder

___.__	(___.__)	Conduct Disorder
		Specify whether:
312.81	(F91.1)	Childhood-onset type
312.82	(F91.2)	Adolescent-onset type
312.89	(F91.9)	Unspecified onset
		Specify if: With limited prosocial emotions
		Specify current severity: Mild, Moderate, Severe
301.7	(F60.2)	Antisocial Personality Disorder
312.33	(F63.1)	Pyromania
312.32	(F63.2)	Kleptomania
312.89	(F91.8)	Other Specified Disruptive, Impulse-Control, and Conduct Disorder
312.9	(F91.9)	Unspecified Disruptive, Impulse-Control, and Conduct Disorder

Substance-Related and Addictive Disorders

The following specifiers and note apply to Substance-Related and Addictive Disorders where indicated:

[a]*Specify* if: In early remission, In sustained remission

[b]*Specify* if: In a controlled environment

[c]*Specify* if: With perceptual disturbances

[d]The ICD-10-CM code indicates the comorbid presence of a moderate or severe substance use disorder, which must be present in order to apply the code for substance withdrawal.

Substance-Related Disorders

Alcohol-Related Disorders

___.__	(___.__)	Alcohol Use Disorder[a, b]
		Specify current severity:
305.00	(F10.10)	Mild
303.90	(F10.20)	Moderate
303.90	(F10.20)	Severe
303.00	(___.__)	Alcohol Intoxication
	(F10.129)	With use disorder, mild
	(F10.229)	With use disorder, moderate or severe
	(F10.929)	Without use disorder
291.81	(___.__)	Alcohol Withdrawal[c, d]
	(F10.239)	Without perceptual disturbances
	(F10.232)	With perceptual disturbances
___.__	(___.__)	Other Alcohol-Induced Disorders
291.9	(F10.99)	Unspecified Alcohol-Related Disorder

Caffeine-Related Disorders

305.90	(F15.929)	Caffeine Intoxication

292.0	(F15.93)	Caffeine Withdrawal
___.__	(___.__)	Other Caffeine-Induced Disorders
292.9	(F15.99)	Unspecified Caffeine-Related Disorder

Cannabis-Related Disorders

___.__	(___.__)	Cannabis Use Disorder[a, b]
		Specify current severity:
305.20	(F12.10)	Mild
304.30	(F12.20)	Moderate
304.30	(F12.20)	Severe
292.89	(___.__)	Cannabis Intoxication[c]
		Without perceptual disturbances
	(F12.129)	With use disorder, mild
	(F12.229)	With use disorder, moderate or severe
	(F12.929)	Without use disorder
		With perceptual disturbances
	(F12.122)	With use disorder, mild
	(F12.222)	With use disorder, moderate or severe
	(F12.922)	Without use disorder
292.0	(F12.288)	Cannabis Withdrawal[d]
___.__	(___.__)	Other Cannabis-Induced Disorders
292.9	(F12.99)	Unspecified Cannabis-Related Disorder

Hallucinogen-Related Disorders

___.__	(___.__)	Phencyclidine Use Disorder[a, b]
		Specify current severity:
305.90	(F16.10)	Mild
304.60	(F16.20)	Moderate
304.60	(F16.20)	Severe
___.__	(___.__)	Other Hallucinogen Use Disorder[a, b]
		Specify the particular hallucinogen
		Specify current severity:
305.30	(F16.10)	Mild
304.50	(F16.20)	Moderate
304.50	(F16.20)	Severe
292.89	(___.__)	Phencyclidine Intoxication
	(F16.129)	With use disorder, mild
	(F16.229)	With use disorder, moderate or severe
	(F16.929)	Without use disorder
292.89	(___.__)	Other Hallucinogen Intoxication
	(F16.129)	With use disorder, mild

	(F16.229)	With use disorder, moderate or severe
	(F16.929)	Without use disorder
292.89	**(F16.983)**	Hallucinogen Persisting Perception Disorder
___.__	(___.__)	Other Phencyclidine-Induced Disorders
___.__	(___.__)	Other Hallucinogen-Induced Disorders
292.9	**(F16.99)**	Unspecified Phencyclidine-Related Disorder
292.9	**(F16.99)**	Unspecified Hallucinogen-Related Disorder

Inhalant-Related Disorders

___.__	(___.__)	Inhalant Use Disorder[a, b]
		Specify the particular inhalant
		Specify current severity:
305.90	**(F18.10)**	Mild
304.60	**(F18.20)**	Moderate
304.60	**(F18.20)**	Severe
292.89	(___.__)	Inhalant Intoxication
	(F18.129)	With use disorder, mild
	(F18.229)	With use disorder, moderate or severe
	(F18.929)	Without use disorder
___.__	(___.__)	Other Inhalant-Induced Disorders
292.9	**(F18.99)**	Unspecified Inhalant-Related Disorder

Opioid-Related Disorders

___.__	(___.__)	Opioid Use Disorder[a]
		Specify if: On maintenance therapy, In a controlled environment
		Specify current severity:
305.50	**(F11.10)**	Mild
304.00	**(F11.20)**	Moderate
304.00	**(F11.20)**	Severe
292.89	(___.__)	Opioid Intoxication[c]
		Without perceptual disturbances
	(F11.129)	With use disorder, mild
	(F11.229)	With use disorder, moderate or severe
	(F11.929)	Without use disorder
		With perceptual disturbances
	(F11.122)	With use disorder, mild
	(F11.222)	With use disorder, moderate or severe
	(F11.922)	Without use disorder
292.0	**(F11.23)**	Opioid Withdrawal[d]
___.__	(___.__)	Other Opioid-Induced Disorders
292.9	**(F11.99)**	Unspecified Opioid-Related Disorder

Sedative-, Hypnotic-, or Anxiolytic-Related Disorders

___.__	(___.__)	Sedative, Hypnotic, or Anxiolytic Use Disorder[a, b]
		Specify current severity:
305.40	(F13.10)	Mild
304.10	(F13.20)	Moderate
304.10	(F13.20)	Severe
292.89	(___.__)	Sedative, Hypnotic, or Anxiolytic Intoxication
	(F13.129)	With use disorder, mild
	(F13.229)	With use disorder, moderate or severe
	(F13.929)	Without use disorder
292.0	(___.__)	Sedative, Hypnotic, or Anxiolytic Withdrawal[c, d]
	(F13.239)	Without perceptual disturbances
	(F13.232)	With perceptual disturbances
___.__	(___.__)	Other Sedative-, Hypnotic-, or Anxiolytic-Induced Disorders
292.9	(F13.99)	Unspecified Sedative-, Hypnotic-, or Anxiolytic-Related Disorder

Stimulant-Related Disorders

___.__	(___.__)	Stimulant Use Disorder[a, b]
		Specify current severity:
___.__	(___.__)	Mild
305.70	(F15.10)	Amphetamine-type substance
305.60	(F14.10)	Cocaine
305.70	(F15.10)	Other or unspecified stimulant
___.__	(___.__)	Moderate
304.40	(F15.20)	Amphetamine-type substance
304.20	(F14.20)	Cocaine
304.40	(F15.20)	Other or unspecified stimulant
___.__	(___.__)	Severe
304.40	(F15.20)	Amphetamine-type substance
304.20	(F14.20)	Cocaine
304.40	(F15.20)	Other or unspecified stimulant
292.89	(___.__)	Stimulant Intoxication[c]
		Specify the specific intoxicant
292.89	(___.__)	Amphetamine or other stimulant, Without perceptual disturbances
	(F15.129)	With use disorder, mild
	(F15.229)	With use disorder, moderate or severe
	(F15.929)	Without use disorder
292.89	(___.__)	Cocaine, Without perceptual disturbances
	(F14.129)	With use disorder, mild
	(F14.229)	With use disorder, moderate or severe
	(F14.929)	Without use disorder

292.89	(___.__)	Amphetamine or other stimulant, With perceptual disturbances
	(F15.122)	With use disorder, mild
	(F15.222)	With use disorder, moderate or severe
	(F15.922)	Without use disorder
292.89	(___.__)	Cocaine, With perceptual disturbances
	(F14.122)	With use disorder, mild
	(F14.222)	With use disorder, moderate or severe
	(F14.922)	Without use disorder
292.0	(___.__)	Stimulant Withdrawal[d]
		Specify the specific substance causing the withdrawal syndrome
	(F15.23)	Amphetamine or other stimulant
	(F14.23)	Cocaine
___.__	(___.__)	Other Stimulant-Induced Disorders
292.9	(___.__)	Unspecified Stimulant-Related Disorder
	(F15.99)	Amphetamine or other stimulant
	(F14.99)	Cocaine

Tobacco-Related Disorders

___.__	(___.__)	Tobacco Use Disorder[a]
		Specify if: On maintenance therapy, In a controlled environment
		Specify current severity:
305.1	(Z72.0)	Mild
305.1	(F17.200)	Moderate
305.1	(F17.200)	Severe
292.0	(F17.203)	Tobacco Withdrawal[d]
___.__	(___.__)	Other Tobacco-Induced Disorders
292.9	(F17.209)	Unspecified Tobacco-Related Disorder

Other (or Unknown) Substance–Related Disorders

___.__	(___.__)	Other (or Unknown) Substance Use Disorder[a, b]
		Specify current severity:
305.90	(F19.10)	Mild
304.90	(F19.20)	Moderate
304.90	(F19.20)	Severe
292.89	(___.__)	Other (or Unknown) Substance Intoxication
	(F19.129)	With use disorder, mild
	(F19.229)	With use disorder, moderate or severe
	(F19.929)	Without use disorder
292.0	(F19.239)	Other (or Unknown) Substance Withdrawal[d]
___.__	(___.__)	Other (or Unknown) Substance–Induced Disorders
292.9	(F19.99)	Unspecified Other (or Unknown) Substance–Related Disorder

Non-Substance-Related Disorders

312.31 (F63.0) Gambling Disorder[a]
Specify if: Episodic, Persistent
Specify current severity: Mild, Moderate, Severe

Neurocognitive Disorders

___.__ (___.__) Delirium

[a]**Note:** See the criteria set and corresponding recording procedures for substance-specific codes and ICD-9-CM and ICD-10-CM coding.

Specify whether:

___.__	(___.__)	Substance intoxication delirium[a]
___.__	(___.__)	Substance withdrawal delirium[a]
292.81	(___.__)	Medication-induced delirium[a]
293.0	(F05)	Delirium due to another medical condition
293.0	(F05)	Delirium due to multiple etiologies

Specify if: Acute, Persistent
Specify if: Hyperactive, Hypoactive, Mixed level of activity

780.09 (R41.0) Other Specified Delirium

780.09 (R41.0) Unspecified Delirium

Major and Mild Neurocognitive Disorders

Specify whether due to: Alzheimer's disease, Frontotemporal lobar degeneration, Lewy body disease, Vascular disease, Traumatic brain injury, Substance/medication use, HIV infection, Prion disease, Parkinson's disease, Huntington's disease, Another medical condition, Multiple etiologies, Unspecified

[a]*Specify:* Without behavioral disturbance, With behavioral disturbance. *For possible major neurocognitive disorder and for mild neurocognitive disorder, behavioral disturbance cannot be coded but should still be indicated in writing.*

[b]*Specify* current severity: Mild, Moderate, Severe. *This specifier applies only to major neurocognitive disorders (including probable and possible).*

Note: As indicated for each subtype, an additional medical code is needed for probable major neurocognitive disorder or major neurocognitive disorder. An additional medical code should *not* be used for possible major neurocognitive disorder or mild neurocognitive disorder.

Major or Mild Neurocognitive Disorder Due to Alzheimer's Disease

___.__ (___.__) Probable Major Neurocognitive Disorder Due to Alzheimer's Disease[b]

Note: Code first **331.0 (G30.9)** Alzheimer's disease.

294.11	(F02.81)	With behavioral disturbance
294.10	(F02.80)	Without behavioral disturbance

331.9 (G31.9) Possible Major Neurocognitive Disorder Due to Alzheimer's Disease[a, b]

331.83 (G31.84) Mild Neurocognitive Disorder Due to Alzheimer's Disease[a]

Major or Mild Frontotemporal Neurocognitive Disorder

___.__ (___.__) Probable Major Neurocognitive Disorder Due to Frontotemporal Lobar Degeneration[b]

Note: Code first **331.19 (G31.09)** frontotemporal disease.

294.11 (F02.81) With behavioral disturbance

294.10 (F02.80) Without behavioral disturbance

331.9 (G31.9) Possible Major Neurocognitive Disorder Due to Frontotemporal Lobar Degeneration[a, b]

331.83 (G31.84) Mild Neurocognitive Disorder Due to Frontotemporal Lobar Degeneration[a]

Major or Mild Neurocognitive Disorder With Lewy Bodies

___.__ (___.__) Probable Major Neurocognitive Disorder With Lewy Bodies[b]

Note: Code first **331.82 (G31.83)** Lewy body disease.

294.11 (F02.81) With behavioral disturbance

294.10 (F02.80) Without behavioral disturbance

331.9 (G31.9) Possible Major Neurocognitive Disorder With Lewy Bodies[a, b]

331.83 (G31.84) Mild Neurocognitive Disorder With Lewy Bodies[a]

Major or Mild Vascular Neurocognitive Disorder

___.__ (___.__) Probable Major Vascular Neurocognitive Disorder[b]

Note: No additional medical code for vascular disease.

290.40 (F01.51) With behavioral disturbance

290.40 (F01.50) Without behavioral disturbance

331.9 (G31.9) Possible Major Vascular Neurocognitive Disorder[a, b]

331.83 (G31.84) Mild Vascular Neurocognitive Disorder[a]

Major or Mild Neurocognitive Disorder Due to Traumatic Brain Injury

___.__ (___.__) Major Neurocognitive Disorder Due to Traumatic Brain Injury[b]

Note: For ICD-9-CM, code first **907.0** late effect of intracranial injury without skull fracture. For ICD-10-CM, code first **S06.2X9S** diffuse traumatic brain injury with loss of consciousness of unspecified duration, sequela.

294.11 (F02.81) With behavioral disturbance

294.10 (F02.80) Without behavioral disturbance

331.83 (G31.84) Mild Neurocognitive Disorder Due to Traumatic Brain Injury[a]

Substance/Medication-Induced Major or Mild Neurocognitive Disorder[a]

Note: No additional medical code. See the criteria set and corresponding recording procedures for substance-specific codes and ICD-9-CM and ICD-10-CM coding.
Specify if: Persistent

Major or Mild Neurocognitive Disorder Due to HIV Infection

___.__ (___.__) Major Neurocognitive Disorder Due to HIV Infection[b]

Note: Code first **042 (B20)** HIV infection.

294.11 (F02.81) With behavioral disturbance

294.10	(F02.80)	Without behavioral disturbance
331.83	(G31.84)	Mild Neurocognitive Disorder Due to HIV Infection[a]

Major or Mild Neurocognitive Disorder Due to Prion Disease

___.__	(___.__)	Major Neurocognitive Disorder Due to Prion Disease[b]
		Note: Code first **046.79 (A81.9)** prion disease.
294.11	(F02.81)	With behavioral disturbance
294.10	(F02.80)	Without behavioral disturbance
331.83	(G31.84)	Mild Neurocognitive Disorder Due to Prion Disease[a]

Major or Mild Neurocognitive Disorder Due to Parkinson's Disease

___.__	(___.__)	Major Neurocognitive Disorder Probably Due to Parkinson's Disease[b]
		Note: Code first **332.0 (G20)** Parkinson's disease.
294.11	(F02.81)	With behavioral disturbance
294.10	(F02.80)	Without behavioral disturbance
331.9	(G31.9)	Major Neurocognitive Disorder Possibly Due to Parkinson's Disease[a, b]
331.83	(G31.84)	Mild Neurocognitive Disorder Due to Parkinson's Disease[a]

Major or Mild Neurocognitive Disorder Due to Huntington's Disease

___.__	(___.__)	Major Neurocognitive Disorder Due to Huntington's Disease[b]
		Note: Code first **333.4 (G10)** Huntington's disease.
294.11	(F02.81)	With behavioral disturbance
294.10	(F02.80)	Without behavioral disturbance
331.83	(G31.84)	Mild Neurocognitive Disorder Due to Huntington's Disease[a]

Major or Mild Neurocognitive Disorder Due to Another Medical Condition

___.__	(___.__)	Major Neurocognitive Disorder Due to Another Medical Condition[b]
		Note: Code first the other medical condition.
294.11	(F02.81)	With behavioral disturbance
294.10	(F02.80)	Without behavioral disturbance
331.83	(G31.84)	Mild Neurocognitive Disorder Due to Another Medical Condition[a]

Major or Mild Neurocognitive Disorder Due to Multiple Etiologies

___.__	(___.__)	Major Neurocognitive Disorder Due to Multiple Etiologies[b]
		Note: Code first all the etiological medical conditions (with the exception of vascular disease).
294.11	(F02.81)	With behavioral disturbance
294.10	(F02.80)	Without behavioral disturbance
331.83	(G31.84)	Mild Neurocognitive Disorder Due to Multiple Etiologies[a]

Unspecified Neurocognitive Disorder

799.59	(R41.9)	Unspecified Neurocognitive Disorder[a]

Personality Disorders

Cluster A Personality Disorders

301.0 (F60.0) Paranoid Personality Disorder

301.20 (F60.1) Schizoid Personality Disorder

301.22 (F21) Schizotypal Personality Disorder

Cluster B Personality Disorders

301.7 (F60.2) Antisocial Personality Disorder

301.83 (F60.3) Borderline Personality Disorder

301.50 (F60.4) Histrionic Personality Disorder

301.81 (F60.81) Narcissistic Personality Disorder

Cluster C Personality Disorders

301.82 (F60.6) Avoidant Personality Disorder

301.6 (F60.7) Dependent Personality Disorder

301.4 (F60.5) Obsessive-Compulsive Personality Disorder

Other Personality Disorders

310.1 (F07.0) Personality Change Due to Another Medical Condition

Specify whether: Labile type, Disinhibited type, Aggressive type, Apathetic type, Paranoid type, Other type, Combined type, Unspecified type

301.89 (F60.89) Other Specified Personality Disorder

301.9 (F60.9) Unspecified Personality Disorder

Paraphilic Disorders

The following specifier applies to Paraphilic Disorders where indicated:
[a]*Specify* if: In a controlled environment, In full remission

302.82 (F65.3) Voyeuristic Disorder[a]

302.4 (F65.2) Exhibitionistic Disorder[a]

Specify whether: Sexually aroused by exposing genitals to prepubertal children, Sexually aroused by exposing genitals to physically mature individuals, Sexually aroused by exposing genitals to prepubertal children and to physically mature individuals

302.89 (F65.81) Frotteuristic Disorder[a]

302.83 (F65.51) Sexual Masochism Disorder[a]

Specify if: With asphyxiophilia

302.84 (F65.52) Sexual Sadism Disorder[a]

302.2 (F65.4) Pedophilic Disorder

Specify whether: Exclusive type, Nonexclusive type

		Specify if: Sexually attracted to males, Sexually attracted to females, Sexually attracted to both *Specify* if: Limited to incest
302.81	(F65.0)	Fetishistic Disorder[a] *Specify:* Body part(s), Nonliving object(s), Other
302.3	(F65.1)	Transvestic Disorder[a] *Specify* if: With fetishism, With autogynephilia
302.89	(F65.89)	Other Specified Paraphilic Disorder
302.9	(F65.9)	Unspecified Paraphilic Disorder

Other Mental Disorders

294.8	(F06.8)	Other Specified Mental Disorder Due to Another Medical Condition
294.9	(F09)	Unspecified Mental Disorder Due to Another Medical Condition
300.9	(F99)	Other Specified Mental Disorder
300.9	(F99)	Unspecified Mental Disorder

Medication-Induced Movement Disorders and Other Adverse Effects of Medication

332.1	(G21.11)	Neuroleptic-Induced Parkinsonism
332.1	(G21.19)	Other Medication-Induced Parkinsonism
333.92	(G21.0)	Neuroleptic Malignant Syndrome
333.72	(G24.02)	Medication-Induced Acute Dystonia
333.99	(G25.71)	Medication-Induced Acute Akathisia
333.85	(G24.01)	Tardive Dyskinesia
333.72	(G24.09)	Tardive Dystonia
333.99	(G25.71)	Tardive Akathisia
333.1	(G25.1)	Medication-Induced Postural Tremor
333.99	(G25.79)	Other Medication-Induced Movement Disorder
___.__	(___.__)	Antidepressant Discontinuation Syndrome
995.29	(T43.205A)	Initial encounter
995.29	(T43.205D)	Subsequent encounter
995.29	(T43.205S)	Sequelae
___.__	(___.__)	Other Adverse Effect of Medication
995.20	(T50.905A)	Initial encounter
995.20	(T50.905D)	Subsequent encounter
995.20	(T50.905S)	Sequelae

Other Conditions That May Be a Focus of Clinical Attention

Relational Problems

Problems Related to Family Upbringing

V61.20 (Z62.820) Parent-Child Relational Problem

V61.8 (Z62.891) Sibling Relational Problem

V61.8 (Z62.29) Upbringing Away From Parents

V61.29 (Z62.898) Child Affected by Parental Relationship Distress

Other Problems Related to Primary Support Group

V61.10 (Z63.0) Relationship Distress With Spouse or Intimate Partner

V61.03 (Z63.5) Disruption of Family by Separation or Divorce

V61.8 (Z63.8) High Expressed Emotion Level Within Family

V62.82 (Z63.4) Uncomplicated Bereavement

Abuse and Neglect

Child Maltreatment and Neglect Problems

Child Physical Abuse

Child Physical Abuse, Confirmed

995.54 (T74.12XA) Initial encounter

995.54 (T74.12XD) Subsequent encounter

Child Physical Abuse, Suspected

995.54 (T76.12XA) Initial encounter

995.54 (T76.12XD) Subsequent encounter

Other Circumstances Related to Child Physical Abuse

V61.21 (Z69.010) Encounter for mental health services for victim of child abuse by parent

V61.21 (Z69.020) Encounter for mental health services for victim of nonparental child abuse

V15.41 (Z62.810) Personal history (past history) of physical abuse in childhood

V61.22 (Z69.011) Encounter for mental health services for perpetrator of parental child abuse

V62.83 (Z69.021) Encounter for mental health services for perpetrator of nonparental child abuse

Child Sexual Abuse

Child Sexual Abuse, Confirmed

995.53 (T74.22XA) Initial encounter

995.53 (T74.22XD) Subsequent encounter

Child Sexual Abuse, Suspected

995.53 (T76.22XA) Initial encounter

995.53 (T76.22XD) Subsequent encounter

Other Circumstances Related to Child Sexual Abuse

V61.21 (Z69.010) Encounter for mental health services for victim of child sexual abuse by parent

V61.21 (Z69.020) Encounter for mental health services for victim of nonparental child sexual abuse

V15.41 (Z62.810) Personal history (past history) of sexual abuse in childhood

V61.22 (Z69.011) Encounter for mental health services for perpetrator of parental child sexual abuse

V62.83 (Z69.021) Encounter for mental health services for perpetrator of nonparental child sexual abuse

Child Neglect

Child Neglect, Confirmed

995.52 (T74.02XA) Initial encounter

995.52 (T74.02XD) Subsequent encounter

Child Neglect, Suspected

995.52 (T76.02XA) Initial encounter

995.52 (T76.02XD) Subsequent encounter

Other Circumstances Related to Child Neglect

V61.21 (Z69.010) Encounter for mental health services for victim of child neglect by parent

V61.21 (Z69.020) Encounter for mental health services for victim of nonparental child neglect

V15.42 (Z62.812) Personal history (past history) of neglect in childhood

V61.22 (Z69.011) Encounter for mental health services for perpetrator of parental child neglect

V62.83 (Z69.021) Encounter for mental health services for perpetrator of nonparental child neglect

Child Psychological Abuse

Child Psychological Abuse, Confirmed

995.51 (T74.32XA) Initial encounter

995.51 (T74.32XD) Subsequent encounter

Child Psychological Abuse, Suspected

995.51 (T76.32XA) Initial encounter

995.51 (T76.32XD) Subsequent encounter

Other Circumstances Related to Child Psychological Abuse

V61.21 (Z69.010) Encounter for mental health services for victim of child psychological abuse by parent

V61.21 (Z69.020) Encounter for mental health services for victim of nonparental child psychological abuse

V15.42 (Z62.811) Personal history (past history) of psychological abuse in childhood

V61.22 (Z69.011) Encounter for mental health services for perpetrator of parental child psychological abuse

V62.83 (Z69.021) Encounter for mental health services for perpetrator of nonparental child psychological abuse

Adult Maltreatment and Neglect Problems

Spouse or Partner Violence, Physical

Spouse or Partner Violence, Physical, Confirmed

995.81 (T74.11XA) Initial encounter

995.81 (T74.11XD) Subsequent encounter

Spouse or Partner Violence, Physical, Suspected

995.81 (T76.11XA) Initial encounter

995.81 (T76.11XD) Subsequent encounter

Other Circumstances Related to Spouse or Partner Violence, Physical

V61.11 (Z69.11) Encounter for mental health services for victim of spouse or partner violence, physical

V15.41 (Z91.410) Personal history (past history) of spouse or partner violence, physical

V61.12 (Z69.12) Encounter for mental health services for perpetrator of spouse or partner violence, physical

Spouse or Partner Violence, Sexual

Spouse or Partner Violence, Sexual, Confirmed

995.83 (T74.21XA) Initial encounter

995.83 (T74.21XD) Subsequent encounter

Spouse or Partner Violence, Sexual, Suspected

995.83 (T76.21XA) Initial encounter

995.83 (T76.21XD) Subsequent encounter

Other Circumstances Related to Spouse or Partner Violence, Sexual

V61.11 (Z69.81) Encounter for mental health services for victim of spouse or partner violence, sexual

V15.41 (Z91.410) Personal history (past history) of spouse or partner violence, sexual

V61.12 (Z69.12) Encounter for mental health services for perpetrator of spouse or partner violence, sexual

Spouse or Partner, Neglect

Spouse or Partner Neglect, Confirmed

995.85 (T74.01XA) Initial encounter

995.85 (T74.01XD) Subsequent encounter

Spouse or Partner Neglect, Suspected

995.85 (T76.01XA) Initial encounter

995.85 (T76.01XD) Subsequent encounter

Other Circumstances Related to Spouse or Partner Neglect

V61.11 (Z69.11) Encounter for mental health services for victim of spouse or partner neglect

V15.42 (Z91.412) Personal history (past history) of spouse or partner neglect

V61.12 (Z69.12) Encounter for mental health services for perpetrator of spouse or partner neglect

Spouse or Partner Abuse, Psychological

Spouse or Partner Abuse, Psychological, Confirmed

995.82 (T74.31XA) Initial encounter

995.82 (T74.31XD) Subsequent encounter

Spouse or Partner Abuse, Psychological, Suspected

995.82 (T76.31XA) Initial encounter

995.82 (T76.31XD) Subsequent encounter

Other Circumstances Related to Spouse or Partner Abuse, Psychological

V61.11 (Z69.11) Encounter for mental health services for victim of spouse or partner psychological abuse

V15.42 (Z91.411) Personal history (past history) of spouse or partner psychological abuse

V61.12 (Z69.12) Encounter for mental health services for perpetrator of spouse or partner psychological abuse

Adult Abuse by Nonspouse or Nonpartner

Adult Physical Abuse by Nonspouse or Nonpartner, Confirmed

995.81 (T74.11XA) Initial encounter

995.81 (T74.11XD) Subsequent encounter

Adult Physical Abuse by Nonspouse or Nonpartner, Suspected

995.81 (T76.11XA) Initial encounter

995.81 (T76.11XD) Subsequent encounter

Adult Sexual Abuse by Nonspouse or Nonpartner, Confirmed

995.83 (T74.21XA) Initial encounter

995.83 (T74.21XD) Subsequent encounter

Adult Sexual Abuse by Nonspouse or Nonpartner, Suspected

995.83 (T76.21XA) Initial encounter

995.83 (T76.21XD) Subsequent encounter

Adult Psychological Abuse by Nonspouse or Nonpartner, Confirmed

995.82 (T74.31XA) Initial encounter

995.82 (T74.31XD) Subsequent encounter

Adult Psychological Abuse by Nonspouse or Nonpartner, Suspected

995.82 (T76.31XA) Initial encounter

995.82 (T76.31XD) Subsequent encounter

Other Circumstances Related to Adult Abuse by Nonspouse or Nonpartner

V65.49 (Z69.81) Encounter for mental health services for victim of nonspousal adult abuse

V62.83 (Z69.82) Encounter for mental health services for perpetrator of nonspousal adult abuse

Educational and Occupational Problems

Educational Problems

V62.3 (Z55.9) Academic or Educational Problem

Occupational Problems

V62.21 (Z56.82) Problem Related to Current Military Deployment Status

V62.29 (Z56.9) Other Problem Related to Employment

Housing and Economic Problems

Housing Problems

V60.0 (Z59.0) Homelessness

V60.1 (Z59.1) Inadequate Housing

V60.89 (Z59.2) Discord With Neighbor, Lodger, or Landlord

V60.6 (Z59.3) Problem Related to Living in a Residential Institution

Economic Problems

V60.2 (Z59.4) Lack of Adequate Food or Safe Drinking Water

V60.2 (Z59.5) Extreme Poverty

V60.2 (Z59.6) Low Income

V60.2 (Z59.7) Insufficient Social Insurance or Welfare Support

V60.9 (Z59.9) Unspecified Housing or Economic Problem

Other Problems Related to the Social Environment

V62.89 (Z60.0) Phase of Life Problem

V60.3 (Z60.2) Problem Related to Living Alone

V62.4 (Z60.3) Acculturation Difficulty

V62.4 (Z60.4) Social Exclusion or Rejection

V62.4 (Z60.5) Target of (Perceived) Adverse Discrimination or Persecution

V62.9 (Z60.9) Unspecified Problem Related to Social Environment

Problems Related to Crime or Interaction With the Legal System

V62.89 (Z65.4) Victim of Crime

V62.5 (Z65.0) Conviction in Civil or Criminal Proceedings Without Imprisonment

V62.5 (Z65.1) Imprisonment or Other Incarceration

V62.5 (Z65.2) Problems Related to Release From Prison

V62.5 (Z65.3) Problems Related to Other Legal Circumstances

Other Health Service Encounters for Counseling and Medical Advice

V65.49 (Z70.9) Sex Counseling

V65.40 (Z71.9) Other Counseling or Consultation

Problems Related to Other Psychosocial, Personal, and Environmental Circumstances

V62.89 (Z65.8) Religious or Spiritual Problem

V61.7 (Z64.0) Problems Related to Unwanted Pregnancy

V61.5 (Z64.1) Problems Related to Multiparity

V62.89 (Z64.4) Discord With Social Service Provider, Including Probation Officer, Case Manager, or Social Services Worker

V62.89 (Z65.4) Victim of Terrorism or Torture

V62.22 (Z65.5) Exposure to Disaster, War, or Other Hostilities

V62.89 (Z65.8) Other Problem Related to Psychosocial Circumstances

V62.9 (Z65.9) Unspecified Problem Related to Unspecified Psychosocial Circumstances

Other Circumstances of Personal History

V15.49 (Z91.49) Other Personal History of Psychological Trauma

V15.59 (Z91.5) Personal History of Self-Harm

V62.22 (Z91.82) Personal History of Military Deployment

V15.89 (Z91.89) Other Personal Risk Factors

V69.9 (Z72.9) Problem Related to Lifestyle

V71.01 (Z72.811) Adult Antisocial Behavior

V71.02 (Z72.810) Child or Adolescent Antisocial Behavior

Problems Related to Access to Medical and Other Health Care

V63.9 (Z75.3) Unavailability or Inaccessibility of Health Care Facilities

V63.8 (Z75.4) Unavailability or Inaccessibility of Other Helping Agencies

Nonadherence to Medical Treatment

V15.81 (Z91.19) Nonadherence to Medical Treatment

278.00 (E66.9) Overweight or Obesity

V65.2 (Z76.5) Malingering

V40.31 (Z91.83) Wandering Associated With a Mental Disorder

V62.89 (R41.83) Borderline Intellectual Functioning

Alphabetical Index of Decision Trees

Aggressive behavior (2.23) (p.116)

Anxiety (2.13) (p.75)

Appetite changes or unusual eating behavior (2.18) (p. 94)

Avoidance behavior (2.15) (p. 83)

Behavioral problems in a child or adolescent (2.2) (p. 25)

Catatonic symptoms (2.7) (p. 49)

Cognitive impairment (2.28) (p. 139)

Delusions (2.5) (p. 38)

Depressed mood (2.10) (p. 61)

Distractibility (2.4) (p. 35)

Eating behavior, unusual, or appetite changes (2.18) (p. 94)

Elevated or expansive mood (2.8) (p. 52)

Etiological medical conditions (2.29) (p. 149)

Excessive substance use (2.26) (p. 129)

Hallucinations (2.6) (p. 44)

Hypersomnolence (2.20) (p. 104)

Impulsivity or impulse-control problems (2.24) (p. 122)

Insomnia (2.19) (p. 99)

Irritable mood (2.9) (p. 56)

Medical conditions, etiological (2.29) (p. 149)

Memory loss (2.27) (p. 135)

Panic attacks (2.14) (p. 80)

Poor school performance (2.1) (p. 22)

Psychomotor retardation (2.12) (p. 72)

School performance, poor (2.1) (p. 22)

Self-injury or self-mutilation (2.25) (p. 126)

Sexual dysfunction in a female (2.21) (p. 109)

Sexual dysfunction in a male (2.22) (p. 113)

Somatic complaints or illness/ appearance anxiety (2.17) (p. 91)

Speech disturbance (2.3) (p. 30)

Substance use, excessive (2.26) (p. 129)

Suicidal ideation or behavior (2.11) (p. 67)

Trauma or psychosocial stressors involved in the etiology (2.16) (p. 87)

Alphabetical Index of Differential Diagnosis Tables

Acute Stress Disorder (3.7.1) (p.225)
Adjustment Disorder (3.7.2) (p. 227)
Agoraphobia (3.5.6) (p. 210)
Anorexia Nervosa (3.10.2) (p. 246)
Antisocial Personality Disorder (3.17.4) (p. 279)
Attention-Deficit/Hyperactivity Disorder (3.1.4) (p. 168)
Autism Spectrum Disorder (3.1.3) (p. 166)
Avoidant Personality Disorder (3.17.8) (p. 284)
Avoidant/Restrictive Food Intake Disorder (3.10.1) (p. 244)
Binge-Eating Disorder (3.10.4) (p. 251)
Bipolar I Disorder (3.3.1) (p. 182)
Bipolar II Disorder (3.3.2) (p. 185)
Body Dysmorphic Disorder (3.6.2) (p. 218)
Borderline Personality Disorder (3.17.5) (p. 281)
Brief Psychotic Disorder (3.2.4) (p. 180)
Bulimia Nervosa (3.10.3) (p. 249)
Communication Disorders (3.1.2) (p. 164)
Conduct Disorder (3.14.3) (p. 266)
Conversion Disorder (Functional Neurological Symptom Disorder) (3.9.3) (p. 239)
Cyclothymic Disorder (3.3.3) (p. 188)
Delirium (3.16.1) (p. 271)
Delusional Disorder (3.2.3) (p. 178)
Dependent Personality Disorder (3.17.9) (p. 285)
Depersonalization/Derealization Disorder (3.8.2) (p. 231)
Disruptive Mood Dysregulation Disorder (3.4.4) (p. 196)
Dissociative Amnesia (3.8.1) (p. 229)
Dysthymia (Persistent Depressive Disorder) (3.4.2) (p. 192)
Excoriation (Skin-Picking) Disorder (3.6.5) (p. 224)
Factitious Disorder (3.9.5) (p. 243)
Functional Neurological Symptom Disorder (Conversion Disorder) (3.9.3) (p. 239)
Gambling Disorder (3.15.2) (p. 270)
Gender Dysphoria (3.13.1) (p. 260)

Generalized Anxiety Disorder (3.5.7) (p. 212)
Hair-Pulling Disorder (Trichotillomania) (3.6.4) (p. 222)
Histrionic Personality Disorder (3.17.6) (p. 282)
Hoarding Disorder (3.6.3) (p. 220)
Hypersomnolence Disorder (3.11.2) (p. 255)
Illness Anxiety Disorder (3.9.2) (p. 236)
Insomnia Disorder (3.11.1) (p. 252)
Intellectual Disability (Intellectual Developmental Disorder) (3.1.1) (p. 162)
Intermittent Explosive Disorder (3.14.2) (p. 264)
Major Depressive Disorder (3.4.1) (p. 189)
Major or Mild Neurocognitive Disorder (3.16.2) (p. 273)
Narcissistic Personality Disorder (3.17.7) (p. 283)
Neurocognitive Disorder, Major or Mild (3.16.2) (p. 273)
Obsessive-Compulsive Disorder (3.6.1) (p. 215)
Obsessive-Compulsive Personality Disorder (3.17.10) (p. 286)
Oppositional Defiant Disorder (3.14.1) (p. 262)
Panic Disorder (3.5.5) (p. 208)
Paranoid Personality Disorder (3.17.1) (p. 276)
Paraphilic Disorders (3.18.1) (p. 288)
Persistent Depressive Disorder (Dysthymia) (3.4.2) (p. 192)
Personality Change Due to Another Medical Condition (3.17.11) (p. 287)
Posttraumatic Stress Disorder (3.7.1) (p. 225)
Premenstrual Dysphoric Disorder (3.4.3) (p. 194)
Psychological Factors Affecting Other Medical Conditions (3.9.4) (p. 241)
Schizoaffective Disorder (3.2.2) (p. 177)
Schizoid Personality Disorder (3.17.2) (p. 277)
Schizophrenia or Schizophreniform Disorder (3.2.1) (p. 175)
Schizotypal Personality Disorder (3.17.3) (p. 278)
Selective Mutism (3.5.2) (p. 201)
Separation Anxiety Disorder (3.5.1) (p. 198)
Sexual Dysfunctions (3.12.1) (p. 258)
Skin-Picking (Excoriation) Disorder (3.6.5) (p. 224)
Social Anxiety Disorder (Social Phobia) (3.5.4) (p. 204)
Somatic Symptom Disorder (3.9.1) (p. 234)
Specific Learning Disorder (3.1.5) (p. 172)
Specific Phobia (3.5.3) (p. 202)
Substance Use Disorders (3.15.1) (p. 268)
Tic Disorders (3.1.6) (p. 174)
Trichotillomania (Hair-Pulling Disorder) (3.6.4) (p. 222)
Unspecified Catatonia (3.2.5) (p. 181)